American Herbalism:

Essays On Herbs & Herbalism by Members of the American Herbalist Guild

Edited by
Dr. Michael Tierra, O.M.D.

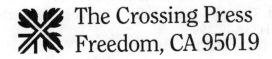

The Crossing Press
Freedom, CA 95019

Library of Congress Cataloging-in-Publication Data

American herbalism: essays on herbs & herbalism/by members of the
    American Herbalist Guild; edited by Michael Tierra.
        p.   cm.
    "Comprised of selected presentations from the first American Herb-
alist Guild Symposium, held at the Lloyd library in Cinncinnati,
Ohio...supplemented with other essays and writing by herbalists
from around the country"—Intro.
    Includes bibliographical references.
    ISBN 0-89594-541-X (cloth).—ISBN 0-89594-540-1 (paper)
    1. Herbs—United States—Therapeutic use. 2. Herbalists—United
States. I. Tierra, Michael, 1939- . II. American Herbalist Guild.
RM666.H33A49 1992
615'.321'0973—dc20   91-44938
                                                         CIP

TABLE OF CONTENTS

INTRODUCTION...vii
   Michael Tierra, O.M.D., L. AC.

OUR HERBAL HERITAGE

A HISTORY OF HERBS AND HERBALISM.............................3
   Jeanne Rose

WESTERN HERBAL MEDICINE - A PERSPECTIVE...................33
   Amanda McQuade-Crawford

INTRODUCTION TO FOLKLORIC HERBALISM.........................37
   Jim Green

FRAGMENTS OF EARTH WISDOM.....................................41
   Feather Jones

HERBALISTS AND HERBAL ELDERS

JOHN RAYMOND CHRISTOPHER:
A LEGACY OF COURAGE..48
   David Christopher

LEAH LISCHNER CONNERS—
PROFILE OF A COMMUNITY HEALER................................60
   Roy Upton

CHARLIE WILL JORDAN: AN HERBALIST WHO
BALANCES BUSINESS WITH NATURE..............................65
   Roy Upton

PORTRAIT OF AN HERBALIST.......................................69
   Jim Green

Herbal Traditions

NVWOTE: CHEROKEE MEDICINE AND ETHNOBOTANY........86
David Winston

FORGOTTEN AND NEGLECTED AMERICAN
MEDICINAL PLANTS..100
David Lytle

THE BENEFITS OF BIAN ZHENG
MORE PRECIOUS THAN ANY HERB.............................108
Dr. Robert Flaws

Herbalists Using Herbs

BOTANICAL TREATMENT OF
CHRONIC GYNECOLOGICAL CONDITIONS
*INFERTILITY, ENDOMETRIOSIS, AND SYMPTOMS
OF MENOPAUSE*..122
Silena Heron

HERBS AND THE MIND...144
David Frawley

OUR EYES—MIRRORS OF HEALTH.............................158
Brigitte Mars

NATURAL REMEDIES FOR EAR AILMENTS.......................162
Brigitte Mars

HERBS FOR CHILDREN...172
Rosemary Gladstar Slick

RHEUMATOID ARTHRITIS: A CASE HISTORY....................193
David Hoffman

HIV POSITIVE: A CASE STUDY................................200
Michael Tierra

SIMPLER SCENTS: THE COMBINED USES OF
HERBS AND ESSENTIAL OILS..............................204
    Mindy Green

HERBALISTS ON THE PRACTICE OF HERBALISM

AN ENERGETIC MODEL FOR WESTERN HERBOLOGY.......212
    Lesley Tierra
HERBAL ENERGETICS IN CLINICAL PRACTICE....................228
    Michael Moore
THE CONTRIBUTION OF HERBALISM
TO WESTERN HOLISTIC PRACTICE............................251
    David Hoffmann
TRADITIONAL EUROPEAN MEDICINE (TEM) AND
TRANSCULTURAL POLYMEDICINE............................269
    Christopher Hobbs
EFFICACY VS. EFFECTIVENESS............................296
    Paul Bergner
HERBAL TOXICITY AND CONTRAINDICATIONS..................303
    Michael Tierra, O.M.D.
APPENDIX............................315

Introduction

MICHAEL TIERRA, O.M.D.

"Who uses those wonderful medicinal plants?" was the question put to me by an Australian herbalist whose materia medica consisted of better than fifty percent North American herbs. During my teaching tour of Australia and New Zealand in 1988 and later in the U.K., I was impressed by the widespread appreciation and use of medicinal plants from North America by practitioners abroad. I began to see that there were perhaps more herbalists in countries as far distant as Australia and New Zealand who knew more about how to use our own herbs than many of us.

While there has always been a lively folk or rural herbal tradition on this continent, official recognition for the practice of herbal medicine has been suppressed by a Western medical, drug-based monopoly. This is not surprising in a country that served as the leading bastion of the industrial-technological age. With our typical fascination for the new, bordering on outright faddism, we traded our "vital roots," as Dr. Paul Lee describes our herbal tradition, for the promise of the quick fix and the glitter of Western scientific medical technology.

People faced with unsatisfactory solutions to their health problems are now resorting more frequently to herbs, often self prescribed. Many are getting incredible results for conditions ranging from cancer, heart disease, depression, infertility, arthritis, and AIDS to chronic headaches, menstrual abnormalities and the common cold. Because of these results, the herbal industry is rapidly growing. Because of this growth there is an increasing need for experienced herbalists to help not only with the herbal products industry, but also with the education of qualified medical herbalists. There is also a responsibility for herbalists to take a more active role as advisors in guiding the evolution of legislation concerning the practice and use of herbal medicine in America.

Following my 1988 lecture tour of Australia, I resolved to take an active role toward the formation of an organization of professional North

American herbalists. Only a few months earlier, at the Breitenbush, Oregon annual herbal retreat, we discussed the need for creating a professional herbalist organization. Therefore, when I sent ten letters to my herbalist friends and colleagues, they responded with timely enthusiasm. The result was the formation of the American Herbalist Guild.

We held our first meeting in Santa Cruz, California on February 18, 1989 with a small gathering (twenty to thirty) of outstanding professional herbalists from various parts of the country. Among the herbalists who attended that first meeting were myself, Cascade Anderson Geller, James and Mindy Green, David Hoffman, Christopher Hobbs, Brigitte Mars, Amanda McQuade-Crawford, Kathi Keville, Dr. Paul Lee, Mara Levin, Lesley Tierra, Roy Upton, and David Winston.

Unlike other Western countries such as Great Britain, for the last fifty years or so the practice of herbalism has been virtually outlawed throughout the United States. As a result, it has mostly been a maverick profession practiced by an assortment of strong-willed and eccentric individuals. With a history of meeting and enjoying each other as friends at various herbal retreats and seminars throughout the country, we tried to accommodate all our individual eccentricities and styles of using herbs and form them into a single organization.

Since we were primarily self taught, many problems that we encountered were new and unfamiliar, involving the articulation of standards of education for new herbalists and the clinical practice of herbal medicine. This was complicated by the fact that we wished to accommodate not only Western medical herbalists, but Ayurvedic, Chinese, Native American, and folk herbalists. Attesting to the timeliness of our meeting is the fact that within the course of two days we were able to formulate nine statements of purpose as follows:

1. To form a professional body to develop, promote, and maintain levels of excellence in herbalism, including individual and planetary health.

2. To strengthen and further the network of communication and support between herbalists.

3. To foster high levels of ethics and integrity in all areas of herbalism.

4. To promote cooperation between herbalists and other health care providers, encompassing traditional wisdom and knowledge as well as current medical models.

5. To establish and maintain criteria and standards of education for the professional practice of herbalism.

6. To promote an ecologically healthy environment and to increase awareness concerning the interdependence of all life, especially the plant-

human relationships.

7. To serve as a liaison with other professional associations and regulatory agencies.

8. To promote further research, education, and study of herbal medicine.

It was decided by unanimous agreement that the guild should include the various traditions of herbalism from around the world. Since most of the herbalists who met were either practitioners or educators, the committee work focused primarily on issues involving these areas of herbalism. There was also a consensus that the guild would serve as an umbrella organization encompassing the full range of herbalism including growing, wildcrafting and manufacturing.

The first interim officers included: David Hoffmann—president, Christopher Hobbs—vice president, Amanda McQuade-Crawford—secretary (later, for logistical reasons, assumed by Roy Upton), Michael Tierra—treasurer, and Cascade Anderson Geller—executive officer.

We decided to organize a yearly herbal symposium to be held at various sites around the U.S. We agreed that the first official meeting and symposium would be in Cincinnati, Ohio, the home of the Lloyd library, one of the finest botanical medicine libraries in the world. It houses the various memorabilia, books, and personal libraries of John Uri Lloyd of Lloyd Bros. Pharmaceuticals, as well as the library of the Eclectic Medical College and the various Eclectic medical doctors from around the country. These books represented the last official medical system to espouse the practice and use of herbal medicine in North America.

This book contains presentations from the first American Herbalist Guild Symposium, held at the Lloyd library in Cincinnati, Ohio, to commemorate the last bastion of medical herbalism in America until the closing of the Eclectic Medical College in 1939. It is supplemented with other essays and writings by herbalists from around the country.

With contributions by many of the country's leading herbalists, this book is intended to appeal to readers with all levels of experience and interest. It is my intention that this book serve as an expression of the current diversity of interest, thought, and range of practice of American Herbalists.

Jeanne Rose has played a leading role in popularizing herbal medicine to the general public. She has seven books to her credit, including the ever popular *Herbs and Things* first published in 1973. Her contribution, which is excerpted from her correspondence course, provides a consummate overview of the history of herbalism from prehistoric to modern times.

Amanda McQuade-Crawford is a medical herbalist, trained in Great Britain. At present, she teaches clinical herbal medicine at the California School of Herbal Studies. Her article, an interpretation of the history of herbalism, may offer some insight as to how we arrived at the present herbal renaissance, with its problems as well as its the promising opportunities for the future.

James Green, author of *The Male Herbal,* is another resident teacher at the California School of Herbal Studies. He and his wife, Mindy, spent several years under the tutelage of and later as assistants to the late Norma Myers in British Columbia. In his introduction to Folkloric Herbalism presented at the symposium, Green argues eloquently for our right to "use Earth's freely given, natural medicines and to do this harmlessly, in harmony with other companion species that make up the wonderful diversity that is the living planet, Earth."

Feather Jones is the first elected president of the American Herbalist Guild. She and her associate, Catherine Hunziker, are founders of the Rocky Mountain Herbalist Coalition, a group which is attempting to set high standards for the wildcrafting of native botanicals. Her contribution is a poetic musing upon the traditional relationships between the Native people of this continent and the society of plants.

David Christopher offers a biographical reminiscence on the legacy of John Raymond Christopher, his father. Dr. Christopher, as we respectfully knew him, served as an inspiration and teacher to many of us today. In literally thousands of herbal seminars throughout the country, he served as a lone, courageous voice in a legally unfriendly wilderness. He espoused and championed the cause of herbalism during a time of great herbal suppression, the period between 1950 and 1975.

Happily, through a paper by James Green, we are also able to commemorate another great herbal elder, *Kwi-tsi-tsa-las,* better known as *Norma Myers*, the "wild woman of the North." Some of us, who were honored to study and work with her, can only marvel at the consummate knowledge she had of Native American medicine and the undaunted, self-giving energy she extended in her dedication to her patients, her students, and the cause of herbal medicine.

Roy Upton is a respected herbalist extensively trained and skilled in the use of both Western and Chinese herbs. Presently he is director of one of the leading herbal manufacturers in the country. He also lectures and offers seminars throughout the country. He has contributed two pieces honoring *Charlie Will Jordan* and *Leah Lischner Conners*, two healers and herbalists who served the needs of their immediate community with compassion and integrity.

David Winston is an outstanding East Coast herbalist with hundreds of students. He knows the principles of Chinese herbal medicine; he also is the only Caucasian to be taken on as a personal apprentice to one of the last surviving Cherokee Medicine men skilled in Cherokee herbalism. The Cherokee Indians are respected by many North American tribes for having the most evolved system of herbal medicine in North America. What David teaches is not only the herbs and the ways of their use by the Cherokee people, but also the spirit in which they are gathered and used. He also recognizes significant similarities in the use of a system of differential diagnosis and the energetic classification of herbs with other traditional herbal systems such as Traditional Chinese Medicine.

David Lytle is a naturopathic doctor currently working on a long-term project of collecting and sorting the 35,000 entries of the *Eclectic Medical Journal* and the writings of John Uri Lloyd. All members in the guild share a profound respect for the Eclectic North American Herbal tradition that flourished from the latter part of the nineteenth through the early twentieth centuries. Mesmerized by scientific technological medicine, few realize that seventy-five to a hundred years ago, there were over 10,000 Eclectic herbal medicine doctors practicing throughout America.

David's article shows the need for us to move away from the overuse and consequent abuse of single herbs such as echinacea, golden seal or lady's slipper. The fact is that the practice of Western herbalism is difficult or impossible with the banning and unavailability of literally hundreds of botanicals which were once part of the standard materia medica. If we are to reinstate the practice of herbal medicine, we must get away from overusing those herbs in the current "Top Ten" category, and focus instead on the specific uses and indications of hundreds of forgotten and neglected herbs which will widen and diversify the range of our materia medica.

Dr. Robert Flaws, better known as Bob Flaws, author of many important books self-published through Blue Poppy Press, is an exponent of Traditional Chinese Medicine. He works in Boulder, Colorado. In his article, he writes about an important Chinese herbal concept that a single herbal remedy can be used for a wide variety of diseases while specific pathologies might require individualized consideration and treatment.

What is implied in his article, at least from the herbalist's perspective, is that there is seldom a specific universal remedy either for cancer or the common cold. For this reason, the art of herbal medicine requires using herbs with broad energetic reactions to gently effect and stimulate systemic organ reactions. I might comment that this traditional view is in contrast to the recent trend of some manufacturing companies to exploit for the sake of scientific one-upmanship, the use of large doses of concentrated standardized[1] herbal extracts. In many cases, these drug-like substances are recommended to be taken without holistic individual considerations. They may be and often are the wrong herb for the individual. When these herbs are taken in a concentrated dosage, they are either ineffective or otherwise unsuitable.

Silena Heron is a registered nurse, naturopathic doctor, and an outstanding herbalist following naturopathic principles of herbalism and the school of British Medical Herbalism. Her piece on the treatment of chronic gynecological conditions offers a clinical herbal protocol for infertility, endometriosis, and menopause.

David Hoffman is a British Medical Herbalist who had a very successful clinical practice in Wales and later at Findhorn in Scotland. Through his teachings at the California School of Herbal Studies and at many seminars around the world, he has earned the respect of his American herbal colleagues and friends. One of his books, *Holistic Herbalism*, describes the principles of treating pathological symptoms as a complex of underlying organic imbalances. Here, David offers a personal case study of his treatment of a patient with rheumatoid arthritis. In another article, he describes his perspectives as an herbalist in "The Contribution of Herbalism to Western Holistic Practice."

David Frawley, author of *Ayurvedic Healing*, is a scholar not only of Western, Chinese and Ayurvedic herbalism. He has taught himself ancient Sanskritand his published translations of the *Rig Veda* are respected throughout India. I am happy to include his essay that establishes the little known use for non-intoxicating effects of herbs on the mind and emotions. In this, he draws parallels between the three gunas or qualities of existence of Ayurveda (sattvas=equilibrium, rajas=destroying equilibrium, and tamas=inertia) and their corresponding energies and properties in herbs.

Brigitte Mars, an herbalist from Boulder, Colorado, has had success in the retail marketing of herbs at Alfalfa's Natural Food Market and in her

---

[1]In standardized extracts the supposed active chemical constituent of an herb is concentrated and reintroduced into a product to guarantee a specific level in each dose.

own line of herb teas. Brigitte contributes two essays on herbal care and treatment for the eyes and ears.

It is hard to imagine an herbalist in recent times who has done more for herbalists than *Rosemary Gladstar Slick.* Besides being the founder of the California School of Herbal Studies, she also founded the yearly Breitenbush, Oregon, herbal retreat that to date has served as a focal point for teachers and students of herbalism throughout the country who gather in the Fall to learn and share their love of herbs with each other. Rosemary has always imparted her joy and heartfelt appreciation to all who have attended her seminars or worked with her. Having moved to the East Coast, she continues to sponsor popular herbal retreats and seminars in that part of the country. We are happy to share a piece from her Healing Ways Series on "Herbs for Children."

Mindy Green is a teacher at the California School of Herbal Studies, the only school where students can receive in-depth training in all aspects of herbalism. Mindy's article about aromatherapy represents an important extension of the herbal movement begun in France. With the possibilities inherent in the combination of essential oils with herbs, even greater therapeutic effectiveness can be achieved.

Lesley Tierra, author of *The Herbs of Life,* is a California state licensed doctor of Traditional Chinese Medicine that includes the practice of acupuncture and herbal medicine. She and I together share a love of native herbs along with Traditional Chinese Medicine. This is expressed in her essay which offers a way to integrate the energetic diagnostic model of Traditional Chinese Medicine with Western clinical herbalism.

Michael Moore is a respected elder of contemporary American Herbalism. His books, *Medicinal Plants of the Mountains West* and *Medicinal Plants of the Deserts and Canyons West,* are universally respected and admired by his herbal colleagues. In his essay, Michael describes a highly individualized and creative approach to the use of Western scientific physiology that is similar to energetic and differential diagnostic systems of Chinese and Ayurvedic herbalism.

It would be difficult to find a more enthusiastic and dedicated herbalist than *Christopher Hobbs.* The opportunity to experience an herb walk with him is a special way to share his voluminous knowledge, experience, and joy of herbs. He has a priceless library of books, ancient and modern, representing the history of herbal medicine. Christopher's article draws comparisons between what he calls Traditional European Medicine (TEM) and Traditional Chinese and Ayurvedic Medicine.

Paul Bergner is the editor of *Medical Herbalism, A Clinical Newsletter for the Herbal Practitioner.* In his article, Paul questions the tenets and methodology of scientific tests and studies as applied to herbs. He argues that a scientifically proven herbal remedy may be ineffective in practice while an herbal remedy that was found to be ineffective or even toxic in scientific studies "may actually be quite valuable in another setting."

Finally, in my contribution, I make a distinction between herbal toxicity and contraindications. In the West, we have had many herbs banned as toxic. Within the context of Chinese or Ayurvedic energetic herbalism, contraindicated herbs can produce toxic reactions which may be cursorily designated as mere allergic reactions. It is part of the traditional herbalist's art to understand and differentiate between the principle of contraindication and toxicity.

This is the first offering from the American Herbalist Guild to the greater world of herbs and herbalists. All royalties from the sale of this work go to promoting the purposes and goals of the organization. It was my intention to achieve a mix of essays reflecting some of the most advanced thinking of American herbalists, together with practical articles dealing with specific issues and protocols for treatment. To my Australian colleagues, the American herbalists, the people struggling to re-integrate herbal medicine as part of the health care system of this country, and the three-quarters of the world's population who continue to depend on the use of herbs for primary health care, I sincerely hope that this book answers at least partially, *"who among us, in fact, does use these wonderful plants."*

Our
Herbal
Heritage

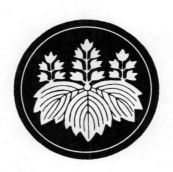

A History of Herbs and Herbalism
JEANNE ROSE

WHO WERE THE FIRST HERBALISTS?

An *herbalist* is a person who collects, studies, *and uses* plants—generally in a medicinal manner (an herb doctor). An *herbologist* (a word, by the way, that does not occur in any dictionary in my possession) is generally meant to be a person who collects and studies the *uses of* herbs/plants. *Herb* comes from the Latin and means grass or green crop and *logy* comes from a Greek root meaning to speak or discourse upon. Currently, many young people casually call themselves herbalists when in fact they are more properly termed herbologists.

Who were the first herbalists? I think it can be said simply that cave women were the first herbalists or herb doctors. Surely these women must have observed animals using certain plants as medicines as we have all seen our modern pets do. Animals sometimes eat large quantities of diarrhea-producing plants in a clear effort to rid themselves of some internal evil. The cave women working alongside their men must have been responsible for the health and well-being of their offspring and administered plants as curatives. This knowledge was passed down from mother to daughter for millennia from the time of foraging to the time when crops were planted.

When people began to settle down, they no doubt planted the medicinal plants they had been picking and using from the wild. Women were the first herbalists treating healing as a natural occurrence having to do with simple observations and knowledge, and nothing whatsoever to do with witchcraft. The wonder of such simple healing, though, must have made these early women curious about a superior being—the one "who gave the plants." Herbalism is indeed the earliest form of medicine. Thus, for humans (man/woman) this knowledge of healing dis-ease using the simple green plants of the fields was probably as instinctive or natural as it was for those animals seeking out appropriate plants for their ills. How did this healing go from these early women into the hands of priests/ magicians and then to the primarily male doctors of our times? This wonderful simple knowledge became the esoteric and secret knowledge of the priest, who in turn was replaced by the academic of the modern-day medical school. The early herb-doctors in every civilized country, at least for the last 5000 years, have regarded healing as a divine art, a gift from the gods. In the ancient herbals, medicine and magic became inextricably linked. I wonder which is the more 'magical'—the witch doctor dancing and shouting, blowing smoke into the various orifices of the patient, and brewing and giving herb teas, or the white-coated man murmuring mild comforting words and dispensing tiny little pills and colored capsules.

Five thousand years ago there were several great cultures practicing herbal medicine: the Chinese, the Egyptians, and the Indians. These cultures used many herbs such as chamomile, ginseng, garlic, opium, and rhubarb and these are still in use today.

E.A. Wallis Budge surmised in his book, *The Divine Origin of the Craft of the Herbalist,* "It has already been said that many ancient nations thought that the gods themselves were the first herbalists, and that it was they who had taught their vicars upon earth how to heal the sicknesses of man-kind by means of certain herbs and plants. More than this, they thought that the herbs and plants which the gods employed in their work of healing were composed of or contained parts of the bodies of the gods. And as the operation or effect of a medicine became more assured, or more potent, if a formula was recited at the time when it was administered to the patient, the god or goddess supplied, according to the general belief, the words which constituted the formula which was recited by the herbalist. Thus the medicine itself, and the knowledge of how to administer it, and its healing effect, came directly from the gods. It is clear that the gods were the earliest herbalists and physicians.

"It is impossible to say exactly which nation possessed the oldest gods of medicine...."

ANCIENT BOTANY AND HERBALISM

EGYPT

3000 BC–2900 BC

In Egypt it is thought that official schools of herbalists existed. The first physician to emerge in this culture that we have a clear picture of is Imhotep who existed around 2980 to 2900 BC. He designed one of the earliest pyramids, the Step pyramid at Saqqarah. He is considered the

Egyptian God of Medicine. He rivaled the Greek god Asclepius or Aesculapius and is sometimes confused with him. Through studying the Egyptian papyrii such as the Ebers Papyrus (circa 2000 BC, translated and named after the 19th century German, George Ebers) which is a list of remedies with the appropriate spells and incantations, our knowledge of Imhotep becomes more clear. According to the heiroglyphs of the Ebers Papyrus, the doctors of Egypt seemed to have practiced a combination of herbalism and faith healing with just a touch of magic thrown in. [The Edwin Smith Papyrus is a treatise on the treatment of injuries and wounds.] In the Ebers Papyrus is that famous folk remedy to cure pimples by washing them with the breast milk from the mother of a newborn boy. (I tried this and found that it worked quite well.)

2500 BC
ISIS AND OSIRIS
These were two of the ancient Egyptians' most important Gods/Goddesses whose origins can probably be traced back to real people who lived during the 4th dynasty, when the Great Pyramid of Cheops was built. Osiris is the God of Agriculture as ShenNung is the Chinese God of Agriculture. Osiris is also the giver of fertility. His twin sister and wife is the Goddess Isis, the Mother Goddess of Herbalism. Osiris and Isis had a son, Horus. Sir E.A. Wallis Budge gives a great account of the sage of Osiris and Isis in his *Divine Craft of the Herbalist,* 1928, now unfortunately out of print. Isis was a great magician as well as a great herbalist, and by means of the "series of invincible spells" which she was taught by Thoth, and by the use of the secret name of the Sungod Ra, she could vanquish every sorcerer, destroy the effect of all incantations, and even raise the dead. Osiris was murdered by his jealous brother Set. Set put him into a wooden casket which he dropped into the River Nile. It floated down to Byblos on the Syrian coast and was found by Isis who returned it to Egypt. Set who was angry and vengeful, found the casket and this time tore the body up into 14 pieces which he "flung" out over the land. Now Isis had her job cut out for her. She set out in a world-wide search. Aided by her tremendous magical knowledge she found all the pieces except his phallus which had been swallowed by a Nile fish of the family Mormyridae, the "Elephant-nosed fish" (a name we hope given to this fish in allusion to the missing royal member). These fish, by the way, were avoided by modern Egyptians well into this century. Isis, with her incredible herbal knowledge, put Osiris' body back together, brought him back to life "by means of the magical touch of her sex," and erected an effigy of the missing

organ. She did such a good job that she was able to conceive as a result of this embrace and bear their son Horus who is represented by the falcon. At this point Osiris also became the God of the Dead.

Sir Wallis Budge says there is good reason for believing that the official schools of herbalists existed in Egypt as early as 3000 BC although all the medical herbals that have come down to us from the Egyptian were written 1000 years later.

CHINA

2700 BC
SHEN-NUNG

As far as we know the Chinese herbalists were the first in recorded history to actually write down the general uses of plants. In 2700 BC there lived a legendary emperor, Shen-nung. He is called the Divine Husbandman and venerated as "The Father of Agriculture," reputed to have tasted all herbs in order to acquaint himself with their value and use. Attributed to Shen-nung is the writing of a catalogue of Chinese herbs, a sort of pharmacopeia called the *PenTsao.* He is said to have lived 123 years and to have had such thin abdominal walls that he could observe the workings of his stomach and what happened to the food and herbs that he ate. For a year he observed the effects of a different plant every day. (One of the plants about which he wrote is ephedra.)

2600 BC
HUANG-TI: THE YELLOW EMPEROR

Ilza Veith in *The Yellow Emperor's Classic of Internal Medicine,* says that Huang-Ti is "one of the most famous of China's legendary rulers. He is said to have reigned 2696-2598 BC and to have been miraculously conceived by his mother, Fu Pao, who gave birth to him on the banks of the river Chi." Huang-Ti authored the *Nei Ching Su Wen,* the classic treatise on internal medicine which is the basis of all Chinese native medicine and *the oldest medical book extant.* This is the book translated by Ilza Veith and which is amazingly enough, available in paperback. The first part of the book is composed of conversations between the emperor and his physician. It is important because "it develops in a lucid and attractive way a theory of man in health and disease and a theory of medicine." The physician at one point says, "The utmost in the art of healing can be achieved when there is unity." After the emperor asks what is unity, the physician answers, "When the minds of the people are closed and wisdom is locked out, they remain tied to disease. Yet their feelings and desires should be investigated and made known, their wishes and ideas should be followed; and then it becomes apparent that those who have attained spirit and energy are flourishing and prosperous, while those perish who lose their spirit and energy.

SUMERIA AND ASSYRIA

2500 BC

Ea, patron of healers, lived in the watery abyss. An herbal was compiled by the Sumerians at some point, probably about 2500 BC. The herbal that is in the British Museum is dated 650 BC, presumably copied from the far older herbal. This copy was originally stored at Ninevah in the library of Ashurbanipal (668-626 BC), the King of Assyria. (A statue of the king, now considered the patron of libraries, resides near the main library in the civic center of San Francisco, 1987.) This herbal seems to have been originally written in the second year of the reign of Enlil-bani, King of Isin, about 2000 BC and "refers to a tradition from the time of the ancient rulers before the Flood." Whether the Sumerians actually discovered the healing arts that they used we do not know, as they might have learned them from another culture. In the medical works of Ashurbanipal's library the remedies are divided into organic and inorganic substances. Plants such as figs, dates, anise, jasmine, juniper, coriander, caraway, and willow have been identified. The Sumerians to have had considerable knowledge of the plants they used and their medicinal properties. The healing arts of the Egyptians and the Sumerians have much in common. It is supposed that the latter learned from the former, although it has also been supposed that both of these civilized cultures borrowed their medical arts from a common source, possibly the highly evolved Asiatic culture rather than the nearer African one. Sir Wallis Budge says of these ancient herbalists, "The herbalist had sufficient knowledge to classify plants according to his/[her] needs, but he does not arrange his plants in the order of modern botanists."

INDIA

2000–1000 BC
AYURVEDA

The earliest concepts of Indian medicine are set out in the Vedas. Filled with magical charms and practices for the treatment of disease and eradication of bodily demons, the Vedas have numerous herbal treatments and treat conditions such as leprosy, abscess, skin disease, coughs, and intestinal complaints. "The Hindus had an extraordinary gift for teaching surgery by operating on vegetables and leaves instead of animals. Their materia medica was even richer than that of Egypt, and the virtues of 750 plants were known to them, garlic and birch bark being particularly praised" (from *The Magic of Herbs* by Leyel). Ayurveda, the science of life, has been practiced in India for centuries. See *Ayurveda for You* by Dr. Chandra-shekhar for a modern treatment of this ancient system.

GREEKS (THE HELLENES)

The Greeks, like the Egyptians and the Sumerians, believed that the Gods were the first herbalists and physicians and that they taught humanity the art of healing. The founders of many of the great Greek schools of medicine owed much of their learning to the Egyptians.

1250 BC
AESCULAPIUS

Aesculapius was the first Great God of Medicine. He was the son of Apollo and the virgin Coronis and was born about 1250 BC. Aesculapius is said to have learned the art of healing from the centaur Cheiron. Cheiron was famous for his wisdom and knowledge of the healing arts and was accidentally shot by an arrow poisoned with aconite (monkshood, *Aconitum napellus*) from the bow of Hercules. Chiron or Cheiron renounced his immortality and at his death was put among the stars by his gods as the constellation Sagittarius the Archer. Aesculapius carries a staff with a serpent* coiled around it, a symbol of renewed life. He was such a success in healing diseases and raising the dead that Zeus became irrationally jealous and killed him with a thunderbolt. The Romans worshipped Aesculapius in the form of a snake around 300 BC. There is no suggestion that he ever authored any works. According to ancient tradition, he was actually an Egyptian healer who wandered to Greece to introduce Egyptian medicine.

Hygieia, the Greek goddess of Health, is the daughter of Aesculapius.

---

*a single serpent = the caduceus of Aesculapius, a symbol of healing; two serpents = caduceus of Mercury or the symbol of trade and business.

1250 BC–600 BC

ASCLEPIADAE

Asclepiadae were a family of physicians and lay herb doctors (ancient barefoot doctors) said to be the cult followers of the hero/god Asculapius and his direct descendants. This group is considered to be the true source of Greek medicine rather than the priests of Aesculapius. These doctors compiled the Greek herbals and wandered from place to place healing the sick wherever they found them. Mrs. Leyel mentions the "magnificent oath of the Asclepiads, which because it represented the ethics of Hippocrates is regarded as part of his teaching." This is the now-called Hippocratic Oath:

"I swear by Apollo the Physician, and Aesculapius, and Hygieia, and Panacea, and all the gods and goddesses, that according to my ability and judgement I will keep this oath and this stipulation—to reckon him who taught me this art equally dear to me as my parents, to share my substance with him, and relieve his necessities if required; to look upon his offspring in the same light as my own brothers, and to teach them the art, if they should wish to learn it, without fee or stipulation; and that by precept, discourse, and every other mode of instruction, I will impart a knowledge of the art to my own son and those of my teachers and to disciples bound by a stipulation and oath according to the law of medicine, but to none others. I will follow that system of regimen which according to my ability and judgement I consider for the benefit of my patients, and abstain from whatever is deleterious and mischievous. I will give no deadly medicine to anyone if asked, nor suggest any such counsel; and in like manner I will not give to a woman a pessary to produce abortion. With purity and with holiness I will pass my life and practice my art. I will not cut persons laboring under the stone, but will leave this to be done by men who are practitioners of this work. Into whatever houses I enter I will go into them for the benefit of the sick, and will abstain from every voluntary act of mischief and corruption; and further, from the seduction of females and males, of free men and slaves. Whatever in connection with my professional practice or not in connection with it I see or hear, in the life of man, which ought not to be spoken of abroad, I will not divulge, as reckoning that all such should be kept secret. While I continue to keep this oath inviolate, may it be granted to me to enjoy life and the practice of the art, respected by all men in all times! But should I trespass and violate the oath, may the reverse be my lot!"

AGAMEDE

Among this group of healers (Asclepiads) is a recognized and famous woman, the herbalist Agamede. She is famous for her vast knowledge of all the plants and their healing powers. Agamede is mentioned in the Iliad, Book XI, "I was the first to kill my man and take his horses—to wit the warrior Mulius. He was son-in-law to Augeas, having married his eldest daughter, golden-haired Agamede, *who knew the virtues of every herb which grows upon the face of the earth."* After Isis this is the only other mention of a woman as herbalist.

600 BC

THALES

Thales was the founder of the Ionic School and a student of Egyptian priests. One of the Seven Wise Men of ancient Greece, he founded the cosmology that water is the basic stuff of the physical universe.

536 BC

JEWISH MEDICINE

"The Jews borrowed very little from the Egyptians. Their physicians were a separate race and their medicine was based on elaborate laws for the prevention of illness. These laws were transmitted by verbal tradition from the time of their Babylonian captivity in 536 BC. Their herbal lore was compiled by King Solomon. The herbal knowledge and a treatise on pharmacy have both perished."

500 BC

Greek medical knowledge advancing. Hippocrates born, he puts medicine on a scientific basis, basing his theories on actual observation, separating fact from fancy.

500 BC

PYTHAGORAS

Pythagoras was the founder of a School of Mathematics at Crotona that stated the earth was not the center of the universe. He was a pupil of Unnefer, an Egyptian priest.

450 BC

HIPPOCRATES

Hippocrates was the Father of Medicine and founder of a system of scientific medicine, the principles of which he learned from the Egyptians. The son of an Asclepiad said to be the 17th in descent from Aesculapius and a midwife who was 18th in descent from Hercules, he was the first to separate magic and superstition from medicine. He used 300-400 mostly plant-derived drugs and medicines and is said to be responsible for the *Hippocratic Collection* which is a series of medical works. He was a teacher with many pupils, many of whom (as healers and practitioners of the healing arts, and while using his remedies), used magical incantations to give greater effect to the cures he taught them. There is no direct evidence that he wrote or put together an herbal. He probably used the lists of plants that were known and used by Thales and Pythagorus when they were in Egypt.

400 BC

First Greek Herbal, compiled by Diocles Carystius, was a list of plants and their habitats with statement about their medicinal attributes (not extant).

350 BC

Aristotle descended from the Asclepiadae. He was a great philosopher, a disciple of Plato, and the teacher of Alexander. He is considered "the first great biologist," and thought to have compiled the work called *De Plantis* which is a list of over 500 plants, although many scholars believe it to have actually been authored by Theophrastus.

325 BC

Theophrastus (372–285) was a pupil of Plato and Aristotle, a native of Eresus in Lesbos. He wrote two books on botany and describes over 500 plants in his *Historia Plantarum.* He also wrote *An Enquiry Into Plants* and possibly *De Plantis* which is usually credited to Aristotle. His knowledge was based on first-hand observation as well as information from caravan merchants about foreign plants. Pure botanical investigation is considered to have virtually ended with his work. He is called the "first scientific botanist." His works, which include parts of the oldest Greek herbals which are lost, are valuable "because they are the most complete biological treatises from antiquity."

300 BC

Herophilus was criticized for administering large doses of vegetable drugs to his patients. He authored a work on plants mentioned by Pliny which no longer exists.

200 BC

Andreus wrote an herbal, now lost, and was physician to Ptolemy IV.

50 BC

Crateuas was a great herbalist, called Crateuas, the rhizotomist. He collected plants and was physician to Mithridates VI (120-63 BC). His herbal shows drawings of all the plants that he discusses as well as their names, descriptions, and medicinal uses. Some of these drawings or rather their accurate copies are of great and continuing interest to botanists. It is said that science owes the "art of portraying the forms of plants exactly and artistically for purposes of identification" (from *The Encyclopedia Britaannica*, vol. 3, p. 653) to him. The first to illustrate the herbal, he is justly called "The Father of Plant Illustration."

30 BC

Niger wrote an herbal, now lost.

300-30 BC

All of the Greek herbals and medical works that were written during this time by the greatest botanists and herbalists of the School of Medicine of Alexandria were based upon the lists of plants and medical works of the Egyptians (from *The Divine Craft of the Origin of the Herbalist* by Budge).

50 AD

Dioscorides was one of the greatest, if not *the* greatest of the ancient herbalists. He served in Emperor Nero's army as physician and collected "a great deal of general information about plants at first hand" (from *The Encyclopedia Britaannica*). His great work, *De Materia Medica*, translated by John Goodyear in 1655 and eventually printed in 1933, was compiled in the first century AD and "has been the chief source whence, for fifteen centuries and more, herbalists of all nations have drawn their inspiration" (from *The Greek Herbal of Dioscorides*). This work was essentially a drug collector's manual, a leading text of pharmacology. A large number of copies of the manuscript have survived the centuries more or less intact. But the *Encyclopedia Brittanica* goes on to say, "this work is ill arranged, almost devoid of general idea and steeped in the errors that must always pursue those who follow purely practical ends without regards to theoretical considerations." From his extensive travels in Greece, Italy, Germany, Gaul, Spain, and other countries, he was able to detail the properties of about 600 medicinal plants, giving the name of the plant, its Greek synonym, a description of it, its natural habitat, directions for its preparation as a medicine, and its medicinal effects. "His Herbal is, in fact, a laborious compilation made from the works of Hippocrates, Theophrastus, Andreas, Niger, Crateuas and many other scientific botanists and herbalists" (from *The Divine Craft of the Origin of the Herbalist* by Budge). The treatise consists of five books: *Aromatics, Oils; Living Creatures; Roots, Juices, Herbs; Herbs and Roots;* and *Vines and Wines.* In Book 3, the common plant *Artemisia vulgaris,* what we now call mugwort*, is mentioned as follows, "Being sodden they are good to be put into womanish insessions for the driving out of the menstrua, and the Embryo. But much of the herb being applied to the lower part of the belly moves the menstrua,...dissolves weariness, and he that bears it on his feet, drives away venomous beasts and devils." It is clear that so many of our modern (!) uses for plants actually originated in the ancient herbals. We can say that in *De Materia Medica* are the beginnings of modern botany.

130 AD
GALEN

The last of the really important Greek herbalists is Claudius Galen in whose work, *De Simplicibus,* the Greek herbal assumed its final form. Galen traveled extensively, studied plants and is said to have authored over 400 works, of which 83 are extant. His herbal contains a list of drugs and their uses. "A paragraph is given to each plant, and after its name come its synonym and its habitat; sometimes Galen gives a description of the plant itself, and he usually ends the paragraph with a statement as to its use in medicine. Galen's work was so complete, and in a way so final,

---

*Wort goes back to the Gothic word for *root* and also to the Anglo-Saxon word, *wyrt,* meaning herb.

that no Greek or Roman botanist attempted to supersede the *De Simplicibus* by a work of his own" (from *The Encyclopedia Britaannica*). Many herbalists based their works on Galen without giving him credit. Actually, until Pliny came along, it was not expected that an author cite those who proceeded him/her and whose work was used.

ROMANS

It was a long time before the Romans could be induced to adopt Greek medicine, or even to regard it as respectable, owing to the sexual intrigues of the Greek physicians with the lecherous Roman women. For about six hundred years the Romans managed without any sort of doctor at all. The universal remedy was cabbage and superstitions (from *The Magic of Herbs by* Leyel).

50 AD

Pliny the Elder (C. Plinius Secundus, 23–79 AD) wrote an immensely popular work in 37 volumes called *Historia Naturalis* and now called *Pliny's Natural History*. The *Encyclopedia Britannica* gives short shrift to his work by describing it as "a mirror of the follies and superstitions of his age" (from *The Encyclopedia Britaannica*). It was more widely read in the Middle Ages than the Bible and many of our worst errors in prescribing herbs in modern herbalism can be traced to this work. Pliny's work, though lacking the respect of modern historians, is truly delightful to read. I have spent many hours puzzling over and giggling over his descriptions of actual as well as fanciful creatures and plants. His work must be read with caution as he was most uncritical in his selection of things to include in the 37 volumes. He includes everything he knows and has heard, the facts as well as the fable. Edward Gibbon is kinder in his evaluation of Pliny and says of these books that they are "an immense register where Pliny has deposited the discoveries, the arts, and the errors of mankind" (from *Natural History Magazine*). Pliny says he mentions 100 authors but actually refers to 146 Latin authors and 327 foreign authors including Homer, Cato, Hippocrates, Theophrastus, etc. He calls Homer a prince of learning and the father of antiquities. Actually, many of the works of antiquity as well as many of the ancient scientists and naturalists we know of only through Pliny's work.

One paragraph that may be of interest to competitive joggers and runners mentions the spleen as the source of laughing: "To hinder a man's running: whereupon professed runners in the race that bee troubled with the splene, have a devise to burne and waft it with a hot iron. An no marveile: for why? they say that the Splene may be taken out of the bodie by way of incision, and yet the creature live neverthelesse: but if it be man or woman that is thus cut for the Splene, he or she looseth their laughing by the meanes. For sure it is, that intemperate laughers have always great Splenes." (from *Pliny's Natural History,* by Pliny).

Pliny was an incredible reader, wasting not a moment of his day lest he lose a minute of reading time. He was read to while he bathed or was massaged, when he ate (he was very corpulent) and when he was traveling. He says, "We sleepe only to satisfie nature, even as much as our health requires, and no more; that whiles we studie and muse upon these things we gain so many hours to our life; for surely we live then only, when we watch and are *awake.*"[6] He constantly had a scribe about him to take down notes. So when he says that he collected from 2000 volumes 20,000 facts, we may well believe him. He was a voracious note-taker and learned much from the early Greeks who had learned from the Egyptians. He felt that no book was so bad that some good could not be gotten from it. He can be described as "the first ecologist" and worried much about the Romans' abuse of their environment. In his only extant work, he delivers a passionate plea against humanity's exploitation of the world. "In fact, in regard to one of nature's elements we have no gratitude. For what usuries and for what outrageous uses does she not subserve mankind?" (from *Natural History Magazine*).

Pliny's *Natural History* became a basic reference work for the medieval scholar. Historically, Pliny's main gift to scientific scholarship was the citing of his reference works by title and author. He says in the preface of the first book, "In the front of these books now in hand, I have set down the verie names of those writers, whose help I have used in the compiling of this: for I have ever been of this opinion, That it is the part of an honest minded man and one that is full of grace and modesty, to confess frankly by who he hath profited and gotten any good: not as many of those unthankful persons have done, who I have alleged as my authors. For to tell you a plain truth, know thus much from me, that in conferring about this work of mine, I have met with some of our modern writers, who word for word have copied out whole books of old authors, and never vouchsafed so much as the naming of them, but have taken their labours and travels to themselves" (from *Pliny's Natural History,* by Pliny).

His life was terminated rather abruptly when Mount Vesuvius erupted August 24, A.D. 79. He sent galleys to the aid of friends that lived at the foot of the volcano. Staying extremely calm, he had the presence of mind to make observations at the scene and in turn to dictate to an ever-present scribe. When he arrived at his friend's house, everything and everybody was in an uproar and terrified at the falling cinders, ash and noxious gas that was everywhere. However, he kept to his routine, soothed everyone's fears and took a nap. He was awakened because houses were rocking from side to side and the people were afraid for their lives.

The galleys were unable to retreat because the winds and waves were high. So Pliny, with a pillow tied to his head, lay down near the shore upon a sail-cloth, drank some water, and died; suffocated, no doubt as his nephew said, "by some gross and noxious vapor" (from *Natural History Magazine*).

130-200 AD
Galen, a Greek, was founder of experimental physiology. He learned anatomy at the Greek School in Alexandria. He was a Greek physician and the most distinguished physician at antiquity after Hippocrates. He is not purely an herbalist. (See previous section.)

400 AD
Priscianus was physician to Emperor Gratian and wrote an herbal.

500 AD
Apuleius wrote *Herbarium* (see the Old Herbals).

600 AD
The Greek Herbals were translated into Latin.

500–600 AD
The important Greek herbals that have been mentioned previously were translated into Latin and used extensively. The works of others were incorporated into these herbals and often names were changed. In Arabia and Syria the herbals of Diosorides and Galen were being translated into the native languages. Those Greek and Roman doctors who were knowledgeable about plant viruses went to these countries and dispersed their knowledge and abilities. These Roman and Greek herbals (based of course on the Egyptian work) became the Arabic and Syrian *Book of Medicines* (*Kethabha dhe Sammane . . .*) that was clearly based on the writings of Dioscorides and Galen. Many of the native prescriptions were taken from the Assyrians and have much in common with the ancient Egyptian remedies. The pre-Islamic Arabs became acquainted with Greek herbs and Greek herbalism through the Jewish teachers of medicine who

had studied at the school of Alexandria.

600–1200 AD
ARABIC HERBAL
The great Greek herbals were translated into Arabic. The great Arab botanist was Abd-Allah Ibn Al-Baitar, born in Malaga and died in Damascus (1248 AD). He compiled the great *Arabic Herbal,* based on the herbals of Theophrastus, Diocorides, and Galen. He studied diligently and amassed great knowledge and was therefore able to correct some of the mistakes of these Greek works. He writes of 800 plants including Indian and Persian ones. Arabic medicine adopted the medicine and treatments of the Greeks but also kept charms and spells and added their own amulets and magic secrets. To the Arabs "we owe the delicious syrups, sherbet and juleps, and the fragrant flavouring waters and conserves of scented flowers" (from *The Magic of Herbs,* by Leyel). because they felt that medicine should not only be effective but should be pleasant to taste and smell as well.

MODERN BOTANY AND HERBALISM

There are two very different ways of looking at the many herbals which lie between their chief source which is Dioscorides and the beginnings of modern botany. We can see science slowly freeing itself from ignorance. The herbalist gave birth to medicine on the one hand and to scientific botany on the other. Another way to look at the herbals and the herbalist is to think them naive, foolish, and antiquated, while considering scientific reasoning to be a recent innovation.

The ancient knowledge of the herbalist was only able to be widely disseminated once the printing press was invented. The ancient herbals were all printed in Latin and not available to most people. Humanity had always used the herbal knowledge of ancestors and parents to cure any problems and the common person's knowledge of plant lore was spread very slowly throughout the civilized world. "With the invention of the printing press in the 15th century the field of Herbal Lore, Folklore, Plant Healing, and Use was given a new impetus."

THE OLD HERBALS

500–1000 AD
The Romans moved up into the northern countries, bringing with them their Greek/Roman herbals as well as many of their native plants. This

knowledge of plants was gradually disseminated among the people who incorporated their own plants and eventually knowledge. Thus we have the *Herbarium of Apuleius, Lacnunga* and *Leech Book of the Bald.*

500 AD
HERBARIUM
The *Herbarium of Apuleius,* a translation of which was used by the Saxons, is perhaps the "first which opened to the English the herbal medicine of southern Europe, and thus connected Britain with the main stream in the history of systematic botany." (from *Herbals: Their Origin and Evolution,* by Arber).

800 AD
DESTRUCTION
During these years there was much destruction of the old herbals and Books of Simples. There are no extant copies from this period. Danish invasions destroyed most of the written works and the Normans destroyed the old Saxon works. The Druidic uses of plants are mostly lost.

950 AD
Leech Book of the Bald is the oldest existing Saxon book dealing with the virtues of herbs. There is a perfect specimen in the British Museum. This book was copied or penned by a scribe named Cild. It is the oldest existing leech (doctoring) book that was written in the vernacular, and is the first medical treatise written in Western Europe. It contains the embryo of modern English medicine. It is probably a copy of an older book. *The Leech Book* is a manual of a Saxon doctor who refers to other doctors or leeches and he combines his herbal knowledge with much Pagan superstition. The herb lore is based not on personal knowledge but on the other, older herb lore.

1000 AD
Lacnunga is an original work and one of the oldest and most interesting of the herbal manuscripts. It is a small but thick volume without illustrations and is considered the most ancient source of Anglo-Saxon medicine.

1250 AD
Bartholomaeus Anglicus wrote the only original treatise on herbs by an Englishman. It is a work of great importance to plant lovers. A great

theologian, he wrote as easily on theology as he did on herbology. A child could understand his herbal wisdom. This book, *De Proprietatibus Rerum* (one of the earliest, if not the first herbal to be printed, first issued in 1470) was the source of information on natural history throughout the Middle Ages. The period 1200 to 1600 AD was an era of great men such as Bacon, Thomas Aquinas, and Albertus Magnus.

There are other herbals and other translations of the older Greek and Roman works under different names. For an extensive discussion of this time, refer to *The Old English Herbals* by Eleanour Rohde or *Herbals* by Agnes Arber. Basically, the knowledge of herbs was disseminated throughout the ancient world by word of mouth. From the very beginning, man/woman had used the knowledge of local plants and their ability to cure, gained from parents to heal ailments and wounds. The plants or rather the way they were used had limited success. Much important knowledge of ancient ways had been lost in this word-of-mouth history. In the middle of the 15th century (1450) the whole field of herbal knowledge was given a new push by the invention of the printing press.

1485 AD
GERMAN
The *Herbarius* is an herbal in which only 350 plants are listed. It contains woodcuts which were much copied and recopied in other herbals. These are the best woodcuts prior to a new period of botanical illustration beginning in 1530.

1491
GERMAN
Ortus Sanitatus. This German herbal was rich in pictures, some of which "display a liveliness of imagination which one misses in modern botanical books" (from *Herbals: Their Origin and Evolution,* by Arber).

1500
FRENCH
Le Grand Herbier (see *Grete Herball*). "Platearius' account of herbs held an important place in the centuries before the invention of printing, and a version of it is believed to have formed the basis of this French herbal which is of special interest to British botanists, since it was translated into English and published in 1526 as *Grete Herball*"(from *Herbals: Their Origin and Evolution,* by Arber).

THE MODERN HERBALS

1525

Bancke's Herbal was the first printed herbal and contained within it a manuscript of exceptional interest, describing the virtues of rosemary. This manuscript, sent by the Countess of Haiault to her daughter Philippa, the Queen of England, is important because it is obviously the original of the very poetical discourse on rosemary in *Bancke's Herbal.* We do not know the author of *Bancke's Herbal;* it was probably based on a medieval English manuscript, now lost. (from *The Old English Herbals,* by Rohde). It is superior to the later and more famous *Grete Herball. Bancke's* gives the impression that it is a compilation from various sources, the author selecting only what pleased him in the older manuscripts. Arber says that this earliest of English printed books is probably a translation of *De Proprietatibus Rerum* (mentioned previously).

1526

Grete Herball has the highest reputation of the earlier English herbals. It was printed by Peter Treveris and seems to be only a translation of the French herbal *Le Grand Herbier.* It is alphabetically arranged, but not with the idea of natural relationships of plants. These relationships were unknown at this time. The *Grete Herball* is very much like the German *Herbarius* but with poor illustrations. Numerous mention is made of magical effects of herbs in amulets and their effects on the mind.** But here we find the first mention of disbelief of the powers of the mandrake (the hoax that it was human-shaped and needed certain conditions to be harvested under or there would be dire results). "Till recently there were at least two survivals of this belief in herbal scents (or aromatherapy)— the doctor's gold-headed cane formerly carried a pomander at the end to ward off the evil effects of the plague and other illnesses and the little bouquets carried by the clergy at the distribution of the Maundy Money in Westminster Abbey" (from *The Old English Herbals,* by Rohde).

1550

Turner's Herbs. William Turner (1510–1568), physician and divine, "the father of British Botany," was the first Englishman who studied plants scientifically. This herbal marks the beginnings of the science of botany. He was a good friend to Conrad Gesner, the famous Swiss naturalist. This work is the only original work of botany written by any Englishman in the 16th century. It contains many beautiful woodcuts, some of which were drawn by the author, the majority being reproductions of the exquisite drawings in *Fuch's Herbal.* He was one of the few herbalists who cautions against excessive use of any herb.

1550

Fuch's Herbal. Leonhard Fuchs (1501–1566) was the greatest of the German fathers of botany. His work is a landmark in the history of natural knowledge and this herbal contains incredible illustrations.

1552

Aztec Herbal was published in 1552. It is also known as *Libellus de Medicinalibus Indorum Herbis* and may well be the earliest treatise on Aztec pharmacology. It was discovered in 1919 in the Vatican Library.*** This book, called the *Badiano Codex,* was written by Martin de la Cruz, an Aztec doctor (who learned his knowledge from the elders of his race) and it was later translated into Latin by Juan Badiano, an Indian doctor from Xochimilco.

1554

Rembert Dodoens (1517–1585) was the first Belgian botanist of world-wide renown. He had an interest in medical botany and wrote an herbal published in 1554 called *Histoire de Plantes* (Cruydeboeck). Dodoens included many of Fuch's woodcuts while adding new illustrations. The most important work of Dodoens, *The Pemptades,* formed the basis of the English herbal known as *Gerard's Herbal* (from *The Magic of Herbs,* by Leyel).

1569

Nicolas Monardes. Mexican knowledge was exported to Spain soon after the conquest of the Aztecs. Monardes, a Seville physician who had never visited Mexico, published a three-volume treatise, *Joyful Newes Out of the Newe Founde Worlde,* concerning the medicinal herbs of the New World. He based his information on oral accounts and also on direct experimentation. Many plants are named after him such as *Monarda fistulosa* (wild bergamot mint) and *Monarda punctata* (horsemint).

1578

Henry Lyte (1529–1607) translated into English from the de l'Ecluse's

---

**About this time the rose and lily were very popular plants and little books were written full of wonderful recipes using the herb and its scent to ward off evil. The herbalists were never weary of teaching the value of sweet scents for the brain.

French version, Dodoens' *Cruydeboeck* (Histoire de Plantes). He called his version *A Nievve Herball* (A New Herball).

1602

Delightes for Ladies was written by Sir Hugh Plat (1552–1608). It is a "Cosmetic 'Simple,'" a reference book on cosmetics that is still in use to this day. He was referred to as a great and learned observer and the importance of the book rests on the fact that it is the "first printed collection of still-room recipes written for the purpose of publication."(from *Golden Age of Herbs And Herbalists*, by Clarkson).

1597 & 1633

Gerard's Herbal. John Gerard (1545–1612) is the second of the great English herbalists (Turner, Gerard, Parkinson). Leyel says his herbal is the work of Dr. Priest. Priest's work was a commissioned translation of Dodoens' *Pemptades* which fell into Gerard's hands when Priest died. Gerard then altered the classification of the plants and added a great deal from his own observations. He was a surgeon, seemingly well-traveled. This book, which he called the *General History of Plants,* was simply titled *Gerard's Herbal,* and has been reprinted in many editions. It was first published in 1597, after which it was corrected and a better version was printed in 1633. Gerard's herbal is plagiarized to this day by amateurs calling themselves "herbalists."

Gerard was a true gardener and often refers to his own seed and garden. He took great pride in being able to grow plants not often cultivated in Britain. He observed the course of his plants' growth and their method of cultivation thoroughly and with detail. He was tireless in tracing down odd plants and observing their virtues and faults as well as the botanical characteristics. He grew over 1000 plants and gives the impression of having personal experience with every plant he describes. Gerard's book is full of errors, however, and we cannot "accept him as a credible witness." One of these errors is his "oft-quoted account of the Goose tree or 'tree bearing geese.' This account removes what little respect one may have felt for him as a scientist—not because he describes it, with utter disregard for the truth, but because he describes it as confirmed *by his own observations*" (from *Herbals: Their Origin and*

***A manuscript text in English is available in holdings of the Newberry Library, 60 West Walton, Chicago, Illinois.

Evolution, by Arber). Even the most cursory reading of the book suggests how much we lose by the lack of the old simple belief in the efficacy of herbs to cure not only physical ills, but also those of the mind and heart. This belief was shared by the greatest civilizations of antiquity, and it is only we moderns who ignore the facts that very wonderful effects may be wrought by the virtues of plants. Gerard had a simple faith in herbs (from *Golden Age of Herbals and Herbalists,* by Clarkson). As a matter of fact, he believed in a new-old system of treating disease, both mental and physical, called Aromatherapy. Aromatherapy treats by the inhalation of volatile oils, treating through the sense of smell and the nasal mucous membranes and also by the absorption of odors through the skin into the circulatory system by using pressure-point therapy.

1606
William Ramn published his own version of Dodoens' work and called it *Ram's Little Dodoens.* It has been used extensively in reference materials but it really is not as good as Lyte's *Dodoen* from which it was excerpted.

1629 & 1640
John Parkinson (1567–1650) was the last of the great English writers who belonged to the true lineage of herbalists.12 His books are *Paradisi in Sole Terrestris* (*A Garden of Pleasant Flowers*) published in 1629, and *Theatrum Botanicum* (*The Theater of Plants*) published in 1640 when he was 73. *Paradisi in Sole* is a speaking garden, a tranquil spacious Elizabethan garden full of loveliness and color and sweet scents. It begins, "Although the ancient Heathens did appropriate the first invention of the knowledge of Herbes, and so consequently of Phy sicke, some unto Chiron the Centaur, and others unto Apollo or Aesculapius his son; yet we that are Christians have out of a better school learned, that God, the Creator of Heaven and Earth, at the beginning created Adam, inspired him with the knowledge of all naturall things....". Parkinson's monumental work, *Theatrum Botanicum,* was intended to be a book of simples, and if he had entitled it so it would have no doubt attained the popularity it deserved, for it is far the superior book to *Gerard's Herbal. The Theater of Plants* is the largest herbal in the English language and was intended to be a complete account of medicinal plants and their virtues. I was the most complete English treatise on plants until the time of Ray. Parkinson mentions over 3800 plants, discards some superstitions while holding onto others, and includes hundreds of recipes for beauty and cosmetics.

1659

Leonard Sowerby wrote *The Ladies' Dispensatory* with many simples and includes the qualities of plants.

1652

Nicholas Culpeper (1616–1654) has been written about by Arber as the "most notorious exponent of the subject of astrological botany." Arber believed that England was badly "infected" with astrological botany. Culpeper was most loved and hated in his time. He believed in the Doctrine of Signatures. He was hated by the College of Physicians because he had the audacity to translate from the Latin and publish in English some of the elitist medical works of the time, notably the *Pharmacopoeia* which he retitled *A Physicall Directory*. This book and its formulas had been an exclusive tome for the elite College of Physicians or anyone who could read Latin and they were most upset that it should be translated into simple English so that anyone could read it and delve into its mysteries. He wrote down in plain and simple English the relationships he believed existed between the stars and herbs. He charged small fees, had an unaffected manner, and his poor West-end patients adored him. He had a garden of English medicinal plants and "scorned the many precious foreign plants that Gerard and Parkinson had collected," for he felt that the poor could not afford them. His book, though scorned by the elite, is the one that has been reprinted over and over again in many editions and has been read by many more people than have ever heard of the other, more important, English herbalists. He was the last public herbalist/astrologist.

1656

William Coles (1626–1662) wrote two books, T*he Art of Simpling* and *Adam in Eden*. He wrote in plain colloquial English. His fame is obscured by the fact that his books are difficult if not impossible to find. He was severely critical of Culpeper, "ignorant in the forme of Simples" and "transcribing out of old works only what was useful" and he scornfully repudiated Culpeper's belief in astrological botany and planetary influence. Coles was considered the most famous simpler or herbalist of his time. "His *Art of Simpling* is the only herbal which devotes a chapter to herbs useful for animals and there is one chapter of plants used in witchcraft." It is a tiny volume, the most readable of all the herbals. It contains no illustrations and no plant descriptions but a series of 33 delightful essays that remark on the various aspects of herbalism.

1686
John Ray wrote *Historia Plantarum.* He is considered a botanist rather than an herbalist.

1710
Herbal of Dr. Salmon was published. This huge book "was the swan song of the great herbalists. He was an astrologer, a chemist and botanist, a prolific writer and a book collector. In this herbal he gives not only the full account of the plants but also the preparations made from them and these preparations are distinguished."(from *Golden Age of Herbs and Herbalists,* by Clarkson).

1722
Miller's Herbal was written by Joseph Miller and is an account of plants that were then used in the Practice of Physick. In the preface of this book, Miller says, "The great number of books already extant upon the same subject, may perhaps, at first view, make this Work appear superfluous," but he goes on to say that the number of herbals available make it impossible for a reader to devote the time and study necessary to distinguish those plants actually used and those that are so exotic as to be seldom used. Therefore this herbal was written to give "a distinct account of all the plants used in the shops, with such descriptions as are necessary for acquiring a true knowledge of them." (from *Miller's Herbal,* by Miller).

1735
Compleat Housewife is an herbal and book of simples that suggests that a woman's first duty is to the health of her family and suggests that women understand herbs and how to use them.

1779
The Toilet of Flora is a collection of recipes subtitled *"the most simple and approved methods of preparing baths, essences, pomatums, powders, perfumes, and sweet-scented waters with receipts for cosmetics of every kind, that can smooth and brighten the skin, give force to beauty, and take off the appearance of old age and decay."*

MODERN HERBALISM

From 1800 to 1900 in both England and the United States, doctors wrote their own herbals and medicinal manuals in which they laid out their treatments both physical and herbal. These books (often called copy-cat herbals), usually included advertisements for their patent medicines—elixirs usually containing a large percentage of alcohol and often made up of highly addictive herbal extracts. Lydia Pinkham's Elixir comes from this time period. In the late twentieth century there came a resurgence of interest in homely herbal medicine. Plants began to be analyzed chemically for their active ingredients. Many of these studies showed what herbalists and believers in folk wisdom knew to be true and what had been proven over the centuries—that herbs/plants had active medicinal components, that plant medicine worked, and that folklore had been based on medical reality. Some of the early 20th century herbalists and herbal books that are unusually interesting are:

1892
American Medicinal Plants, compiled by Charles F. Millspaugh. This book is considered to be the definitive study of American medicinal plants; 180 native and acculturated plants are discussed in terms of curative and adverse effects along with nomenclature, description, history and habitat.

1900
Potter's Cyclopedia by R.C. Wren is a source of herbal remedies.

1900
Sebastian Kneipp (1821–1897), a priest, wrote *My Water Cure* and had it published in 1886. This book is considered a classic in the health field. Devoted to curing all ailments with water therapy, it includes a second part dealing exclusively with herbal medicine. Currently (1985), Kneipp's formulas are used to make aromatic as well as cosmetic products that are notable for their excellence and therapeutic value.

1911
Herbs and Weeds is a useful booklet on medicinal herbs by Father John Kunzle who was a Swiss herbalist, former country parson, and pioneer of the science of medicinal herbs. He was born September 3, 1857 and died January 9, 1945, a simple, humble man unaffected by fame and with a direct naturalness that all herbalists should aspire to.

1928
The Divine Origin of the Craft of the Herbalist was written by Sir E.A.

Wallis Budge (1857–1934), an Englishman who was an acknowledged expert on Egyptian antiquities.

1920–1950
Eleanour Sinclair Rohde (1882–1950) is an acknowledged expert in the history of the herbal and her *The Old English Herbals* is one of three basic reference works used. She wrote many, many books during this period, all about gardens, herbal history and herbal usage.

1930–1980
Edmond Bordeaux Szekely was a philosopher, health advocate, herbalist and expert on many cultures and in many languages. He has over 70 books to his credit, including the matter of his philosophy as well as water therapy, nutrition, herbal therapy, food therapy, etc.

1926
Joseph Meyer (1878–1950) wrote *The Herbalist*, a book still in use for its herbal knowledge. He founded the Indiana Botanic Gardens in the U.S. which is still in operation at this writing and run by his family.

1900–1957
Hilda Leyel (1880–April 15, 1957), writing as Mrs. C.F. Leyel, was the author of six major herbals. She also wrote many minor herbals and cooking books. She is the editor of Grieve's *Modern Herbal*. Among her works is *The Magic of Herbs,* published in 1926, the first book to be a history of the use of herbs in medicine and pharmacy. She founded the Society of Herbalists and in the author's introduction to Grieve's *Modern Herbal* says, "I have always experimented in the innocent alchemy of scent blending and cooking but it was not until I had written my first book on herbs that the idea came to me to found the Society of Herbalists and since 1926 I have done nothing else but research work in herbal medicine." She also opened Culpeper House, an establishment devoted to the manufacture and sale of herbal products from medicine to cosmetics. She is indeed one of our greatest herbalists.

1931
A Modern Herbal was written by Maude Grieve. This book, edited by Mrs. Hilda Leyel, is an extremely useful source book with few drawbacks. It is truly a modern herbal, bringing up to date the history, folklore, usage, and abuse of herbs listing medicinal, cosmetic and culinary applications.

1939

Back to Eden is Jethro Kloss's (1861–1946) interesting herbal, subtitled *A Human Interest Story of Health and Restoration.* Unfortunately, this quite unique volume full of recipes and information has been used as a 'bible' of herbal healing by the subculture. This book has a number of drawbacks, notably incorrect naming of plants, but is important as a source of the historical uses of herbs, though not necessarily their correct or current use.

1940

The Golden Age of Herbs and Herbalists was written by Rosetta Clarkson (1892–1950) who wrote several other books on herbs and herb use. Her work is eminently readable.

1950–1970

Herbal Handbooks on various subjects were written by several authors, some of whom will no doubt become renowned historically. These include:

Juliette de Bairacli Levy, a modern herbalist and student of Edmond Szekely, the famous and great Hungarian doctor, whose subject matter has included herbal medicine for children, dogs and farm and stable animals;

Nelson Coon, who wrote several books detailing the use of wayside plants and planting for fragrance;

Maurice Messegue, a Frenchman who gave new and interesting ways to use plants and claimed to have all the royalty of Europe as clients;

Richard Lucas, who has several books to his credit; and

Jean Valnet of France who has written several interesting books including *Phytotherapie* and *Aromatherapie.*

1970–1988

Authors of note include Jeanne Rose, termed the "grande dame" of modern herbalism with seven books to her credit; James Duke, *Handbook of Medicinal Herbs;* Tisserand, writing about Aromatherapie; Paavo Airola, many books to his credit with much information repeated from one to the other; Michael Tierra, with an interesting book combining Western and Eastern herbs; John Lust, who wrote *The Herb Book* and Christopher's rather important work; and Michael Moore, author of *Medicinal Plants.*

ANCIENT HERBS STILL IN USE TODAY

SUMERIAN, THROUGH GREEK AND ARABIC

apricot	almond	cherry
cypress	flax	lupin
mulberry	mandrake	poppy

EBERS PAPYRUS, 2000 BC
EGYPT

onions	dates	pomegranates
caraway seeds	poppy	gentian
squills	castor oil plant	elderberry
mint	aloes	myrrh
colchicum	lotus flower	chamomile
licorice	henna	camphor
honey	olive oil	palm oil and leaf
flax seed	raisin or grape	elder berries
papyrus	mandrake	wheat

SOME HERBS USED BY HIPPOCRATES (300 BC), STILL IN USE TODAY

absinthe	almond	alum
anchusa	anemone	anise
asphodel	balm	basil
brier	bryony	burdock
cabbage	capers	cardamom
carrot	cinnamon	cloves
coriander	cress	cyclamen
elder	fennel	fig
garlic	hawthorn	heather
hellebore	hemlock	henbane
horehound	ivy	juniper
laurel	lettuce	mallow
mandragora	mint	mugwort
myrrh	myrtle	narcissus
oak	olive	onion
pennyroyal	peony	pomegranate
poppy	quince	rose
rosemary	rue	saffron
sage	sesame	squills
tarragon	thistle	thyme
turpentine	verbena	violet
wild cucumber	willow	

ASSYRIAN HERBAL, FROM LIBRARY OF ASHURBANIPAL, KING OF ASSYRIA (667–626 BC)

dates	figs	anise
juniper	coriander	jasmine
oleander	willow	colewort
caraway		

ANCIENT HINDUS (750 PLANTS WE CAN IDENTIFY)

garlic	birch bark	rhubarb
ginseng	opium	

THE YELLOW EMPEROR CLASSIC (2500 BC, CHINA)

thyme	millet	wheat
rice	beans	apricot
plums	dates	mallows
onions	leeks	mandrake
ginseng	licorice	ephedra
ginger	cinnamon	mugwort
clove	water lily	ferns
banyan	figs	loquat
gardenia	geranium	cotton
ginseng	witch hazel	sunflower

PLINY'S NATURAL HISTORY (1ST CENTURY)

wild cucumber	radish	parsnip
chervil	onion	elecampane
leek	garlic	wild lettuce
beets	endive	sea coleworts
parsley	rocket	rue
wild mint	garden mint	pennyroyal
nepeta	cumin	panax
marjoram	dill	poppy
coriander	mallow	dock
sorrel	horehound	thyme

AZTEC HERBS (IN USE IN 1552)

dioscorea	euphorbia	manzanita
artemisia	copal tree	ipomoea
saponaria	mezquite	ephedra
nettle juice	rue	chile
storax	cotton plant	chia
nasturtium	corn	fennel

Western Herbal Medicine: A Perspective

AMANDA MCQUADE-CRAWFORD, B.S.C.

When I was doing my homework for giving an overview of Western herbalism in fifteen minutes or less, I saw too many interconnected chains of events. I realized any overview I could speed read to you in fifteen minutes would not be worth having. I could do Egypt and Hammurabi, 18th century BC Middle East, Mediterranean and Europe up to the 10th century AD in five minutes, then spend five minutes on Medieval and Renaissance Western herbalism through the Age of Reason to the New World, and do five minutes of Western herbalism in the Americas, North and South through the 1800s until meeting in Cincinnati today at the end of the twentieth century. But many herbalists and interested persons already have a grasp of the heritage from Dioscorides, Avicenna, Paracelsus, Samuel Thomson, Maud Grieves and the unsung healers of Western herbalism during its ebb and flow for the last 1000 years at least. When I was trying to distill Western herbalism down to say something true and worthwhile, there was one clear common pattern repeated in many historical settings:

1. Western herbalists in the past always have prospered because they successfully addressed the health needs of a large number of people.

2. Our cyclical swings in popularity are in proportion to the failure perceived in conventional, allopathic medicine.

3. Herbalists in the West have often welcomed the anonymity, even invisibility of being the quiet, compassionate, ever supreme healthcare modality existing under—but not submissive to—established, regulated medical practice.

4. Western herbalists, when they have felt this underground status to become unhealthy, have attempted self-government, self-improvement and some vision of legal self-defense.

5. Western herbalism has a pattern in the past of consistently failing to

achieve its goals as a profession, through allowing internal disagreements to lay the therapy wide open to external pressures instead of acknowledging diversity and unity. Good ideas have been fragmented fairly consistently down the centuries through egos striking antagonistic postures about petty pecking orders. The bitter debate about gentle art versus hard science, tea over standardized herbal tablet, the human tendency to rise up in the eyes of authorities by distancing from and knocking those seen as directly below you—these are a common thread woven into the fabric of Western herbalism's past; but we can choose now to stop this back and forth dance and start a new dance, which accords better with the conscious herbalism I've already heard articulated at this inaugural meeting of the American Herbalist Guild.

We often point out that herbs were orthodox medicines until the 1920s or 1930s, but the issues regarding Western herbal practices and the current medical monopoly go way back. These days there is an increasing pressure in modern professional herbalism to justify ourselves again, but it's an old battle we can win only by not buying into the whole war. This war takes form now as an increasing pressure among gentle natural healers to publish or perish, competing against each other to be seen as the most scientific or authoritative, *or* as the most natural—who's more organic than the next herbalist, who's commanding more at the box office, who's the best. While upgrading quality is appropriate, we have some timely lessons to learn from our historical pattern of scrambling to the top in such a fashion as to pull all of us down. The current mood affecting us in 1990 happened to Medieval Western herbalism as well as the Eclectics and countless other waves of herbal medicine. There are dangers now in becoming dedicated to the cause of herbal medicine. The cause is not that of herbalism. The only cause is that of the people that we serve and the planet that we walk. This necessarily includes ensuring that herbs of the highest possible quality are widely available in wilderness areas, preserved for their value in and of themselves, as well as for conscious medical use. This can be according to *our* criteria, created with our consensus. We all know herbalism has a timeless gift of simplicity and elegance which our late twentieth century requires, just as we require a new balance of personal success with right livelihood and service to the whole.

We all know that not all herbs are safe because they are natural, but herbalists—unlike doctors—rely on observation of whole plant/whole human interactions recorded over centuries of similar use. Good herbalists know how and why to gauge a safe and effective dose. Even Britain's

1964 Medicines Act agreed to accept as proof of safety and efficacy the fact that an herb had been in use for a long period without giving any ill effects. This wise judgment from the Ministry of Health was only due to a professional body of herbalists who finally organized the massive resource of their loyal, satisfied patients to help make their legal voice heard. So we in the West have sometimes had tenuous, fragile claims to legitimacy, but we are not out of the woods yet. The FDA, the Gras lists, the EEC legislation in progress, all smolder with group memory of official hostility and misunderstandings common to us herbalists who are human as well as authorities. Even the American Herbalists Association (AHA) of respectable gardeners disavows any medical use for herbs in case they are tarred and feathered with the same brush as our AHA and the rest of us mountebanks and dangerous eccentrics. The real danger to public health is not from herbalists getting somewhere with a valid therapy, but from knee-jerk closed-mindedness of nervous bureaucrats who find it more comfortable to uphold the expert researchers who can be notoriously haphazard, even dishonest, when paid to prove what they want to believe anyway. Any good herbalist can tell you what the problems facing scientific analysis of herbs are. Now that we are learning how to accomplish plant research that we might trust, wholistic nature cures are still going to be hard to patent and, for a lot of people, Western herbalism will still appear tedious, gradual, strange-tasting and inconvenient for those who are not ready to change their lives to integrate healthy personal and planetary ways; thus, conventional plant research has been a dead-end career for much of this century, but that may be changing now, as the whole Western hemisphere, not just herbalism, is reawakening to simple concepts like wholeness and compassion.

Too many "normal" people are speaking about herbs now for it to go quietly back underground from current pressures. Too many species, especially humans, need the message of wholistic health choice inherent in Western herbalism, from Beijing to Boise. The vision of the people cannot be squashed, although it may be turned aside a few more times before it finds its mark. Whether we want to deregulate or create our own appropriate structure, this historic dance of tea versus tablet, of ideas fragmented by personalities, this need not go back and forth forever. We can avoid the divisive squabbles among our strongly held opinions by now, can't we? Don't we have a responsibility to change old patterns for the common good? From the Russian folk medicine to the science of Dr. Brekham, with Herboriste of France and Italy being vindicated by the plant research of Germany, with Medical Herbal Consultant of England, Australia, and New Zealand, and the Herbal practitioner of any tradition in North America, there is promise of unity with diversity. Let us hope we in the West have learned our lessons well.

Introduction to Folkloric Herbalism*

JAMES GREEN

At this historic event, I have the honor and the overwhelming chore of introducing folkloric herbalism. I'm pursuing this task not as an expert, but rather as an heir and a participant; a grateful heir and an avid participant. Folkloric herbalism is not easily interpreted or defined. My knowledge and words are appropriately humbled as I stand here before you attempting to impart some unique understanding of an art and science of herbalism that I personally value above all others, and yet, intellectually, that I realize I know so little about. Like many herbalists, I feel our folklore deep within my being. Its nature is infused in my spirit, but to express these feelings in words is difficult.

What is the essence of folkloric herbalism? (I recycled many a piece of scrap paper with notes and outlines searching for an answer to this question; an answer that could serve as an adequate introduction to this immense, though highly illusive concept and practice. Yet the definition of folkloric herbalism, in most part, remained a mystery to me.)

I could not readily isolate the active ingredient, so to speak, that makes it special to an herbalist's soul, the mysterious constituent that renders it profoundly different from its companion—Western scientific herbalism.

I kept asking myself...
What mystery does it hold?
What mystery does it hold?
What mystery it holds.
What mystery!

---

*As presented in Cincinnati to the American Herbalist Guild Symposium 1990

From behind a slowly dispersing mist it came to me... What makes folkloric herbalism so uniquely splendid is the mystery it holds, and the profound mysteries of creation that it conveys for our daily use. The enduring tenacity of the marvelous mystery that has entwined folkloric herbalism throughout the ages—and to this very moment—is what renders it so timeless, so undying and so relevant to human beings who live every moment enshrouded in mystery.

Folkloric herbalism reaches out and cares for humanity directly from the world of wonder. It's not difficult to understand why folkloric herbalism is ignored, as much as possible, by our Western rational science. Western science simply does not assimilate mystery very well. Its nature must know *how;* and it must know *why.* What it can't prove by its peculiar methods of investigation and manipulation, it tends to impulsively invalidate.

And on top of this, our current western society has great difficulty dealing with the shadows of life. Folkloric herbalism is rich with mysteries and whole with its shadows. It's alive with the use and activities of incense smoke, healing, curanderos, herbal energetics, shamans, empirical evidence, drumming, amulets, charms, witches, plant and animal allies, potents, medicine people, fairies, rituals, chanting and prayer.

In most Native American folk healing the word *medicine* signifies a complex of ideas, rather than merely a remedy or treatment alone. What Western rational therapists speak of with the word "medicine" the Native American calls "mysterious," meaning that which is beyond his or her power to account for; the inexplicable.

The Native American called the horse, medicine dog; the gun, medicine iron; alcohol, medicine water; and the medicine man, healer and mystery man, a worker of magic. "Medicine" was accepted and used in the sense of the magical, the supernatural, the unaccountable. I healed with great power.

In contrast, the Western scientific mind thinks of medicine in terms of drugs (standardized herbal and mineral drugs), ointments, serums, cathartics and so on which will act on the body in a predictable fashion...or at least, usually they do.

Practicality and wisdom are deeply embedded in folkloric herbalism. The mystery and ritual of its remedies cushion and preserve the patient's hope; and hope is the ultimate placebo. The placebo effect is the primary healing agent in all medicines, be they western, eastern, northern or southern medicine. Modern Western placebo research has confirmed this fact many times over, but this is not widely publicized.

For those individuals who wish, folkloric herbalism supplies the knowledge, the language and the simpler's tools which allow each person to empower himself and herself to thrive independently and tend to their own basic nutrition and health maintenance.

Intimately conjoined with the elemental laws and pulses of Earth, folkloric herbalism shows great respect for all Her plants, animals and minerals. For the nature of these wonderful beings is also deeply mysterious to the folkloric practitioner. Each of these companion beings has profound, unseen medicine power.

This power is called *mana* by the Melanesians; *orenda* by the Iroquois; *wakan* by the Dakota. This is the power of all life, whether in action or in passive endurance. To folkloric consciousness, even the commonest sticks and stones have a spiritual essence which must be revered as a manifestation of the all-pervading mysterious power that fills the universe. This respect is evidenced throughout the mythology, the folkloric ceremonies and the prayers of ancient people, our wise ancestors.

> *We return thanks for all herbs,*
> *which furnish medicines for the cure of our diseases.*
> *We return thanks to the corn, and to her sisters,*
> *the beans and squashes,*
> *which give us life.*
> *We return thanks to the bushes and trees,*
> *which provide us with fruit.*

This is a simple Iroquois prayer. It would be good medicine to see this folkloric prayer on the walls of our local supermarkets and our local drugstores.

Folkloric herbal science is heir to a wealth of practical, empirically proven knowledge and skills which were contributed by the perception and conscious intelligence of our ancestors. This has been bequeathed to our generations by ancestral actions and patient teaching. It is no wonder that folkloric herbal traditions openly honor and care for their elders. The ancestors of each one of us has contributed to this gift of plant knowledge. It is an all-encompassing science, a modern expression of the cumulation of all the healing sciences known to humanity. It is at once the most ancient of sciences and the most advanced, for it embraces all healing science known to us. Folkloric medicine is forever now in the making. There are no experts in folkloric herbalism; there are myriads of participants, and we are forever students. We are all contributors and we are all heirs to its wisdom and its practicalities.

Currently in this culture, we consider most things to be disposable, but our myths and folklore are not disposable; their extinction will cause our culture to die. We must not allow this. We can revive our genetic memory and refocus on our planetary connections, honor and nourish them and relearn to utilize and enhance the timeless folkloric knowledge of our elders.

The science of folkloric herbalism encourages the empowerment of each person to use Earth's freely given, natural medicines and to do this harmlessly, in harmony with the other companion species that make up the wonderful diversity that is the living planet, Earth.

Fragments of Earth Wisdom
FEATHER JONES, C.H.

The traditional Native Americans approach medicinal herbs from the basic understanding that all healing comes from within the individual through a reconnection with the Great Spirit. The Mother Earth is seen as sacred and her children, the plant people, are beings with much to teach us. When an herbalist starts on the medicine path, either through the Wise Woman, the holistic, or the shamanic traditional ways, one of the first lessons given is a simple concept that when the body or spirit is stressed beyond its capacity for self-restoration, the plant which corresponds to the lost function will "teach" the body or spirit how to take up the job again. In this way, we develop a kinship and appreciation for the botanical realm.

With this traditional viewpoint, respect for the plants is a reflection of our respect for nature. Never does one just go to an area and start harvesting in a rape and pillage fashion. This is a teaching. The spirit of the plant is recognized and called forth in communion and appreciation. The medicine person asks permission to gather through use of ceremony, and describes the purpose of the taking. An offering of cornmeal or tobacco is given, not so much in exchange for the plant, but to act as a sacred covering to the empty spot on the earth now left by the vacant space of a newly dug hole.

The traditional people tell us each plant has a purpose to its life and has inherent intelligence to fulfill that purpose regardless of its environmental struggle. Sometimes the purpose will be instrumental in the healing of a human being.

Judith Whitesinger, a Mandan-Hidatsa medicine woman and pipe holder, lives on one of the Plains Indian reservations in North Dakota. As one of my earlier teachers, she taught me how to gather plants whose medicine power and personality are the strongest. This does not necessarily correspond to a plant's color, brightness, or sturdiness in a stand, but rather to its calling and subtle characteristics.

A lesson that I continually learn on deeper levels is that plants are entities that carry vibrations many of which are compatible to humans. People vibrate on different energy frequencies depending on their thoughts, emotions and state of health and disease. Certain plants correspond to various energy frequencies of people when they are sick and teach the body how to heal itself through the power of their medicine. To give an example, I was visiting at a time when the mother of a young man on the reservation came to see Judith for some doctoring. Her son had broken his leg. He was an athlete at school and needed to get back on his feet as soon as possible. Judith took me with her to a nearby field to collect poultice herbs. We passed the comfrey in her backyard, the arnica on the hillside and the St. John's wort by the ditch. Trying to sound intelligent, I immediately started telling her the virtues of these plants for internal wounds. I remember her tolerant gaze as she waited for me to finish my herbal computer printout. She said I would have to set aside my previous experience and knowledge of these herbs and listen to the plants in the field. They would speak to me if I could turn off the internal dialogue long enough to hear them. I briefly closed my eyes thinking some plant would pop into my consciousness waving leafy arms. Instead when I opened my eyes and scanned the field, I saw a group of very tall Mullein stalks. The one that came into my view was a stalk that had a strange curvature in it. It had a 90 degree right angle halfway up the stalk and then resumed its normal upward growth pattern. It looked just like a fractured bone where the two ends of the break do not meet. The meadow was a "clean" area away from any roadside or powerlines, so I ruled out toxic or electrical mutations as the cause of its unusual form. I asked Judith if this was the plant. She smiled and said it was. We collected the whole plant, the leaf being used as a poultice to decrease swelling and bruising and the flowers as a tea to drink for pain. The results were quickly noticeable as no pain killers were needed and swelling went down right away.

The traditional herbs such as comfrey would have worked, she said, but not as well. She explained this by saying its subtle energy field was not harmonizing to this person's needs. Again, she said each plant is born with an internal code to know its life's purpose through some inherent intelligence, be it wild life fodder, compost, food, seed producer, nectar or medicine. It will fulfill its purpose with intent. If one makes prayers and a connection to the plant, using intuition balanced with intelligence, one can never wrongly harvest and it will be the strongest medicine obtainable. If looked at from this perspective, laboratory validation of herbs and standardized measures of strength move down considerably on the priority list. It's hard to place a value on such teachings, as the measure of value is within oneself.

We all have the intuitive ability to know what herb or formula is going to work best, but like any talent that isn't used, it becomes dormant. We have to cultivate our intuition to gain accessibility.

SOME NATIVE PLANTS USED IN MEDICINE AND CEREMONY:

Juniper, Western Cedar (*Juniperus communis*). This plant is used for smudging and sweatlodge smoke. Smudging is the burning of sacred herb and fanning the smoke to oneself. This simple cleansing ritual, through use of ancient aromatherapy, purifies one's energy field, clears the mind, stimulates hypothalamic recall and, as the Mandan people say, "it frees up the Spirit." When this sacred plant is burned in the sweatlodge on the rocks and smoke rises to fill the earthen womb, our prayers are sent to the Great Spirit. Cedar invokes the Spirit keeper of the Western direction, and with the smoke, prayers are sent to this direction. Clinically, we know it as an antiseptic and urinary disinfectant. Being aromatic, the properties are excreted into the lungs which dilates the bronchioles and acts as an expectorant. Native people chew about a handful of the berries, breathe deep several times and spit them out. It is also used in vapor baths for coughs and colds.

Silver Sage, Wormwood (*Artemesia* spp.). Besides smudging and sweatlodge use, the body of one who is seeking a vision is rubbed with the herb, and the person in this way becomes the offspring. In the Sun Dance, we use wreaths of sage upon our heads and around our wrists as a sign that our hearts and minds are close to Wakan Tanka. The wreath represents the things of heaven, the stars and planets which are mysterious and holy. For a medicine, it is used in the bath for rheumatism. As a hot tea, it will induce sweating; as a lukewarm tea, it is good for gastrointestinal worms and diarrhea; as a cold tea, it is a bitter, helping with indigestion.

Sha, Bear Medicine, Chuchupate (*Ligusticum porteri*). A sacred plant among the Arapahoe and Pawnee, she is used to induce sweating before purification rites and sweatlodge ceremonies. It is called bear medicine because in early spring after hibernation, the bears dig the plant root for food. Claw marks can be seen on rotten fallen trees moved out of the way. The Arapahoe would send runners through the mountains as messengers. These people would stop to pick and chew the roots for increased stamina. It is worn around the neck in medicine pouches and around the ankles to ward off rattlesnakes. Clinically, it is a bronchiole dilator and expectorant. It strengthens resiliency of alveolar sacs, increasing CO_2 and H_2O transport, and supports elastic properties of the septum to prevent further deterioration and scarring in emphysema. We know it as a strong antiviral and diaphoretic with action upon the lungs, urinary tract and immune system.

Chokecherry, Wild Cherry (*Prunus virginiana*). The bark is used in fasting ceremonies to pray for a vision, branches are put to the four directions with a bed of sage in the middle and lit to pray. This tree is considered sacred and represents the universe. The fruits are red like our life blood. It is also used in hoop and medicine wheel making. The Navajo use the wood in their dance implements to pray to the northern direction. All native people understand its virtues as a cough medicine for colds and feverish conditions. Clinically, we know it's a respiratory depressant. It is used to soften up bronchiole mucus, making it easier to get fluids in and out of the lungs. It is proven beneficial for bubbly sounding congestion as well as a dry, raspy cough. It slows cardio-pulmonary excess, so it is good for hot conditions. It softens the pulmonary vein by increasing fluids to the membranes and keeps the lungs from drying out.

Aspen (*Populus tremuloides*) and Willow (*Salix* spp.). These two trees are used interchangeably in construction of the sweatlodge frame. Twelve to sixteen young willows are soaked in a stream until they become soft and bendable without breaking. Then they are made in such a way that they mark the four quarters of the universe, so the lodge is an image of the universe and everything is contained within it—people, four-leggeds and all things of the world. This is set up in a ceremonial way with songs, invocations, prayers and chants while being constructed. People are smudged before making the lodge and all medicine objects that go into the lodge are smudged in the Lakota tradition. The door faces the east. The lesson the willow teaches us is in the fall the leaves die and return to the earth, but in the spring they come to life again. People die to live again in the real world of Wakan Tanka. The sweatlodge provides this opportunity to be reborn within Mother Earth's womb in a ceremonial way. Medicinally, the bark tea is used internally for rheumatism, headaches and to bring down a fever. The twigs are chewed to numb a toothache. The sticky buds of early spring are combined with tallow to make a salve. This is rubbed into the nostrils and the strong aromatic vapors relieve congestion. Clinically, we know willow and aspen contain salicin and populin, similar to aspirin. These properties are anti-inflammatory and control prostaglandin imbalances and act to turn down the internal thermostat.

These plants and many more have strong healing benefits not listed in any clinical text. What is required from us is the frame of mind that recognizes their subtle power.

The native people use ritual to bring forth the spirit of the plants. It is hard to describe in words that which is conveyed through ritual and prayer. Ritual allows one to make a shift in consciousness. This freeing up of the Spirit creates a vision where the wind blowing through the trees is the song of the land, and the ripened seed pod is the rattle of rhythm. When White Buffalo Calf Woman came to teach the pipe ceremony to the people, she brought her wisdom. This smoking of sacred herbs is still the same and invokes the potent healing forces of the Spirit Keepers.

Without discrediting the modern day clinical approach to plant medicines, our "new age" herbalism with its reliance on technology is quite often only seeing part of a picture. If we take the time, if we care to listen, we can walk in the backyard or to the woods and learn the songs of the plant people. Besides holding intuitive abilities, we gain a stronger connection and deeper understanding of earth medicine. "Mitakuye Oyasin" in the Lakota language means we are all related.

Herbalists &
Herbal Elders

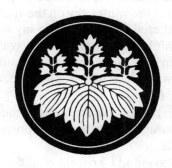

John Raymond Christopher: A Legacy of Courage*

DAVID CHRISTOPHER

INTRODUCTION

Snow drifted high along the drive, and the icy spindles of bare branches seemed to scrape against the winter sky on the stark morning of February 11, 1983, when we gathered to memorialize my father. Five days earlier we had stood around his bedside—my mother, who had come to tuck the hand-stitched quilts around his shoulders; his children, who stroked his magnificent mane of white hair with gentle care; and his grandchildren, who scampered at our feet.

We held him in our arms, warm against the chill of winter, as he slipped peacefully through death into the presence of One who had guided him through life.

My father, John Raymond Christopher, did not die before the age of thirty-five, as the squadrons of physicians had predicted. His gentle practice of natural healing helped him overcome the chronic conditions he was born with—as well as the life-threatening injuries he sustained as a young adult. He succumbed instead at the age of seventy-three to complications of a severe head injury. He had slipped on the treacherous ice outside his beloved Covered Bridge Canyon home, nestled in the mountains outside Spanish Fork, Utah.

Hundreds of mourners packed the church where we held his funeral—the same building where, a year earlier, he had stood for the last time to conduct his choir. The performance had been electrifying. There had not been a dry eye in the house that Sunday afternoon; there was not a dry eye now among those who crowded into the chapel for a chance to

*An excerpt from "Master Herbalist" by David Christopher, 1991, Christopher Publications, P.O. Box 412, Springville, Utah 84663

bid him farewell.

Family members spoke to the congregation that gathered there. Friends shared their fondest memories. A profusion of little ones named Ray, John, and Christopher abounded, their parents let us know that they were named after my father—without whose herbs they would never have been conceived. A church leader remembered my father's uncommon dignity, painting for us the reflection of dad mowing the lawn in his pin-striped suit. He shared the podium with the then vice-president of the prestigious National Health Foundation.

How had such acclaim been earned by a man who had started out his life abandoned in an orphanage—a man who had been ridiculed in the courts and had been jailed? The acclaim was just. My father was considered the nation's number-one authority on herbal medicine. Tens of thousands of people owed their health and even their lives to his work.

If I were pressed to remember anything in particular about my father, it would be his extraordinary happiness. He hid his physical suffering with good cheer, making countless journeys into the blackness of night on his famed "house calls." I often wondered where he found such happiness. I know now it was from the people whose lives he touched. It was from the six-month-old blind baby whose sight was restored…and from the elderly asthmatic who was able to sleep in a bed for the first time in four decades.

My father's abiding happiness seems even more exceptional when I reflect on all the reasons he had to be *un*happy. His life's work was dedicated to helping others, yet he was slandered by the judicial system that should have protected him. He was incarcerated on a number of occasions, left to grovel in the meanest of circumstances while those of us who loved him waited patiently for his release. Once, in what I am convinced was an effort to harass, a judge levied $50,000 bail for a licensing infraction…yet I cannot erase from my mind's eye the gentle kindness of my father's perpetual smile.

He never retaliated against those who did him harm. He was counseled early in his life to love his enemies—and to pray for those who cursed him and persecuted him. That counsel became his clarion cry. I have never seen greater love emanate from any man.

We, as his children, were fiercely loyal to him, but he never coaxed any of us to follow in his footsteps as herbalists. He loved us deeply and he knew only too well of the abuses and persecutions we might endure. I quietly came into the practice on my own—partly, I guess, out of my love for him and because I watched first-hand the way his teachings changed people's lives.

He is gone from among us, but he leaves behind a legacy that will never be forgotten. He created more than fifty herbal formulas that have exacted almost miraculous healings; he spearheaded the School of Natural Healing, which found its way overseas to England. He authored many works on herbs, some of which are considered to be classics in their field.

I struggle daily to live a life that would make him proud. I cherish my memories of him and I hold dear the hundreds of letters that still pour in, almost a decade after his death, thanking him for life itself. They come from every state in the union and some from remote areas of the world, a poignant reminder of his powerful influence. Yes, he is gone...but he will never be far away.

As his son, I share his love and concern with all of those he so cared for—people he had never seen, but whose lives he prayed fervently for. I hope that this brief biography will stand as a fitting tribute to him.

—David Christopher

"I'M GOING TO BE A DOCTOR"

The fiery golds and scarlets of autumn had reluctantly given way to winter, which had crept almost unnoticed that year into the serene Salt Lake Valley, pocketed among the rugged peaks of the Rocky Mountains. It was fitting that John Raymond Christopher, a pioneer in the art of natural healing, should be born in this valley, which had been settled first by a courageous hand of humble pioneers more than half a century earlier.

He was born November 25, 1909, in Salt Lake City, Utah, to Jean Ramone and Lorena Roth Raymond, whose homes were listed on the birth certificate as Loraine, Switzerland, and Paris, France, respectively. For reasons that only these European travelers could have known, they left their infant son and his older sister at the Salt Lake City Orphanage. Shortly after his birth, they moved on from the shelter of the magnificent Rockies.

It was the custom at the orphanage, when prospective parents called, to arrange available children in a line; from that line of hopeful faces, the couple could make their choice. One early summer afternoon, Leander and Melissa Ann Craig Christopher assumed their anxious station in front of such a line. Their fervent hope was to adopt a child—and they prayed they could find a son.

Suddenly and without invitation, a baby clad only in a diaper and a thin undershirt toddled out of line, crawled onto Melissa's lap, and settled comfortably into her shoulder with a hug. Melissa's misty eyes met those of her husband as she exclaimed, "This is our son!"

The Christophers left the orphanage that day with not only the son they had prayed for, but also with his sister Ruby as the blood parents had stipulated. The little family settled into the home Leander had built in Salt Lake City's historic avenues district, a house still listed with the Utah Historical Society. Later the family moved to a comfortable home on Highland Drive—now a teeming metropolitan area, but then a "country" neighborhood characterized by fields of hollyhocks in the summer and lanes of deep snowdrifts in the winter.

The first glimpse the Christophers had of Raymond's extraordinary future came one wintry night in that house on Highland Drive. Young Ray lay critically ill with croup; his anxious parents paced the floor, cradling his fevered body in their arms and praying with all their might that he would have the strength to catch another breath. Suddenly a knock came at the door; Leander, startled because of the late hour, answered.

Standing on the porch was a bearded man in shirt sleeves, with no coat to protect himself against the bitter cold. He announced to Leander that a young child was ill, but was not to die; that he had an important mission to perform. With a sense of awe, Leander listened as the stranger gave explicit instructions on how to cut the phlegm and stop the croup.

Anxious to save the life of his choking child, Leander turned to do the stranger's bidding; when he turned back to thank the man and invite him to warm himself against the winter cold, the man was gone—without a trace. There were no footprints in the deep snow to mark his passing.

With the instructions left by the bearded stranger and the loving faith of his parents, Ray recovered. It was an experience the Christophers would not soon forget, and Ray always remembered that his life somehow held great purpose.

It is ironic that Ray's "mission" involved healing; the wintry croup crisis and his ensuing brush with death were far from the only health problems he suffered. Born with advanced rheumatoid arthritis, he endured excruciating pain; even as a child, he sometimes walked with a cane or was confined to a wheelchair. He also developed hardening of the arteries. Doctors of his day proclaimed that he would never reach the age of thirty.

Most children suffering this kind of pain would become depressed or gloomy—but not John Raymond Christopher. He radiated good cheer;

early in life, he developed a great love for the music that lifted his spirits through years of trying adversity.

His love for music grew as he traveled every Tuesday night on an old streetcar with his beloved mother to her practices with the famed Mormon Tabernacle Choir. Each Tuesday night he sat with rapt attention on the step next to his mother's seat in the alto section. His presence became such a trademark that at the age of fourteen he became the youngest person ever invited to become a member of the choir. He sang with the choir for another eleven years.

Ray's "mission" of healing was all the more appropriate in light of his mother's condition: Melissa Craig Christopher, the woman upon whose lap he had snuggled that afternoon in the orphanage, endured the quiet desperation of diabetes and dropsy. Hers was a chronic and debilitating condition. At first it confused the little boy, who suffered himself with crippled feet and the wheelchair that had become his prison. Later it tore at his heart as he sat, helpless against the diseases that ravaged her and unable to ease her agony.

Once as he was playing among the fragrant blooms of the garden on Highland Drive, his mother watched him with unusual interest. At last she knelt beside the spot where he worked the imaginations of youth and asked, "Raymond, what are you going to be when you grow up?"

"I'm going to be a doctor!" he announced, without hesitation.

"Oh, Raymond!" she laughed. "How can you be a doctor? You can't stand the sight of blood. You've never been able to slay the rabbits you raise for food, and you run from the kitchen whenever I raise the old butcher knife to a chicken. What kind of doctor would that be?"

There was a moment's pause before he answered this time, and a look of intent unusual in a child his age. "Mother, I will be able to heal people without cutting them up," Raymond replied. "There will be natural ways of doing it." His musings in the garden that day became a prophetic statement that would describe his life's passion.

With the hope of becoming a doctor, young Raymond watched with interest as various practitioners treated his mother. One visit from a health practitioner proved to be especially noteworthy to the sixteen-year-old. One day his mother drew him aside with quiet determination and told him, "Son, a doctor's coming to visit me today—but he's a new type of doctor, different from any of the others who have treated me. I thought you might like to see him."

At the appointed hour, Ray eagerly answered the door—and the young man noticed that the doctor glanced nervously up and down the peaceful neighborhood street before stepping across the threshold. As he introduced himself to Melissa, she offered, "Let me tell you what is wrong with me."

"No," the doctor urged emphatically. "*I* will tell you what is wrong with you." Fascinated, Ray watched as the man looked into his mother's eyes and recited with pinpoint accuracy the conditions for which she had sought medical help over the span of many years—and the conditions for which she had taken countless prescriptions of orthodox medications.

Ray listened to every pronouncement the doctor made, absorbed with curiosity about his gentle efficiency. He took mental notes as the doctor prescribed wholesome changes in diet and pressed a collection of herbal remedies into Melissa's hand. As they bid the doctor goodbye and watched him travel down Highland Drive, Ray told his mother, "*That's* the kind of doctor I'm going to be when I grow up."

Several months later when Ray tried to locate the man, he had his first glimpse of what would prove to be a foreshadowing of his own future: the doctor had been arrested for practicing medicine without a license and had been jailed. Ray tucked his ambition away temporarily and worked to finish his high school studies.

After graduation, news accounts and magazine articles about a Canadian practitioner caught Ray's eye: this man, the accounts said, massaged people's feet and effected remarkable healings. His treatments were in such demand, in fact, that people stood in long lines—even pitching tents for weeks at a time—in order to see him. Ray knew that this man could ease his rheumatoid arthritis; but, even more important, he yearned to study under him, to learn his natural way of healing. Cautiously, he approached his parents with his plan.

They could feel his excitement for his plan, but did their best to discourage him. The Depression had tightened its grip on most of the families living along Highland Drive and there was no extra money to finance a trip to Canada. Ray pleaded. "I'll find a way," he promised. "I'll thumb rides—I'll do whatever I have to do. Somehow, I'll make the trip." Just as he was completing his preparations, his enthusiasm was crushed: news filtered from Canada to Utah that the practitioner had been arrested. It was a definite blow, and Ray temporarily abandoned his ambition to study medicine.

In his twenties, Ray was involved in a devastating automobile accident that left him paraplegic. He was once again directed into natural procedures which restored his mobility. Finally, back on his feet after the accident, it wasn't long before his lifelong nemesis, arthritis, crept back and again complicated his life.

One morning, confined to a chair with the pain of arthritis, he picked up *The Doctrine and Covenants*, a volume of scripture published by The Church of Jesus Christ of Latter-day Saints. It fell open to the eighty-ninth section—more commonly known as the faith's "Word of Wisdom," it spells out the church's health code in a few brief paragraphs.

Ray had read the passage many times before, but this time several words jumped out at him as if lighted with neon: the words *sparingly* (in regard to meats) and *wholesome* (in regard to grains and vegetables) struck him so hard they seemed to have power enough to knock him out of the chair. He vowed to follow the health code strictly and developed for himself a diet of fruits, vegetables, grains, nuts and seeds.

The improvement in his health was staggering: within a few months, he gained weight, began sleeping soundly at night and started enjoying enough energy to allow for a full day's work. In 1939 he authored *Just What Is the Word of Wisdom?*, a thought-provoking booklet that described his experience and articulated his thoughts about diet and health.

As he pursued his studies he began lecturing. At one such lecture he met Wendella Walker, whom he married on August 19, 1944. Della became an avid supporter of his ideas and practice. This new marriage began in the middle of a tumultuous decade and the world was at war.

One afternoon a few months after he was married, the war invaded Salt Lake City. It came in the form of a draft notice on the Christophers' doorstep and it reflected wartime's dire circumstances: they had drafted a nearly thirty-five-year-old man who had divorced and remarried, and who had *two* families to support.

When he reported for service, Ray requested the status of conscientious objector. With a dedication to preserving life instead of taking it, he had included a section about the taking of life in his *Word of Wisdom* booklet. He carried it with him to the examiners, presenting it as evidence of his unwavering beliefs.

"I'll serve my country with pride on the front lines," Ray told the examining officer. "I'll carry stretchers that can save people, but I will not carry a gun. I cannot kill another human being." Reluctantly, the examining officer assigned him the status of conscientious objector, along with a permanent rank: as long as he served in the army as an objector, he could never achieve a rank higher than that of private.

Ray's commitment to principles proved to be one of the trademarks of his military service. Once during his brief stint in basic training an officer ordered that he carry a gun on night watch. "I do not carry guns,"

Ray replied. "As you can see from my papers, I'm a conscientious objector. I will not handle guns that kill."

The commanding officer shrugged his shoulders and thrust a night stick at the young private. Ray slowly shook his head; "I refuse to carry a night stick, too, because you could kill a man with a night stick."

The commanding officer reacted with anger and ridicule, confining Ray in quarters under guard until the next morning, when he was tried for his stubborn rebellion. The officer hearing the case slapped his palm sharply on the table and shouted, "This is one of the most ridiculous things I've ever heard! A conscientious objector who won't carry a night stick? What if everybody in the world felt as you do?"

"Then," replied Ray, with words that flooded suddenly into his mind, "there would be no war."

The examiner quietly sized up the young father and husband who sat before him. "That's the answer I needed," he said, scratching his signature across a small card. "You are a *conscientious* conscientious objector; this card shows that you have my approval. Carry it with you always, and no one will challenge you again."

From Fort Douglas, Utah, Ray traveled to North Fort at Washington's Fort Lewis, where he was assigned to supervise a medical dispensary. It seemed to be a comedy of errors. John Raymond Christopher, a lowly buck private, issued orders to master sergeants who were pharmacists and staff sergeants who were therapists. Even the cleaning boy outranked him—he was a corporal! Under Major Shumate's direction, they all took commands from the private at the dispensary.

At first, Ray felt frustrated and angry. He had been plucked from a situation in which he taught hundreds of people the benefits of a wholesome diet and natural healing methods, yet here he was allowed to use only orthodox medicines for people he knew he could help much better in other ways. His knowledge of wholistic healing had become extensive by the time he was drafted and he desperately wanted to use that knowledge to help the soldiers he served with. Each time he tried to approach Major Shumate about herbal healing, however, he was firmly denied.

As frustrated as Ray was, he began to see some purpose behind his time at the dispensary. First, he was able to see first-hand the effects of orthodox medications—and the futility of treating symptoms instead of causes. But most important, he had the chance to treat a soldier for a supposedly incurable condition—and it was a treatment that literally changed the course of Ray's life.

It happened one Monday morning, when the supervisors of the eight dispensaries were holding their regular meeting; they gathered that morning at Ray's dispensary and settled down with notepads to discuss the various cases they were faced with.

"I want all of you to see one man before we release him from the army," Major Shumate told the dispensary heads. "I worked as a private dermatologist in New York for years, and I've never seen a case of *impetigo contagioso* as severe as this one." Shumate explained the man's history: he had been hospitalized nine times with the condition. Each time it ran its course of thirty to thirty-six days, gradually clearing up, only to flare up again within days. Specialists from the eastern United States's most prestigious hospitals had treated the man with every known remedy but nothing had worked.

With that, Shumate opened the door and gestured for the soldier, who was ushered in under guard. The other dispensary heads gasped with horror when they saw the soldier, whose head had been shaved as much as possible, Wherever the stubble of hair grew, the man's scalp was covered with a crusty scab nearly an inch thick.

Ray had treated quite a few cases of impetigo but never one this bad. As he visually examined the man, he muttered, quietly, "What a *beautiful* case of impetigo!"

Shumate, who overhead his remark, slapped him on the shoulder good-naturedly. "You must be a natural doctor," he told Ray. "That's just how I see it—as one of the most amazing things I've ever seen. But, unfortunately, we have to release this man from the army."

At that the soldier, who had maintained a demeanor of embarrassed silence, spoke up with passion. "I *object* to that!" he cried. "I came into this army a clean man. I caught this thing while I was here," he said, pointing at his blackened, crusty scalp. "Now you're asking me to take this filth home to my wife and children. *I won't do it!*"

"I'm sorry, but there's nothing more we can do," Shumate responded, quietly. "We've done everything possible. We've used every cure medical science has to offer and nothing has worked. We have to give you a release—but we'll make it an honorable discharge."

"Wait," Ray interjected. "That man can be healed."

Shumate whirled to face Ray. "Not some of your blasted herbs!" he spewed. The other dispensary heads rolled their eyes and started to laugh.

"I should have something to say about this," the soldier cried. "I don't care if he puts horse manure on my head—as long as he heals me!"

Shumate paused, studied the man's scalp again, and agreed that Ray could try his treatment—if the soldier agreed to sign legal papers releasing the government and the army from any liability. With papers signed, the soldier was checked into Ray's dispensary and placed under twenty-four-hour military police surveillance to guard against escape. As the meeting broke up, the other dispensary heads were curious.

"When will the big unveiling be?" one of them jeered.

"Monday morning!" Ray snapped back, without even thinking. Then reality settled in: he had a week. Just one week. He was far from home, impossibly removed from the herbs he usually used. And in that week far from home, he had to heal the worst case of impetigo he'd ever seen.

Immediately he called a friend in Salt Lake City, a professor at the University of Utah whose backyard was sheltered by the spreading branches of a majestic black walnut tree. Ray explained his dilemma—even though the ground was covered with a blanket of snow, the professor agreed to gather the husks, take them to the army air depot and have them transported overnight to Fort Lewis.

The next morning Ray cradled the walnut husks as if they were pure gold. They were sopping wet when they arrived—not the best situation. And that wasn't the only handicap Ray faced. He had to put them in a base of 70 percent rubbing alcohol, because grain alcohol was not available through the army medical system. Moreover, instead of allowing the tincture to age for fourteen days, as he had been taught, he figured he only had about forty-eight hours. He made the best of it, shaking the tincture vigorously every time he walked past it during those two days.

At last he strained the tincture and made a compress that fit over the soldier's head like a football helmet. He secured the compress with adhesive tape. Then he instructed his aides that the compress had to be kept wet with the black walnut tincture twenty-four hours a day for the rest of the week. He wrote out a prescription—this time to the mess sergeant—that prescribed wholesome foods for the soldier to eat.

Monday morning arrived all too quickly—and with it one of the most harrowing times of Ray's life. The commanding officers and the dispensary heads met and they sat on the edges of their seats, ready to ridicule the failure they knew would meet their eyes.

"Everybody ready?" Shumate asked in a mocking tone. He turned to Ray and asked, "Are you ready to show us your miracle?"

"I'm ready," Ray responded with quiet determination. "I haven't seen him yet, but we'll take a look."

The soldier was ushered in again by the guards, and Ray worked quickly but carefully to cut away the adhesive tape. As he lifted the compress off, the scab came off with it—and the soldier's scalp was as clean and pure as a baby's. The impetigo was gone and had left no scarring.

The men gasped loudly; Major Shumate struggled to catch his breath. "I've never seen anything like this in all my days of practicing medicine," he cried. As the soldiers crowded around to get a better look, he took Ray aside.

"I've misjudged you, Private Christopher," he admitted. "From this day on, you have my permission to use herbs. In fact, you can set up a laboratory here. You're free to do anything you want with herbs as long as you are under my jurisdiction at Fort Lewis." With that proclamation, Ray became the only practicing herbalist in the United States Army during World War II.

Ray's black walnut tincture gained a widespread reputation and he continued to use it to treat impetigo. He also used it in the treatment of two other stubborn conditions: fungus infection and jungle rot. When word spread that Private Christopher knew how to cure jungle rot, his patient load multiplied tenfold. Ray eventually found that the black walnut hulls exacted an almost miraculous cure against a variety of other stubborn conditions, including scrofula, eczema, ringworm, shingles and chronic boils.

At last Ray's military obligation was over. Despite an invitation from Major Shumate to spend another tour of duty in the dispensary and to let the Army pay for his medical education, he declined and eagerly headed home to Olympia, Washington, to join his wife. John Raymond Christopher took with him a distinguished service record and the proud knowledge that he had helped countless soldiers who had been failed by the orthodox medical community. He also brought home with him the determination to learn all he could about herbs—and to make the practice of herbology his life's profession.

At the age of forty-five, *a full decade beyond his predicted life expectancy*, he was required to undergo a physical examination in order to enhance his life insurance coverage. The doctors who conducted the physical were astounded. Despite his early history, he had the blood pressure of a healthy teenager. Almost three decades later, just a few years before his death, a physician who examined him proclaimed that at seventy years of age he had the blood pressure and circulatory system of a vibrant young man in his twenties.

He was prolific in his final years, adding nine works to his original booklet on the Word of Wisdom. Those interested in the art he practiced can read his words in *Dr. Christopher's Three-Day Cleansing Program and Mucusless Diet*; *Rejuvenation Through Elimination*; *The Cold Sheet Treatment and Aids for the Common Cold*; *The Incurables; The School of Natural Healing*; *Herbal Home Health Care*; *Capsicum*; *Regenerative Diet* and *Every Woman's Herbal*. At the time of his death, he had begun work on several other volumes; his family is working to finish them in his memory.

The "Doc," as he was affectionately called, touched all of us. He healed many of us. His legacy is his students, his formulas and the love he left behind. With uncommon valor and unequalled compassion, he gave himself to all of us...and we, with him, are the winners.

Leah Lischner Conners:
Profile of a Community Healer

ROY UPTON

There are people in the healing professions who become well known nationally and internationally for the work they do in relieving the suffering of humanity. Then there are people who remain anonymous within their communities but provide no less valuable a service. Leah Conners is one of these people.

Leah Connors' mother was a Russian, Jewish immigrant who suffered from pernicious anemia. She was told not to have another child but one year later Leah came into the world. She was born on Delancey Street, New York, on June 30, 1899.

By the time Leah was born, her brother, who was to raise her, was a medical doctor specializing in Homeopathy. His name was Dr. Hyman Lischner. She was delivered by another Homeopathic physician, Dr. Imodene Wilcox, who had steered her brother into this special branch of medicine and theosophy. This professional and philosophical direction would guide Leah throughout her life.

Sickly as a child, Leah was unable to walk well until she was four years old. The experience of being nursed to health by her brother and Dr. Wilcox, eventually led to her training as a nurse and to a practice of her own that spanned almost thirty years. Leah notes that "at that time, Homeopathy was at the forefront of medicine."

"I was never vaccinated, brother didn't believe in it. Whenever we were sick, brother gave us echinacea and sometimes goldenseal. When nursing, I would have kids with whooping cough, and adults, veterans from World War I, coughing in my face, but I never got anything. All's I ever remember getting as a child was measles."

Some herb teachers say that is better to know a few herbs intimately than a little about a lot of them. Leah is an example of one of these teachers. When actively working in her health food store in Clearlake, California, she used only four herbs predominantly and another scant few occasionally. I watched her successfully treat everything from crippling rheumatoid arthritis to cancer with these herbs, common sense dietary rules, a handful of vitamins and some Homeopathic remedies.

In fact, she herself had rheumatoid arthritis when she first arrived in Clearlake. She was in her sixties—"these days, it's hard to remember." She was told by the doctors that she would never walk normally again. "I remember my sister Pauline used to rub my legs. I was in such pain you wouldn't believe. I changed my diet, stopped eating heavy meats, eliminated acid foods like tomatoes, peppers, citrus and strawberries. Oh! And I loved strawberries, but they were one of the worst. I kept eating chicken and fish but cut out most other animal protein. At the same time I started taking apple cider vinegar and honey in a cup of piping hot water every day. Within three months there was a dramatic change in my condition. I was no longer in pain, much of the stiffness was gone, and now, thirty years later, I only have a touch in my hands. I still take apple cider vinegar and honey in hot water every morning. That and a daily shot of brandy keeps this old body going."

"I have never taken any drugs or antibiotics. I had a major surgery once but, rather than take the morphine after it was over, I controlled the pain with Homeopathic Calms. These days if my hands bother me, I take the Calms. Last year I began to take an aspirin occasionally, but I figure at ninety-two it's not going to kill me."

Leah lived in New York as a child and came to Point Loma in the San Diego area with her brother. Dr. Wilcox was a student and devout follower of Madame Helena P. Blavatsky and of theosophy. She came to California to start a theosophy center and Leah's brother followed. Leah attended grammar school in Roseville, graduated from San Diego High School, began her nurse's training in Los Angeles General—"but the smog got to me"—and finished her R.N. in San Diego County General. From there, she went on to study nutrition at 5th Avenue Hospital in New York.

"The smog was terrible back then. Brother had a sanitarium on 123 acres of land in the country. We would take care of lots of tuberculosis patients. Many of them had been gassed in the war and the pollution made it worse. We grew alfalfa. We nurses would have to grind it and squeeze it by hand into cups to give to patients. There were newspaper headlines all over saying, 'San Diego Physician Finds Cure for Tuberculosis.'"

"Everyone in San Diego knew us. At the sanitarium, I had a small pig. The patients named him Dynamite. We didn't slaughter him, we used him to get rid of the garbage. One day I drove to town to shop. My Overland had no side windows in it. I saw my brother's car down the road. His had windows, so I put Dynamite in his car while I shopped. Well, everything went fine and I picked Dynamite up later. When I got home, I got a call from brother. He went to get something from his car, Dynamite jumped out shocking brother to kingdomcome, and there he was, a distinguished, well-dressed physician with a gout, chasing a little piglet down the street. He acted like he was angry, but I think inside he was really laughing. I wish I could have seen it or at least had a picture..."

"The tuberculosis patients were always melancholy and miserable. I used to have them write something every day to pass the time away. This was one of their first 'works':

> Her teeth are so pearly and white,
> they said someone made them but that isn't right.
> Her cheeks are so rosy and full of charm,
> they say it's from whiskey, don't do her no harm.
> So dainty and small her feet are each time,
> that the man charges her double when getting a shine.
> When dealing with men, it sure is a sin;
> it never fails she drives them to gin.
> Her nose is turned upward, I can't tell you why,
> but if she followed it always she'd land in the sky.
> When dealing with patients, she's never a bore,
> but when it comes to sleeping, boy can she snore.

Before too long, I think they had a line for every part of my body."

"One of my favorite moments in my life was when I met Evangeline Booth, the founder of the Salvation Army. I spent two hours with her in a suite at the Biltmore Hotel in Los Angeles. We had tea and she held my hand most of the time. That was one of the best two hours I ever spent in my life. I felt I was in the presence of a great soul."

"I nursed according to brother's Homeopathic philosophy. If people couldn't pay, we would care for them anyway. I believe we are our brother's keepers. I squeezed carrot and alfalfa juice till the cows came home, but Irish moss was one of my favorites. We would take well-rinsed Irish moss and cover it with a little more than just the right amount of water, let it soak overnight, and cook for a while in a double boiler the next day. When it was done we added pure grape juice, a little bit of honey and a touch of lemon, and put it in the refrigerator. This makes one of the tastiest and most nutritious desserts you can imagine. Besides that, it is fabulous for anemia and equally good for people with cancer. From the sea we came, to the sea we will return."

"Through the years, I have seen a lot of people with cancer. I believe it to be a disease of the soul. Everyone with cancer you see has strong emotions behind it. Mostly emotions like anger, hatred and jealousy. Jealousy is a bad one—it stabs at the soul—but hatred is the worst. It attacks the spirit."

"Working at an Air Force base as a hematologist, I saw a lot of cancerous cells under the microscope from radioactive testing. I was fired because I wouldn't keep my mouth shut. I always was a rebel. They hauled me into court for selling a cancer cure. I ended up winning a $42,000 judgment. They asked me if I would settle for $5,000. I said, 'Make it $10,000 and you've got a deal.' A few weeks later I got a $10,000 check."

Leah settled in Clearlake, one of the largest senior citizens' communities in the state of California, and began working in health food stores, eventually starting her own. She also traveled to health food stores and conventions promoting an herbal formula of her brother's. During this time, she served for many years on the board of directors of the community hospital.

"When brother died, he willed the formula to his son who then passed it on to me. We used it for a lot of things and it made me a decent living. I did it to get out of the L.A. smog." Originally, it was only available in pharmacies, but "Old Man" Hain got it into the health food stores.

In her store, Leah would work with dozens of people every day. She would counsel them on proper diet, talk to them about changing their lifestyle, and seemingly perform miracles sometimes with good down-home advice.

She was still driving at eighty-seven years of age, and at eighty-nine, she traveled to Haiti to be part of a mission relief orphanage for starving children. "I was there a year. We all starved together. Things were really tough. When I came back I was all skin and bones. I am still a little weak. I figure I must be getting old. But I loved the children and they loved me. I still get letters asking me to come back."

Leah, now at ninety-three, resides in Santa Cruz, California. The herbs she used were the fluid extracts of echinacea, goldenseal, hawthorn berry, calendula, and, once in a while, B and B extract and valerian.

Charlie Will Jordan:
An Herbalist who Balances
Business with Nature

ROY UPTON

Santa Fe herbalist Charlie Will Jordan has two consuming passions: to preserve the folk traditions of wildcrafting and herbal healing, and to promote environmentally and ethically conscious methods of growing, collecting and distributing herbal products.

In a 1990 article in a local Santa Fe newspaper called *Crosswinds,* Charlie discussed his views regarding these two issues with writer Annie Woods. We received permission to use this article, feeling that it is important to get Charlie's message across to herbalists and herbal manufacturers throughout the country.

"I'm a traditional herbalist" related Jordan, "I'm vertically integrated which means I am a direct link from the raw product to the consumer and I take that responsibility very seriously."

A great part of that responsibility is to practice "bioregional herbalism," which Charlie defines as "the practice of herbal medicine as it pertains to a local environment and its community."

Charlie is particularly unhappy with how the escalating interest in herbs for alternative healing has fostered a "big business" attitude toward this simple folk tradition. "I see people caught up in the *business* aspects who have never even seen the herbs," he says with a sigh; "I want to see them involve themselves in the responsibility to the environment and the community—for their own health, for the concern of the plants and for the welfare of the planet."

Jordan is a man who acts on his opinion. He now lives on a small farm in a town high in the mountains near Vallecitos, New Mexico. At this site, he will realize a dream to put the principles of bioregional herbalism and permaculture into action. In a small village near Abiquiu, Charlie still employs a local person in his wholesale business, providing herbs and herbal extracts to the community at wholesale or for trade.

"Permaculture is the regeneration of the land in a way that respects the way nature regenerates," he explains. "It sets up a microcosm that allows all forms of life to flourish. As an herbalist, I have a responsibility to *regenerate* the land, not *degenerate* it."

Charlie had his "profound calling" to herbalism after the fast track of a successful business career on the West Coast pushed him into "value shock." This spurred a move to Santa Fe where, in 1981, he attended The Institute of Traditional Medicine. He plugged into an intense curriculum of twenty-six credit hours per semester in herbalism plus courses in several other disciplines such as kinesiology, nutrition, Chinese medicine, physiology and massage. He also studied under the renowned herbalist Michael Moore.

His business, Dragon River Herbals, was established in 1983 with a small line of herbal extracts made from wildcrafted herbs. Charlie's line now includes 160 single herbal extracts, plus thirty-four combinations with specific remedies for both body and mind. He collects his herbs in New Mexico, Colorado, Kansas and Arizona with occasional ventures into Texas, Oklahoma and Utah. Once a year, he journeys to both the East and West Coasts, and to Mexico. He chooses only organic-quality plants for their freshness and "energetic stability." Although one wall in his shop is filled with jars of fragrant dried herbs, Charlie prefers to work with the raw plant because "the fresh extracts best preserve the particular healing quality of the plant."

Charlie says he introduces people from all walks of life to herbal healing through education, not by prescribing. "Once you take your health issues into your own hands and get involved, you set yourself up for healing all aspects of your life," he believes.

As if to illustrate this point, a large burly man wearing a Harley Davidson cap enters Charlie's shop and heads for the valerian tincture (valerian is well known for its calming and tranquilizing properties). During a brief and colorful conversation, the man reveals he is a Vietnam veteran who "used to do what Jimi Hendrix used to do." In order to get off drugs when he returned to the states, the man said, "I took what the government gave me—Valium—to come off the shakes." Not surprisingly, the man became addicted to Valium. A sobering car accident caused him to re-evaluate his life and this gentle giant of a man turned to alternative healing. Now he helps friends, particularly other

Vietnam vets, kick drug habits by using valerian and other herbs.

"It works," says the man bluntly. "It's good for the shakes. It's good for cocaine." As an afterthought when heading out the door he adds, "And it helps you quit cigarettes, too!"

Charlie says he sees a lot of stress-related illness which he believes is related to the fast pace of modern life. "Our accelerated lifestyle leaves us open to illness," he says. "In the past fifty years, we've accelerated so fast that we now live in one week what people used to live in three months. And genetically, we haven't changed that much." Not surprisingly, he sells a lot of tinctures for stomach and immune problems.

"The nature of our business is to listen and try to help people help themselves," says Jordan. "And we will refer people to other practitioners if necessary." Such willingness to *cooperate,* not *compete,* has put Charlie in touch with many local chiropractors, acupuncturists and medical doctors. Word of mouth, referrals by practitioners and private individuals have cultivated a successful small business that needs little advertising to sustain itself.

Charlie also feels it is important to donate a percentage of his earnings to organizations such as Greenpeace, World Wildlife Fund, the Wilderness Society, Environmental Defense Fund, National Audubon Society and the Native Plant Society—organizations dedicated to preserving the natural environment for generations to come.

When he's not working his retail and wholesale business, Jordan is putting the word out about bioregional herbalism. He feels the time has come to replace business hype with an ethical regard for both plants and planet. Charlie presented a paper at the first American Herbalists Guild-sponsored Symposium of Herbal Medicine in 1990. His paper carried the message that many of the herb companies who adopt "big business"-type policies block cooperation in trade, replacing it with competition, alienating herbalists from their true purpose—to be caretakers of the land.

"We, as herbalists, have lost our true purpose and connection with the Earth," he writes. "We push products, we create enormous loads of brochures and fliers claiming we promote herbal health, when in fact we create needless pollution. We are working against universal cooperation and partnership using monetary gain and self-purporting fame as reason to justify our actions. Competition only breeds alienation."

Charlie admits his views may not sit well with some of his colleagues but he is adamant. "It's scary to think of some companies with no real connection to the Earth and the plants that come from the Earth. Our purpose as herbalists is to keep things harmonious and integrated. We are on the front lines—the direct link between plants and people."

Kwi-tsi-tsa-las:
Portrait of an Herbalist

JAMES GREEN

Dedicated to Symphytum O.
...throughout these difficult times when your ancient
pyrrolizidine alkaloids are so eloquently stylized by our
fashionable paranoiac accolades.

PASSAGEWAY OF A HERITAGE...

I stepped through the doorway of the North Island Senior Secondary School faculty lounge in search of a little solitude and lots of strong coffee. Mentally preoccupied with the art and English lessons I was scheduled to teach in the following hours, I failed to notice another presence in the room. "Would you hold this cloth for me, so I can strain my tea through it?" were the first words of a relationship destined to radically alter the future direction of my life.

I accept full responsibility for the ensuing cataclysmic changes. All the woman requested was some momentary assistance. It was I who asked to taste the aromatic brew of twigs and berries and leaves. It tasted atrocious to me at the time, and I had a class to get to, so I left the room as quickly as I had entered. But some inner pulse lying previously dormant in my spirit had been quickened; my tongue's bitter flavor receptors had been strangely touched and curiously seduced by an infusion of wild-plant parts; and two kindred-spirit, green-dragons had shared tea. That's all it takes sometimes to initiate a fellow herbalist.

It was 1970 in British Columbia, Canada, and Gertrude Norma Myers had been employed by School District #85 (Vancouver Island North) to teach biology and other life sciences. But the facts and figures presented in high school science can be interpreted to envision infinitely diverse beliefs about the reality of our shared universe, and Norma's expressed vision was vastly different than the educational system's standard and preferred lesson plans. The young students thrived on the fresh air that

Norma's consciousness freely let into their science curriculum, and, as you can imagine, the kids deeply appreciated her for this. Of course they also poked fun at her eccentricities and you can imagine the frequently derisive remarks that circulated amongst the teaching staff and within the administration's supervisory back room parleys. Norma was notably a unique human being; she tried to appear ordinary, but despite her valiant endeavors, the resilience of her earthy green-spirit prevailed.

The second time I saw Norma was through a window; she was outdoors, wearing the acceptably conservative dress and feminine accessories of a proper high school teacher with, however, the added touch of a pair of large, floppy, black rubber, fisherman's gumboots and heavy cotton sweatsocks over her nylon hose. The soles of the boots at this moment were caked with fresh mud, and Norma, shovel and rake in hand, was teaching her ninth grade biology pupils the steps required to build a successfully active compost pile. She was already teaching recycling back in the '70s and the young students were eagerly participating in the task. The class was being held outside on wet earth during a light North Island drizzle.

Norma had no personal agenda or specific mission to save the world through high school studies; she simply perceived and participated in life from a practical, unorthodox perspective and from a Native American-oriented lifestyle. She definitely taught biology from a point of view closer to that of the living plants and animals themselves than from one that habitually perceives plants and animal cadavers through multi-powered lenses with dissecting probes.

Midway through the school term, the administrative overseers of scholastic status quo recognized their initial misjudgment of Norma's unique expression of normalcy and arranged appropriate documentation to relieve her of her teaching position. She was not offered a contract to return to the faculty a second year—something to do with her failure to get raw test score data into the principal's office by some crucial deadline. Norma was understandably disconcerted and upset by this action, for she put her heart into her work and looked forward to further communication with young souls about their living relationship with wildlife and the environment.

I met Norma at the beginning of my second year of teaching at this high school. By this time I was already bumping my head on the creative ceiling constructed by the school system and I could clearly see that a teacher's systematic salary increases or administrative rank was about all I had to look forward to. So, with ears deaf to an avalanche of unsolicited advice, I refused the third year contract and automatic salary increase offered me. At the conclusion of the school year, I too departed from the public school system. But all this was merely the physical-social processes of our lives unfolding as we wished them to; the true changes had been voluntarily arranged in our subtle realms. My subconscious decision to move on had been made the moment I perceived the intriguing root bark and berries steeping in Norma's pot of tea.

Even before the school year celebrated its final day, Norma had outlined an initial inventory for an ensuing herb and healthfood store. She had connected with natural food and herb distributors who agreed to extend us credit; procured a small electric grain mill and a reliable source of organic whole wheat, oats, corn and rye; manifested some excellent bread, cinnamon roll and matrimonial cake (date squares) recipes and discovered a small bakery that was up for sale by two gentle old souls who had chronically debilitated themselves with their own white flour and white sugar baked goods. A week after the school's year-end commencements, we bought the tiny establishment and its mysterious bakery equipment (I had never baked bread before; I hadn't a clue what all the machinery was designed to do). By St. John's Wort harvest we were ready to open the *Sun & Seed Natural Food Store,* organic whole grain bakery and herb dispensary. Now this type of food store is no big deal today, nor was it even then in locations like Vancouver, B.C. and coastal California. But opening an herb store anywhere on the northern half of Vancouver Island in 1970 and locating it across the street from the local pub and neighborhood supermarket, in the midst of a community composed predominantly of fishermen, loggers and copper miners who thrived on meat, potatoes and fermented beverages and who had never heard of (or gave a damn about) organic grains, nutritional yeast, raw honey and medicinal herbs, confronted us with a serious marketing problem. But that's another story. My partnership and apprenticeship with Norma initiated me as a student of the mysterious and intensely beautiful coastal lands and forests of the Pacific Northwest.

The building that for three years housed the *Sun & Seed,* sat at waterside, next to the fisherman's pier, about a country mile down island from Norma's cedarwood house. The doors of our bakery and herb store opened onto a narrow, windswept road that serviced our village. The village's name was Alert Bay and it was located on Cormorant Island, a charming but typically overlogged land form jutting up in the midst of the Queen Charlotte Strait, between Vancouver Island and the B.C. mainland. While working as a teacher, I had bought a small abandoned farm which sat near Donegal Head on the neighboring Malcolm Island. To tend our new business, my family and I would routinely commute to Alert Bay from our waterfront dwelling by means of an antiquated government-run passenger ferry. But the channels' winter currents were dangerously swift, the sinister gale winds were highly unpredictable and the ferry's posted arrival & departure schedule was usually irrelevant, so frequently during the winter seasons, my family and I inhabited a minute but cosy attic room at Norma's house.

To say the least, living on Norma's turf was simple and captivating. At least that was my experience. My wife and our two toddling daughters might have selected different adjectives to reveal their experiences, but I lived there happily and contentedly. The ambiance of Norma's home was filled with the jolly spirit of many generations of Native American ancestors who had been born, lived and died in this family dwelling. Somehow this energy was as strangely familiar to me as was that first taste of herbal tea. Norma had been married to her husband, Carey, for forty years, and this house had belonged seemingly forever to their clan. A wood burning heater and an upright piano, two handwoven cedarbark baby carriers, time worn family photographs hanging on the wall, a lumpy chesterfield and two sensual overstuffed chairs adorned the modest living room. But upon entry, these household items were not what demanded one's attention. Surrounding and intermingled with these furnishings was an accumulation of herblore the likes of which I have never seen since in one abode. Like a Chinese herb shop salient with its scores of unmarked herb-filled drawers, Norma's living room was filled with orderly arranged yet mostly unlabeled containers of dried herbs. And Norma knew what was contained in each paper sack and in each tin box and where any herb she might need was located. Every herb in Norma's living room pharmacy was fresh and vital; her medicinal stash consisted almost entirely of current harvests. This is the way it is when one picks, prepares and dispenses their own herbal medicines. There were also shelves and tables laden with glass jars inside of which macerated recently wildcrafted plants. Intermingled with all this sat assorted trays and jars of freshly sprouting seeds: sunflower and soy, mung bean and chia, radish, mustard, wheatgrass and broad bean (sprouted as special food for her cancer patients). The conspiracy of herbal aromas that seduced one's sense of smell in Norma's home was unlike anything I had experienced before. And I loved it. The attic space next to our room was full with furniture that previously occupied the living room but which had to be relocated to make room for Norma's herbal pharmacy. Norma and Carey's house sat on the waterfront looking out over the Queen Charlotte Strait; seagull, raven and eagle, orca and salmon passed by their front yard. Wild and cultivated herbs, garden vegetables, assorted compost piles and the irrepressible blacktail deer thrived in their backyard. A mellow, robust German shepherd dog named Jake and a couple hobo kittens were animal companions who lived within the house. Norma was an avid gardener, herbal medicine-maker and culinary alchemist; Carey was a fisherman. They ate well and simply. Everyone who visited or lived in Norma's house ate well—the food was homegrown or wild and deliciously prepared. Norma's Native American name, Kwi-Tsi-Tsa-Las, translates "woman who feeds you when you come to her home."

It was a joy to accompany Norma's spontaneous liberation, ignited by our departure a deux from the public school system. Like a bewildered female deer (or maybe more like a female buffalo) whose hooves can never find amicable footing on the city's paved roads and concrete sidewalks, Norma leaped back onto her natural turf, back into the forestland. Resuming her work in the Pacific Northwest bush dynamically refurbished her spirit. She had great heart and she was never tamed; she functioned poorly in the cages of normal domestication. At school as a teacher, she too occasionally set aside science's newly discovered knowledge and technology and, with her students, would look out the open window and dream on warm spring afternoons. She would teach the value of wild places and wild things. These are the traits that disturbed the public school employers, but these are the matters of the heart that innervate herbalists. Norma was at home in the wilderness and the wilderness occupied a major portion of her spirit. Norma's husband, Carey, used to look at me with his warm mellow smile and slowly shake his head back and forth whenever Norma got on her high horse about civilization's continued destruction of the wilderness and the wildlife; he knew there was no changing her. He wouldn't even try. He knew that she was right and that it was breaking her heart to witness it.

The woman did not lack a shadow self; none of us do. But in tribute to her wholeness, I must say she neither denied the existence of her shadows nor overly repressed their expression. Norma had high visions. Her primary vision was to establish a residential herbal college but she wasn't interested in starting small and building. She wanted to initiate it in grandiose style, and her attempts to do this carried a substantial cost. With heart and eyes set on this accomplishment, Norma often got herself into difficult situations with other people, as her means sometimes blindly pursued the noble end. She devised innumerable complex plans which required the assistance of many individuals, some who failed her, others who helped her with wholehearted dedication and she failed them. In good faith, she made sincere promises for a return on people's contributed energy, but some of these promises she was not able to fulfill. A couple times she asked me to mortgage my farm for money to help her follow through with a crucial step of a plan in process. She was always very gracious when I denied her these requests and receptive as I explained why. In our relationship, she taught me about herbs and nutrition, and I helped bring her plans back down to earth. We understood each other. I valued what was in her heart and she valued my insights. We worked well together and maintained good friendship.

Norma was an herbalist and a healer through and through. Although practicing herbal therapeutics and dispensing herbal preparations as healing medicine is outlawed in Canada and the USA, this was the essence of her life. She was my first herbalist teacher. She shared an ancient human heritage with me. She taught me the ways of the forest and shoreline plants. She taught me how to pick stinging nettles without using gloves; how to follow the Devil's club plant back to its grandparent stock whose roots give the strongest medicine (the roots of the younger generations supplying us with milder extracts when needed); and how to patiently coax these dragon-claw-like roots out of the dense forest mud. She taught me how to extract burdock's medicinal seeds from their needle sharp casings and how to harvest a tree's inner bark without harming the tree. She was the first person I ever wildcrafted with; she built with me my first compost pile. She showed me how to apply a comfrey poultice and prepare Balm-of-Gilead salve. She was the first person I ever dropped out of high school with. She was a companion and a professional herbalist ally, therefore she was a fellow outlaw. But as Tom Robbins once wrote, "When freedom is outlawed, only outlaws will be free."

WORKING WITH PATIENTS

Of Irish and Scotch ancestry, married into the native Kwakiutl community, Norma became the proverbial local herbalist. The native community held profound respect for this woman who used the forest plants for medicine. Norma was renowned as a medicine woman in the Native village portion of Alert Bay and was revered as such by much of the Native American population in the Vancouver/Victoria area of B.C. She nursed and nourished many a small child, old man, cancer patient, diabetic, pregnant woman in distress and Indian grandmother back to health.

Those very sick who didn't revive while in her care usually departed at least pain free. Norma knew that herbs were the primarily planetary source of healing, for this was her experience, but she also knew that human touch and caring worked miracles. She shared her daily life (and chores) and her home with many of her patients. They drew healing from her dedication and from her indomitable attitude that anyone could do better, especially with timely help from another.

Using her herbal remedies and her intimate knowledge of nutrition, Norma nursed her husband, Carey, back to health from a major stroke and paralysis. His brother was taken down similarly at the same time, but the brother didn't survive his hospital care. After Carey's recovery, Norma continued to monitor his diet, and he continued to put up with the nasty-tasting herbs and other supplements. He knew she had saved his life, had helped him regain good health and that she could help him retain it. With the aid of Norma's care and skill, her husband returned to the hard working life of a fisherman. The Indian community witnessed this re-markable accomplishment and respected Norma as a "Pakwhala," an Indian healer who used plants, and her bitter Indian Herb Formula became a legend (at least its flavor did). Members of the local native community frequented the village doctor and hospital for medical care, but when the situation was grave, Norma was visited, usually on the advice of someone's grandmother or aunt.

Norma possessed a remarkable understanding of the intricate process of human digestion and metabolism; a practical knowledge superior to that of anyone I have since worked with. Norma used breakfast, lunch and dinner as medicine. She prepared each patient's meal differently, each especially designed for that individual's needs. She blended flavors, aromas and nutrients in her meals, though she seldom taught this ver-bally. One learned by eating and gardening with her at her house. Her meals were always delicious, simple, fresh garden-grown with a portion of bitter greens or a small cup of bitter tea to accompany it all. No one needed much added sweet, for the bitter contrast made many foods taste satisfyingly sweet naturally. And there was always plenty of food; she had a refrigerator in the kitchen, crocks filled with homemade sauerkraut and other perennially fermenting fruits and vegetables in her pantry. Two more refrigerators sat fully stocked on the outdoor porch. Employing an exotic century-old Russian yogurt starter, Norma made quarts of yogurt from fresh goat's milk (two lactating French Alpine goats named Char-lotte and Angel Eyes and a prepubescent Nubian named Pennyroyal lived beneath the front portion of her hillside house). Dessert was a bowl of this homemade yogurt sprinkled with sliced, lightly roasted almonds and a little Montreal maple syrup; I still experience the nurturing feelings of meals at Norma's home each time I eat this dessert.

Norma had cancer in the bones of the right side of her face. During the ten years that I worked with her, she kept this in remission with the Indian Herb Formula, fasting and dieting. The pain of this condition would return whenever she became stressed or was required to work outside her element. The year of her teaching experience in the public school system was a difficult one for her; she was often in pain due to this condition. With her patients she employed mild fasting and herbal enemas as vital components to cleanse the body, reduce pain and enhance health, and they did well in her care. She fasted herself, too, when she thought she should; however, her self-discipline was sometimes suspect. It was not a rare experience for Norma to visit our home and say something like, "I'm on the fifth day of a ten-day fast, do you have any cheese?" You had to grow fond of the woman; she was so openly human.

A quaintly characteristic scene I often observed upon walking into Norma's kitchen was that of a large pot of bitter herb tea steeping on the stovetop, the kitchen air humid with the steaming aroma of the day's stewing potherbs, and a necktie with the coat and vest of some person's urban three-piece suit thrown casually over the back of an old wooden straight back chair next to the woodheat stove. Usually there would be heard the sound of Norma's voice coming from outside in the backyard garden. Walking to the kitchen window one could view her instructing a slightly bewildered middle-aged man on how to dig Jerusalem artichokes or fresh beet roots and greens or some other garden vegetables for the day's upcoming lunch and dinner—the man's once shiny leather shoes comically smeared with garden mud, his white shirt sleeves rolled up to his elbows, a glow of newly generated circulation showing on his cheeks, his city-molded body a bit awkward on the irregular surface of the garden turf but his spirit responding excitedly to its sudden recommunion with the earth and fresh country air. This person (just as often a woman) was usually visiting Norma, seeking an alternative means for healing a diagnosed cancer or a heart condition or some other health problem. Norma was showing him where to begin.

Norma taught her patients to identify and harvest their own medicines. She took them with her into the forests and seasides or into her garden to see and harvest. When they stayed at her house, she didn't change her lifestyle to accommodate them, rather she took them along with her to educate them. If they were too sick, she gave them her bedroom and served them until they regained their strength. Often a patient's family members would stay at Norma's house too. Norma asked them to help and they were usually fascinated and eager to work. Predominantly, Norma worked with and helped cure those who suffered from the seriously debilitating conditions—the cancers, arthritis, diabetes, chronic skin conditions and the other degenerative diseases that the medical profession could not heal with their medicine.

MATERIA MEDICA

Norma used an herbal repertory of approximately 300 herbs. She made extensive use of trees as sources of herbal medicine: broad leaf maple, white poplar and apple tree (or wild crabapple) barks for liver cleansers and tonics (also apple bark with pine and garlic for normalizing high blood pressure); the red alders which grow like weeds in B.C. blended with willow bark for "brain energy" to counter brain fatigue; and alder bark combined with basil and mugwort to help overcome the effects of drug use; arbutus leaves and white poplar (with marigold, wild rose and cineraria) for eye nutrients and for eye washes; the buds of the trembling aspen and the cottonwood poplar with pine pitch and elder flowers—prepared as an ointment to treat serious burns; white pine, wild cherry and bitter cherry, alder and black elder for treating the throat, bronchials, lungs and the skin; hawthorn flowers and berries for the heart; alder, propolis (bee-gathered tree resins), pine pitch, black walnut and oak for treating infection. white poplar and (imported) slippery elm for stomach; Douglas fir, balsam, hemlock, pine, birch and walnut in poultices, foot baths and sitz bath hydrotherapy when treating arthritis, infection and a variety of other conditions.

She used the evergreens that grew near her home—Oregon grape, uva ursi, sword fern (*Polystichum munitum*) and licorice root fern (*Polypodium glycyrrhiza*). She picked the salal berry, thimbleberry, wild huckleberry, rose hips and the fruit and flower of the Oregon grape plant to use for high vitamin/mineral food. She included yarrow to strengthen heart and circulation in a majority of her formulas and Devil's club root bark extensively when treating cancer, diabetes and arthritis; She used licorice root fern for stomach, adrenal gland, colds, sore throat and arthritic conditions and sword fern fronds as pain relievers. Often she would pursue her tasks with these fronds sticking out randomly from beneath her hat to help relieve the discomfort of facial pain or headache. She also covered the mattresses of patients' beds with these ferns (spreading the bottom sheet over the ferns) to help relieve aches in the bones and joints of their bodies. Norma used mostly local herbs, primarily those she wildcrafted and the medicinal garden perennials she grew and harvested as needed. Of course, she also used medicinal plants that came her way from other sections of the country, arriving via visiting herbalists and students. But primarily she dispensed and taught about her local medicinal flora.

Norma didn't appear to harvest wild plants with the ceremony and outward show of gratitude and respect that I felt they warranted. One time, when we were harvesting Devil's club roots in the shadowy crevice of a cedar forest, I called her on this issue. She stood upright and wiped some sweat from her cheek, replacing the sweat with twice as much muddy earth from her glove, and asked me to be quiet and quit interrupting her conversation with the plant. She was not a maudlin woman and she possessed practical knowledge about these plant medicines that I never found in the books. These conversations were obviously a one-way dialogue from plant to Norma. She listened a lot while she worked in the forest.

INDIAN HERB FORMULA

About every two or three years, at least when I first met her, Norma would embark on her Indian Herb pilgrimage, traveling around the country harvesting the herbs that she would use to prepare this bitter herbal formula. She traveled to Michigan, Wisconsin and Northern Saskatchewan to pick specific herbs at special harvesting sites. She told me she learned this formula and the special places to find the best herbs from a Mohawk medicine man. It was her trump card for healing the chronic ills, cancer in particular, that resisted orthodox medical techniques and other therapies.

Norma used this formula as a foundational formula to which she added other appropriate herbs for treating an individual's symptom picture.

When treating cancer, Norma first cleared and detoxified the individual's bowels using herbal enemas prepared from burdock leaf, tansy, marigold and thimbleberry leaf and a laxative herbal infusion (2 parts each of: star anise, buckthorn, caraway, dandelion, fennel, fenugreek, flaxseed, psyllium seed combined with 1 part each of: cascara, coltsfoot, ground ivy, licorice and chickweed) given as a tea. This greatly, if not completely, eliminated the patient's physical pain and also improved brain function, uplifting depression when it stemmed from toxic bowels and pain. She healed the bowel walls with a soothing cupful of blond psyllium seed and marshmallow root cold water infusion taken after the evening meals. Norma wold employ *mild* fasting when appropriate, but only if the person was strong enough. Next, Norma would work to rebuild and support the liver. This enhanced the detoxification of the body and improved blood quality. The Indian Herb formula was used predominantly for this phase (she also relied a lot on the actions of Oregon grape root) as well as an organic food and whole grain (for essential B vitamins) diet to rebuild the nutrient foundation. Frequently, castor oil fomentations were applied over the patient's liver to help draw out toxins through the skin. Along with liver care, Norma attended to the individual's endocrine system. She used high doses of Vitamin C supplements (1000 mg 3 times daily) along with Vitamin C-containing herbs (young needles of fir trees, rosehips, violet leaves, etc.), sea vegetables, uva-ursi with licorice root "to relax the adrenals," devil's club, blueberry leaf, the Bach Flower Essences and prescribed rest as some of the primary tools for this particular care. Norma would then concentrate directly on improving the condition of the blood. To accomplish this she used variations of her blood conditioning formula [3 parts each of: burdock, red clover, calendula; 2 parts each of: yellow dock, blue violet, wood betony, periwinkle (vinca minor), anise, flaxseed, hops combined with 1 part each of: blue flag, European mistletoe, chaparral and devil's club]. The amount of chaparral and devil's club used varied depending on how much the patient could take at first (the devil's club root bark of the young plants she used for weaker patients. She would not use devil's club or chaparral for very weak patients until they had been built up nutritionally first). In addition to these herbs Norma used nutritional supplements—Vitamin A and potassium, in particular—for elimination of excess mucus production and retention (she used supplements to help revive their health, then she took them off the regime), and she employed the actions of enzymes to assist the function of the pancreas for digestion of proteins.

Norma found cancer to be a very complex and difficult disease to cure, and she stressed preventive lifestyle above all else. She displayed tremendous empathy for her cancer patients, for she realized that they needed help and that many of them were depressed, had lost their job and had little money. She knew that for them to survive, they required knowledge, time, energy, money and compassionate friends. Payment was seldom assured for her care and teaching.

I asked Norma to give her Indian Herb formula to me, so it could be shared with others after she died. She died May 27, 1988. Norma may also have given the precise details for preparing this formula to other students in later years. We eventually parted company around 1980 and went our separate ways as our work required. She did give me the formula, and I am pleased for this opportunity to share what she taught me with my peers. I hope it will assist you in your healing work as it did Norma. It is prepared as follows:

HERBAL INGREDIENTS
Burdock (*Arctium lappa*)
> Use the large leaves, root of the first year plant and the seeds.
> (Norma considered this plant to be the heart of this formula, especially when treating cancers.)

Horse Mint (*Monarda fistulosa*)
> Use the leaves and flowers.
> (This plant is also commonly known as bee balm and wild bergamot.)

Tansy (*Tanacetum vulgare*)
> Use the leaves and flowers.
> (Norma also used this plant singly as a hot wash for external suppurating cancer sores and as a fomentation to assist the healing of sprains and varicose veins.)

Calamus (*Acorus americanus*, also *A. calamus*)
> Use the rootstock.
> (Norma indicated that this plant must be included or the other herbs won't work well in this formula.)

Trembling Aspen (*Populus tremuloides*)
> Use the inner bark of this tree.
> The inner bark of the cottonwood poplar (*Populus candicans*) can be used as a substitute.

Wormwood (*Artemisia absinthium*)
> Use the cultivated leaf.

[Other herbs Norma added to this formula were: marshmallow root and red clover when treating stomach cancer; comfrey leaf when treating bowel cancer; yellow dock, periwinkle (*Vinca minor*), red clover and stinging nettle when treating cancer of blood and/or lymph tissue.]

METHOD OF PREPARATION
(Precisely as dictated to me by Norma, and as we prepared it)
To make 6 gallons—

Mix a large handful each of leaves, flowers and seeds; a medium size piece of calamus root which is about 1-1/2 inches thick; a large burdock root (2 or 3 roots if you wish); and a strip of the bark (10 to 15 inches).

1st brew: Cut all the herbs into small pieces. Drop these into boiling water which has been taken off the fire. Use a porcelain pot (never use metal, especially not aluminum). Let this steep for 20 minutes (don't boil). Strain out the tea infusion, press the mash and place the mash into a second pot.
Filter this entire first brew and divide it equally into 6 gallon jugs. This first brew is the most precious part; take care.

2nd brew: Cover mash with water and boil for one minute; turn off fire. Let sit for 20 minutes. Pour off liquid, filter and divide equally into the 6 jugs, adding this to the first brew. This brew is the second most precious part.

3rd brew: Cover the mash again with water and boil it like hell for 20 minutes to one hour. Strain, filter and divide this equally into the 6 jugs, adding it to the other two brews. Now fill each jug to its full gallon capacity with pure water. Add 1 teaspoon of salicylic acid dissolved in boiling water to each jug as a preservative. Refrigerate when the tea has cooled.

GENERAL INSTRUCTIONS FOR USE

Take 2 ounces, 4 times a day, 1/2 hour before meals and at bedtime, plus water if desired.

TEACHING AND OTHER TEACHERS

During the years I worked with Norma she wrote very little about her experiences; she was too busy treating patients, struggling to make a living and contriving to establish her herb school. Toward the end of our partnership, she did write ten chapters of a correspondence course as an aspect of her Greenvale Herbal College, and she prepared a formal submission for a proposed Herbal Act in British Columbia, submitted from the Coastal Society for Herbal Enlightenment in B.C., a society which she organized and founded.

Norma did teach classes however, and she assisted many students to get a foundation in practical herbalism. I used to refer to her as a tangential teacher, for in the midst of discussing a specific topic, her illustrative stories of personal experiences often stampeded in directions far removed from the original topic of discussion. These were notoriously wild stories, and few listeners tried very seriously to round her back to the original topic; she eventually got back to it on her own, and we all enjoyed the ride. Norma didn't normally teach in the vernacular of reductionist medical science, although she was quite knowledgeable and conversant in the language and concepts of this school. Her exacting knowledge of the physiology and biochemical alchemy of the digestive process in the human body combined with her ebulliently shared knowledge of plant medicine was the gemstone of her herbal instruction. Norma had the memory vault of a comprehensive herbal and medical encyclopedia, however the entries were not always arranged in alphabetical order. Often when I asked her a question, I would get no immediate answer on my chosen topic (she might have been suggesting that I figure it out for myself), but she would always get back to me eventually with either precise information or a relevant, thought provoking comment.

To my memory, Norma never spoke much about her human teachers, other than the Mohawk gentleman who gave her the Indian formula. I know she sincerely considered just about everyone her teacher and she quickly assimilated all that she heard. And of course, like most herbalists, she possessed a home library flagrantly abundant with herbals and myriad notecards filled with formulas and botanical information.

STUDENTS AND VISITING HEALERS

Norma was usually accompanied by young students who were attracted to her novel lifestyle and unique method of teaching. Through the years she influenced and brought together many present day professional herbalists. I believe Norma was one of the first to bring students and herbalists together for extended herbal seminars. She hosted healers who traveled long distances to participate in her gatherings: Dr. Christopher, Rosemary Gladstar, Michael Tierra, a grand teacher named Gabriel (I wish I could recall his last name) and Sun Bear and Wabun of the Bear Tribe, to name just a few. This is how I met and began working with Dr. John Christopher, my second most inspirational herbalist teacher, a jolly lion of a man, who would travel from his home in Utah to visit for a week at a time teaching his skills and telling his stories. The stories of his experiences stampeded as swiftly and wildly as Norma's did, but they thundered their hooves over a different terrain and he entertained and inspired his audiences for hours at a time.

Norma and Dr. Christopher are two of the grandelders whose images are fondly pictured in the minds and memories of many of today's herbal practitioners, teachers and medicine-makers. Precursors of the present generation of inspired herbalists who are continuing to usher in today's North American herbal renaissance, these elders were the solitary, courageous, self-empowered, visionary beings of their era that helped reclear a path for those of us who work as herbalists today and who in turn continue to tend and re-seed this herbal pathway. Other healing elders of Norma and Dr. Christopher's era include Ella Birzneck, Elvin Rasmasson, Dr. Bernard Jensen, Dr. A. Vogel, Dr. Nowell, Dr. Edward Shook, Dr. Edward Bach, Dr. Otto Mausert and Jethro Kloss, to name merely the individuals that I either knew personally or whose writings strongly influenced me and my peers.

A WOMAN WARRIOR SPIRIT

I must add that when provoked, Norma Myers was a warrior and clever adversary (especially when challenged by an autocratic bureaucracy that threatened her work as an herbal therapist). A number of Norma's peers had been harassed and incarcerated in the '60s and '70s for the innovative work they were doing, but Norma proved too clever to be trapped and prosecuted for practicing as a 'non-licensed' healer. Yet she treated and helped heal hundreds of beings who were sick and asked for her help. She regularly evaded the bureaucrats and government regulators by simply manipulating their rules more cleverly than they, outmaneuvering them within their own regulations. Once Norma understood the rules of the game, she was a brilliant contender; her ability and inclination to research these rules were uncanny. She successfully treated cancers, diabetes, arthritis and all the other conditions that are strictly reserved by legislative decree for licensed members of the mainstream medical establishment. She wasn't inhibited by any of this foolishness and it delighted me to accompany her and watch her in action.

CLOSING WORDS

In closing, I leave the reader with a taste of Norma's words and ideas. She felt strongly about issues that affected her community, her human companions and her plant and animal allies; her life clearly reflected an indomitable Spirit. Her life was a portrait of an herbalist. The following collection of paragraphs has been taken from the introductory section of the Herbal Act that Norma wrote and submitted to the B.C. provincial government:

"Herbalists traditionally use natural methods. By natural methods we mean the return to common knowledge *and* practice of those things that were well known to many of our ancestors; the importance of sunshine for the prevention of calcium deficiencies and arthritic problems; the importance of hard work and exercise in the fresh air to increase body oxygen levels, as well as health of circulation, heart, lungs, liver, kidneys and bowels; the necessity of eating coarse, unrefined foods and raw vegetables for stomach and bowel health and more fruit to increase potassium levels (to clear out abnormal muco-proteins deposited because of present day Vitamin A deficiencies). Also, to eat lightly from time to time to give our systems a break (even to eat half the quantity we presently do), and to have what we do eat of the highest quality and purity possible; to exhibit better understanding and discipline in our daily schedules of sleeping, eating and exercising (e.g. not allowing Edison lights, modern TV or present day urban activities to put us in the position of modern day hens who have the lights turned on to make them lay more eggs, which in turn greatly shortens their lives); to return to the use of God-given natural herbs which our grandparents knew well on the pioneer farms and homesteads as well as in the Indian villages of Canada."

"This preventive health philosophy is what the provincial health promotion program is all about (and the federal program as well). To deny the utilization and appropriateness of herbal therapy today is tantamount to denying the very rational for the government's own health promotion program."

"The wisdom that herbalists bring to the task of helping to restore people to health is based on their knowledge of the interaction of the energies of the biological world. The human body is a natural system. Particular plant materials have demonstrable properties for restoring bodily health."

"A shift is going on in the public's consciousness of personal responsibility for health. The support for herbal therapy today is practical. Thousands of individuals are turning to herbalist for assessment of health problems and counseling about lifestyle issues."

"Herbalists are performing the valuable service of educating the public. Self-care is a viable alternative to surgery and drugs."

And from *Walking with Trees*, a recording of an herb walk with Norma Myers through the remaining forests that stood behind her home in Alert Bay:

"It is not enough for us to heal ourselves. It is not enough just for us to heal others. We cannot do this job unless we also become herbal gardeners and herbal farmers. Therefore, we have to know about seeds. We have to collect seeds; and we have to know the actual way of seeding of every single tree and plant that grows in our region or that could be introduced into our gardens for our benefit without harming the ecology of our area. We must work hard to protect and increase the sources of our wonderful herbal medicines."

Herbal Traditions

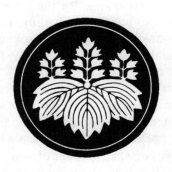

Nvwote: Cherokee Medicine and Ethnobotany

DAVID WINSTON

Cherokee medicine is an ancient system of medical/spiritual knowledge and practices that developed over the last 3,000-5,000 years. This system (*Nvwoti*) is still practiced in the mountains of North Carolina. Although there has been tremendous change for the Cherokee over the past 300 years, a core of indigenous belief and plant use remains.

When the world was still young, the Cherokee (*Ani Katuah*) received much of their traditional medicine and ceremony from two sources. Stone Clad (*Nvyunuwi*), an ancient wizard (*ada'wehi*), showed the people the dual nature of life. First he preyed on the Cherokee, then later when they killed him, he gave them their songs, ceremonies and formulas. The other source of Cherokee medical knowledge was the plants themselves.

This is a story my uncle told me when I was a boy: In the beginning of this world when life was new, all manner of new creatures came into this world. There was Awi the deer, Yvna the bear, Justu the rabbit, Gili the dog, Suli the buzzard and many others. Last of the creatures born was a strange new animal called man. In those days every living thing could communicate with one another because all spoke a common language. People could talk to animals or the water, the plants, the fire or the stones. All beings respected & understood each other, taking only what they needed to live. But gradually within man something began to change. People forgot they were a part of one Great Life: they would take more than they needed and showed disrespect for other creatures. Instead of taking one deer, they would kill an entire herd, taking only the choice meat and leaving the rest to rot. They poisoned whole pools of fish instead of taking a few. They trampled insects and other small creatures through dislike or carelessness. As people continued to separate themselves from the rest of the Great Life and disregarded the Laws of Nature they forgot how to speak the original language. When the animal nations came together in council, they would ask "What do we do about the problem of man?" The bear nation held a council and the Great White Bear asked his people this question. Their answer was to declare war on man. To give themselves a chance against the more numerous and aggressive man, they decided to make themselves a bow and arrow. When it was made, one of the warrior bears drew back the bow and fired. The arrow flew wildly landing nowhere near the target. The bear offered to chop off his claws so he could be a better bowman, but the Great White Bear stopped him, reminding the bears that the Great Life had provided the bears with their claws and teeth to feed and defend themselves. If they tried to change what they were, then they became no better than man. Hearing this, all the bears agreed and the council disbanded.

Over the years other animal nations held their councils but they too could come to no conclusion about what to do with the problem of man. Finally the creeping, crawling nation—the insects—held a council and they decided to give man disease. As they shouted out the name of each disease—liver disease, heart disease, pain in the joints, fever—these illnesses came into the world. Every man, woman and child was afflicted and many died, but a few began to recover. So in order to rid themselves of man completely, the chief of the insects, the White Grubworm, went to the chief of the Green People, Grandfather Ginseng. He asked Grandfather Ginseng to help the insects totally destroy mankind. The plants are a patient people and the ginseng plant asked for four days to pray and think about the decision. After four days Grandfather Ginseng said, "We have heard your words and there is much truth in them. People have hurt and abused us as much or more than they have you. But we also understand that man is still young and foolish and we are all part of the same Great Life. So we have decided that if people come to us in a good way, a sacred way, we will help them by giving them the cure for every disease which you, the insects, have made."

This is a promise made to us by the Green People and to this day they honor their pledge by providing us with food and medicine. It is still a common practice among Cherokee herbalists to walk through the woods allowing the needed medicine to announce itself by unusual shaking or other obvious signs.

The botanical diversity in Western North Carolina is extensive; it is estimated that in times past the average Ani Katuah would have been familiar with 100-200 plants and a medicine person (*didaganiski*) might know as many as 800 useful plants. From this tremendous quantity of available plants, many commonly used Cherokee medicines made their

way into American medical practice. We can thank the Cherokee and
other Eastern native peoples for introducing many of our most popular
botanic remedies. (see table 1)

COMMON NAME	LATIN BINOMIAL	TRADITIONAL CHEROKEE USE
Black Cohosh	*Cimcifuga racemosa*	rheumatism, anodyne, emmenagogue, backache
Bloodroot	*Sanguinaria canadensis*	coughs, fungal infections, antiseptic
Blue Cohosh	*Caulophyllum thalictroides*	nervine, parturient, anodyne, rheumatism
Butternut bark	*Juglans cineria*	laxative, liver tonic
Collinsonia	*Collinsonia canadensis*	swollen breasts, sore throat
Ginseng	*Panax quinquefolium*	adaptogen, bitter tonic, nervous problems
Goldenseal	*Hydrastis canadensis*	stomachic, bitter tonic, antiseptic
Lobelia	*Lobelia inflata*	emetic, antispasmodic-palsy, expectorant
Mayapple	*Podophyllin peltatum*	laxative, cathartic
Passionflower	*Passiflora incarnata*	liver pain, earache, nervine
Pink Root	*Spigelia marilandica*	vermifuge
Pleurisy Root	*Asclepias tuberosa*	expectorant, heart trouble, bronchitis, pleurisy
Poke Root	*Phytolacca americana*	rheumatism, skin conditions, as poultice for swollen breasts
Prickly Ash	*Xanthoxyllum spp.*	arthritis, joint pain

Sassafras	*Sassafras albidum*	skin problems, rheumatism, eyewash, carminative, gout
Slippery Elm	*Ulmus fulva*	bulk laxative, diarrhea, sore throat, heartburn
Tobacco	*Nicotiana rustica*	antiseptic, expectorant, emetic, antispasmodic, tetanus, snakebite
Wild Indigo	*Baptisia tinctora*	emetic, purgative, as poultice for inflammation and gangrene
Wild Yam	*Dioscorea villosa*	heart pain, intestinal pain, menstrual pain
Witch Hazel	*Hammamelis virginiana*	sore throat, bath sores, bruises, rheumatism, tuberculosis

Parallel to the Chinese system of energetics, the Cherokee had their own methods for matching herbal medicines to a specific person and illness. The Ani Katuah developed a simple but effective system that combines the use of colors, tastes and energy (hot, cold, drying, slippery and symbolism or spiritual energy). With these techniques a medicine person can easily discern the specific herbs needed in each situation. Yellow herbs and roots (Goldenseal, Yellow Root, Barberry) are used for "the yellows" (*dalanigei*) and other common liver disorders. Red herbs and roots (Bloodroot, Sumach berries, Gerardia) are used for illnesses relating to the blood. Blue and Violet flowering herbs (Scullcap, Hercules Club berries, Passion Flower) are used for their effects on the nervous system and the psyche. Hot, pungent herbs (Prickly Ash, Ramps, Spikenard) increase digestion, circulation, expectoration from the lungs, and stimulate the menses and diuresis. Cooling bitters and sours (Balmony, Dogwood Bark, Tulip Tree) reduce fevers, normalize digestion and bowel function and protect the heart from high fevers. Sweet, slippery herbs and barks (Slippery Elm, Sweet Cicely, Violet Leaves) are laxative, nourishing and soothing to the mucous membranes, lungs, stomach, vaginal tract and the bowel. Dry, astringent herbs (Witch Hazel, Oak Bark) check excess secretions and are used for excessive mucus discharge, bleeding, diarrhea and prolapsed uterus. Herbs growing in damp, marshy environments would be more appropriate for similar conditions in the body, i.e. head colds, damp pneumonia, dull, achy arthritis. Water plants (Cattails, Calamus, Lizard's Tail) are useful for excessive fluid in the body. Plants found on the dry, hotter northern ridges (Lady's Slipper, Chimaphila, Trailing Arbutus) are generally more appropriate for hot, irritable conditions.

The Cherokee concept of plants is broader than the dominant culture's concept. To the Cherokee, a plant is much more than its chemical constituents. Each plant has a personality which includes not only its physical constituents but also abilities to heal the mind and spirit as well. Every herb has a quality of its personality that is unique and gives insight into the subtle use of the plant. An example would be wild grape vine's ability to cling; it is used in love conjuring to bind broken hearts and relationships. When a plant is gathered in the proper season and dried carefully you preserve its chemical constituents. Only by ceremonially harvesting a plant (asking permission, offering tobacco, in some cases doing specific ceremonies and always leaving a healthy viable community behind) do you preserve its subtle healing abilities.

In any Cherokee herb formula there exists a combination of medicines. Some herbs are utilized for their chemical activity, others have a homeopathic basis (like cures) and one acts as a catalyst to stimulate the patient's inner doctor (will to get better, immune function). Interestingly enough this last medicine was usually ginseng, an effective adaptogen and immune potentiator.

While many plants became widely used by herbalists and physicians, others were underutilized or totally neglected. Today, many herbalists limit their materia medica to a small variety of herbs. This over-reliance on a few plants has contributed to the decimation of many wild plant populations (i.e. ginseng, lady's slipper, goldenseal, bethroot, and more recently *Echinacea angustifolia*, lomatium, and helonias). Are we using these plants with respect? The Cherokee use a great variety of medicines not only to prevent overutilization of species, but also because they believe that every plant has its specific use in relationship to human ailments.

CONTRIBUTIONS TOWARDS A CHEROKEE PHARMACOPOEIA

Each plant in this obviously partial listing is an effective medicine and, equally important, is abundant throughout large areas of the U.S.

Balmony (*Chelone glabra*) Taste - bitter; Energy - cool, dry; Part Used - herb; Western classification - aperient, anthelmintic, bitter tonic, cholagogue.

Balmony or turtlehead is a beautiful herb with either white or pink flowers (*C. lyoni*). It grows in damp deciduous woods and is frequently found along side of small branches (creeks). Balmony is an effective digestive bitter stimulating saliva, gastric, liver and gall bladder secretions. It is especially useful for people with poor fat metabolism, usually accompanied by gas, nausea, belching and a chronically sluggish bowel. Associated skin problems (psoriasis, eczema or acne) and non-hepatitis jaundice respond to its effects as well. Mixed with other anthelmintics (Elecampane, Garlic, Wormseed, Quassia) it is useful in treating pinworms and giardia.

Dosage: herb tea - 1 tsp/8 oz. water, steep 1 hour. 4 oz. before meals. Extract: 30-40 drops, 3 times per day.

Bearsfoot (*Polymnia uvedalia*) Taste - pungent, bitter; Energy - cool, dry; Part Used - herb, root; Cherokee Name - *Gadeti*; Western Classification - anodyne, emmenagogue, laxative.

Another resident of moist woodlands, Bearsfoot has a peculiar flower (often missing its rays) and an even more peculiar odor. Just by handling and smelling this sticky resinous herb, one is aware of its strong medicinal nature. Used by the Cherokee for liver pain and swollen breasts, the Eclectic physicians refined its indications noting its prominent effect upon "full flabby tissue, with poor circulation, atonic impairment of function and glandular enlargement". Internally it is most often used for Hepato- and Spleenomegaly, Metritis and a feeling of fullness in the pelvis. Externally, as a poultice or bath it is very effective for rheumatic pain, mastitis, bursitis and first degree burns.

Dosage: leaf tea - 1/2 tsp./8 oz. water, steep 1 hour. 4 oz. 2 times per day. Extract: 5-10 drops up to 3 times per day.

Bellwort (*Uvularia perfoliata*) Taste - bitter, acrid; Energy - cool, moist; Part Used - root; Cherokee Name - *Tsusaleti*; Western Classification - demulcent, nervine, sub-astringent..

Perfoliate Bellwort is a small herb, usually found along dry hillsides under heavy shade. This species, along with most other Uvularia species, is utilized as a substitute for the increasingly scarce Lady's Slipper (*Cyprepedium* spp.). Somewhat milder in action, it is never the less useful for insomnia, tension headaches, grouchy irritability and for anxiety associated with chronic nervous debility. Externally, Bellwort Root is used as a poultice or ointment for boils, herpes, snake bite (preferably non-venemous), mastitis and erysipelas.

Dosage: root tea - 1 tsp/8 oz. water, decoct 15 minutes, steep 1 hour. 2 - 3 cups per day.

Devil's shoestring (*Tephrosia virginiana*) Taste - sweet,acrid; Energy - warm, dry; Part Used - rhizome; Cherokee Name - *Distayi*; Western Classification - alterative, cathartic, diaphoretic, vermifuge.

Tephrosia, a member of the Fabiacae family contains many highly active compounds including Rotenone. Long used as a fish poison and vermafuge, it is equally effective for lice and other skin parasites. Used as a substitute for the scarce pink root (*Spigelia*), this rhizome can be used for pin and round worms. The Cherokee also use devil's shoestring internally and externally (as a wash) for pain caused by arthritis, bursitis and shin splints.

Dosage: root tea - 1/4 tsp/8 oz. water, steep 30 minutes. 2 oz. 3 times per day.

Dogwood (*Cornus florida*) Taste - bitter; Energy - cool, dry; Part Used - bark, flower, berries; Cherokee Name - *Kanvsita*; Western Classification - anodyne, antiperiodic, antispasmodic, astringent, bitter tonic.

The dogwood is a small shrubby tree, with lovely early spring flowers. The white flowers (they are actually sepals) have been used as a substitute for Chamomile for colds, colic and flu. The bark was once substitued for quinine for malaria and other periodic fevers. It is still useful for many chronic low grade fevers, especially if accompanied by diarrhea or muscle aches. Lower back pain, prolapsed uterus and muscle spasms (legs and feet) all respond to regular use of the tea. Mixed with Butternut Bark, Dogwood is effective for pinworms in children. Externally the bark poultice can be used as a wash for bed sores and ulcers.

Dosage: Bark Tea - 1/2 tsp/8oz. water. Decoct 15 minutes, steep 1/2 hour. 4 oz. 3 - 4 times per day.

Dwarf ginseng (*Panax trifolium*) Taste - sweet, bitter; Energy - cool, moist; Part Used - root, leaf; Cherokee Name - *Yunwi Usdi*; Western Classification - adaptogen, carminative, nutritive.

The small, delicate dwarf ginseng is a common spring ground cover in eastern deciduous woods. The small bulbs are edible (rather bland and starchy) and can be cooked in winter stews to strengthen the lungs and resistance to colds. The leaves (which contain ginsenosides) are added to almost any traditional herb formula to increase its effectiveness and activity. The dwarf ginseng, like its larger relative, is used for fatigue, nervous exhaustion, allergies, anorexia and depleted conditions such as chronic fatigue syndrome, TB and mononucleosis.

Dosage: Leaf Tea - 1 tsp/8oz. water, steep 1 hour. 2-3 cups per day.

Figwort (*Scrophularia nodosa, S. marilandica*) Taste - bitter; Energy - cool, dry; Part Used - herb, root; Cherokee Name - *Guniqualisgi Utanu*; Western Classification - alterative, bitter tonic, diuretic.

A large vigorous herb most often found in partial clearings. Its squared stems and odd brown flowers make it simple to identify. The root or the leaf can be used; I prefer a combination of the two. It is an excellent remedy for chronic swollen lymph nodes or cystic breast disease and it combines well with burdock, red clover or violet.

Scrophularia is also used extensively for chronic skin conditions (eczema, psoriasis, acne), arthritis, edema and chronic non-infectious liver disease. Externally, figwort makes an excellent poultice for mastitis, hemorrhoids and boils.

Dosage: leaf/root tea - 1 tsp/8 oz. water, decoct 15 minutes, steep 1 hour. 2 -3 cups per day. Extract: 20 - 30 drops, 3-4 times per day.

Gerardia (*Agalinis* spp.) Taste - bitter; Energy - cool, dry; Part Used - herb; Cherokee Name - *Dilastesti usdi*; Western Classification - astringent, diaphoretic, cardiac tonic, sedative.

Most gerardias are inconspicuous herbs that could be easily overlooked, except for their small but showy blossoms. Also known as false foxglove, this herb is usually found in fields and meadows. The herb tea is used as a mild cardiac tonic and is especially useful for palpitations, angina and shortness of breath if they are induced by stress. The Cherokee also use this plant for fevers with agitation, high blood pressure, anxiety attacks and to protect the spirit from shock.

Dosage: leaf tea - 1/2 tsp/8oz. water, decoct 15 minutes, steep 45 minutes. 4 oz. 2 times per day.

Goldenrod (*Solidago* spp.) Taste - sweet, pungent; Energy - warm, dry; Part Used - leaf, root; Cherokee Name - *Unestala*; Western Classification - antiseptic, astringent (root) carminative, diaphoretic, diuretic, nervine.

Often thought of as a source of allergy causing pollen, the large *Solidago* genus rarely causes allergy problems. There are dozens of common species in the southeast; for medicine I prefer the sweeter tasting *S. graminifolia* and *S. tenuifolia* . The leaf tea makes a pleasant beverage and is frequently used for colds, fevers, coughs, stomach aches, headaches and menstrual cramps. The tea or extract is also effective for chronic urinary tract infections, especially if mixed with sweet birch bark (*Betula lenta*). Many older people in Snowbird Community use the leaf tea for high blood pressure. Although this treatment is somewhat effective, I believe it's effectiveness is mostly due to its diuretic action. Goldenrod root is utilized for diarrhea, dysentery, thrush, apthous stomatata and chewed for toothache.

Dosage: leaf/flower tea - 1-2 tsp/8oz. water, steep 30 minutes. 1 -2 cups per day. Extract: 20 - 30 drops, 2-3 times per day.

Hercules club (*Aralia spinosa*) Taste - pungent; Energy - warm, dry; Part Used - bark, fruit; Cherokee Name - *Utsegeda*; Western Classification - anodyne, carminative, diaphoretic, emetic.

Hercules club is a shrubby member of the Araliaceae family that frequently has been used to adulterate Prickly Ash. Spiny in appearance and pungent in taste, there is some similarity in action between the two herbs. The bark of the root or stem is often used to move "stuck energy" in chronic arthritis, paralysis and painful joints. The tea is also taken for sore throats, fevers, toothache and skin problems. Externally a poultice is used for skin ulcers and bathing in the decoction increases its effects for paralytic conditions. The purple-blue fruit is abundant and can be used as a substitute for the bark; it is in fact stronger in action than the bark but has a short shelf life (dried) of only 2 - 3 months.

Dosage: bark tea - 1 tsp/8 oz. water, steep 2 hours. 4 oz. 2 -3 times per day. Extract: 5 -20 drops, 2 -3 times per day.

Indian pipe (*Monotropa uniflora*) Taste - bitter; Energy - cold, dry; Part Used - root, fresh herb juice; Cherokee Name - *Unesdala;* Western Classification - anodyne, antispasmodic, diaphoretic, sedative.

Indian pipe or ice plant is a small saprophyte that is usually found in the acid humus of mature forests. It especially likes pine woods, but can be found in mixed hardwood forests as well. The root of Indian pipe is unlike any other that I have ever seen. It is a round mass that easily crumbles into sand-like particles. The fresh root extract or a tea of the recently dried root is an excellent remedy for pain, muscular spasms and irritability. Once touted as a substitute for morphine, this plant does create a sense of separation from pain without narcotic side-effects. The

Cherokee have traditionally utilized this herb for petit mal epilepsy, bells palsy, tic douloureux, fevers with irritability or convulsions and as a pain reliever (usually mixed with black cohosh, lobelia or willow bark). The fresh plant juice mixed with salt water is an excellent remedy for conjunctivitis and irritation of the eye.

Dosage: Extract - 15-20 drops, 3-4 times per day.

Rabbit tobacco (*Gnaphalium obtusifolium*) Taste - sweet, bitter; Energy - cool, dry; Part Used - herb; Cherokee Name - *Katsuta equa*; Western Classification - astringent, carminative, diaphoretic, expectorant, nervine.

Common in fields and clearings, rabbit tobacco is frequently found in Cherokee homes as a remedy. The tea is used for colds, flu, coughs, diarrhea, strep throat and children's fevers. Mixed with other medicines it is also used for colitis (with wild yam and catnip), asthma (with lobelia, wild cherry bark and occasionally datura) and vaginal candidiasis (with yellow root). Externally the tea is applied to cuts, sore muscles and bruises. The leaves are chewed by some people in preference to tobacco, others mix the two to moderate tobacco's emetic qualities.

Dosage: herb tea - 1-2 tsp herb/8 oz. water, steep 40 minutes. 2-3 cups per day.

Rattlesnake weed (*Hieracium venosum*) Taste - bitter; Energy - cool, dry; Part Used - leaf, root; Cherokee Name - *Awi Tati Gigagei*; Western Classification - astringent, expectorant, vulnerary.

Rattlesnake weed is a low growing member of the Asteraceae that is usually found in dry, open areas. Its red veined leaves are its most prominent feature and easily suggest full, sluggish blood vessels. The root and/or leaf tea are utilized for hemorrhoids (as a tea and a wash), diarrhea, colitis, menorrhagia, nosebleeds, varicose veins (as a poultice), blood poisoning and snakebite (as a tea and as a poultice). The fresh sap is applied to slow healing wounds and as a cure for warts.

Dosage: herb tea - 1 tsp herb/root/8 oz. water, steep 30 minutes. 2-3 cups per day.

Solomon's seal (*Polygonatum gigantum, P. biflorum*) Taste - sweet; Energy - cool, moist; Part Used - root; Cherokee Name - *Uganasta Equa*; Western Classification - demulcent, immune tonic, nutritive, vulnerary.

The Great Solomon's Seal and its smaller relative grow in moist, deciduous forests. The rhizomes with their namesake leaf scars (seals) are a highly regarded Cherokee medicine. The tea is taken as a remedy for weakness, general debility and for hot, irritated lungs (bronchitis). The rhizomes (which contain diosgenin) are considered to be a women's tonic and are used for menorrhagia, menopausal discomfort, irregular menstruation and infertility.

Externally the roots are heated and applied to boils, staph infections and ingrown toenails.

Dosage: root tea - 1 tsp rhizome/8oz. water, decoct 15 minutes, steep 1-2 hours. 1-2 cups per day. Extract: 30-40 drops , 3 times per day.

Sourwood (*Oxydendron arborum*) Taste - sour; Energy - cool, dry; Part Used - leaf; Cherokee Name - *Udoqueya*; Western Classification - antiseptic, astringent, diuretic, nervine.

Sourwood with its racemes of white bell-like flowers is a favorite pollen source for mountain bees. The honey from this source is famous for its unique taste and fragrance. In contrast to the honey's sweetness the leaves are tart and drying. The leaf tea is an effective urinary tract antiseptic primarily due to its arbutin content. Chronic UTIs with burning urine respond well to its soothing action. The tea is also frequently used for apthous stomatata, thrush, edema, chronic prostatitis, diarrhea, nervous stomach and frazzled nerves (a nice hot cup of the tea with a generous dollop of sourwood honey works wonders!).

Dosage: leaf tea - 2 tsp. herb/8 oz. water, steep 40 minutes. 2-3 cups per day.

Spicebush (*Lindera benzoin*) Taste - pungent, sweet; Energy - warm, dry; Part Used - bark, leaf, fruit; Cherokee Name - *Nodatsi*; Western Classification - antiseptic, carminative, diaphoretic, emmenagogue, expectorant.

Spicebush is one of the most common understory shrubs throughout second or third growth eastern forests. Early in the spring it is covered with small yellow flowers which perfume the air. Every part of spicebush (aka spicewood) is medicinal; the tea of this herb is used extensively for colds, flu, coughs, nausea, indigestion, croup, flatulence and amenorrhea. The inhaled steam is used to clear clogged sinuses and the decoction of the twigs makes a soothing bath for arthritic pain (some of the tea is also taken internally). Spicebush is also commonly used as a beverage tea and the fruits can be used as a spice in baking.

Dosage: bark/herb tea - 1 tsp herb/8 oz. water, steep 1 hour (covered). 2 -3 cups per day.

Spikenard (*Aralia racemosa*) Taste - pungent; Energy - warm, dry; Part Used - root; Cherokee Name - *Yanuniyesti*; Western Classification - antiseptic, diaphoretic, emmenagogue, expectorant.

Spikenard is a large herbaceous member of the Araliaceae family. Growing in moist shaded hollows, it prefers deep rich humus and is usually found near bloodroot, ginseng and black cohosh. Spikenard, like many members of its botanical family, has long been used as a tonic for weakness and tired blood. Its mild adaptogenic qualities are usually overshadowed by its strong effects on the uterus and lung. Cherokee midwives still use spikenard mixed with blue cohosh for stimulating labor and expelling the placenta. Spikenard is also used for amenorrhea, menstrual cramps and feelings of fullness in the pelvis. As a lung remedy this herb is effective for "damp asthma," croup and coughs (with profuse clear or white mucus). A poultice of the root is useful for cuts, bruises , sore muscles and rheumatic pain. Dosage: root tea - 1 tsp/8 oz. water, decoct 15 minutes, steep 1 hour. 2 -3 cups per day. Extract: 20 -30 drops, 3 times per day.

Sumach (*Rhus glabra, R. copallina, R. typhina*) Taste - sour; Energy - cool, dry; Part Used - berry, bark; Cherokee Name - *Qualagu*; Western Classification - alterative (bark), antiseptic, astringent, diuretic.

Sumachs are small shrubby trees that have highly visible clusters of bright red berries each autumn. It's toxic relative poison sumach (*R. vernix*) has white fruit and prefers swampy areas instead of the dry open environment where other sumachs are found. Sumach berry tea is highly effective for urinary tract infections (it acidifies the urine), thrush, apthous stomatata, ulcerated mucous membranes, gingivitis and some cases of bed wetting (irritated bladder). The fruit tea can be taken hot or chilled as a refreshing beverage similar in taste to hibiscus or rose hips. The bark is a strong astringent (used for diarrhea, menorrhagia) and it has a pronounced effect on the female hormonal system. Traditionally the bark is used for alleviating menopausal discomfort (hot flashes, sweating) and as a galactogogue. Externally the berry or bark tea has been used as a wash for blisters, burns and oozing sores.

Dosage: berry tea - 1 tsp fruit/8 oz. water , steep 30 minutes. 2 - 4 cups per day. Bark tea - 1/2 tsp/8 oz. water, decoct 15 minutes, steep 1 hour. 4 oz., 3 times per day.

Sweet Cicily (*Osmorhiza claytoni*) Taste - sweet; Energy - warm, moist; Part Used - root; Western Classification - carminative, demulcent, expectorant, immune tonic, nutritive.

Sweet Cicily is a small herbaceous member of the Apiaceae family. Growing in moist woodlands, it is easy to overlook until you sample its sweet anise-tasting root. Cherokee have long considered this root to be an important medicine for increasing strength, weight and resistance to disease. The tea can be used for colds, sore throats, coughs, flu and digestive disturbances (gastritis, nausea, gas). Sweet Cicily strengthens what the Chinese call the *wei qi*, making it useful for preventing colds and other external pernicious influences. The root can be used as a substitute for licorice or astragalus with many similar applications.

Dosage: root tea - 1 tsp/8 oz. water, steep 2 hours (cooking 3-4 hours is even better). 2-3 cups per day.

Sweet gum (*Liquidambar styraciflua*) Taste - pungent, bitter; Energy - warm, dry; Part Used - resin, bark; Western Classification - antiseptic, astringent, carminative, diuretic.

A large tree fond of moist soils, it has become more common since the decline of the previously dominant chestnut. Sweetgum has rough bark, in which its fragrant resin can occasionally be found, and spiky fruits that children love to throw at anything that makes a good target (as a child, dodging "sticky balls" was a constant occupation). The tea of the inner bark is helpful for diarrhea, dysentery, UTIs or menorrhagia, as are most antiseptic astringents. In addition to these uses, it has been used as a bath and tea for rheumatic and muscular pain. The decoction of the resin can be used similarly, plus it is excellent for strep throat, herpes sores, bedsores, cracked nipples and mixed with Wild Yam for heart pain. A poultice of the inner bark or resin makes a good drawing plaster for splinters and boils and can also be applied to wounds, cuts and local infections.

Dosage: bark tea - 2 tsp/8 oz. water, decoct 20 minutes, steep 1 hour. 1 - 3 cups per day. Resin tea - 2 tsp/8 oz. water, decoct 45 minutes. 4 oz., 3 times per day.

Tulip tree (*Liriodendron tulipifera*) Taste - bitter; Energy - cool, dry; Part Used - bark; Cherokee Name - *Tsiyu*; Western Classification - anodyne, astringent, bitter tonic, febrifuge.

Tulip tree or tulip poplar is a large, straight growing member of the Magnolia family. Its yellow, green and orange flowers are large and showy and they mature into a densely packed cone of winged seeds. The smooth young bark harvested in the spring makes a wonderful basket perfect for gathering herbs or berries. This same bark is used as a medicine for periodic fevers, diarrhea, pinworms, as a digestive aid and for rheumatic pain. The decoction is used as a bath for fractures, sprains, hemorrhoids and is applied to snakebites received in dreams (if left untreated, traumatic arthritis will often develop in the area bitten).

Dosage: bark tea - 1-2 tsp/8 oz. water, decoct 20 minutes, steep 1 hour. 4 oz. 3 times per day.

Yellow root (*Xanthorhiza simplicissima*) Taste - bitter; Energy - cool, dry; Part Used - root; Cherokee Name - *Dalanei*; Western Classification - antibacterial, antifungal, antiseptic, bitter tonic, cholagogue.

Yellow root is a shrubby berberine containing plant that is found growing along branches and springs. It is abundant throughout the southeast and is regularly substituted for the increasingly scarce golden seal. *Xanthorhiza* is milder than Hydrastis but is more appropriate for long term use. It is especially effective as a digestion/liver bitter for people with sluggish bowels, a tendency towards hemorrhoids and faulty fat digestion. Mixed with fresh black walnut hull extract and spilanthes, yellow root is an effective treatment for local (thrush,vaginal candidiasis) and systemic candidiasis. The tea makes a soothing gargle for strep throat, apthous stomatata, ulcerated mucous membranes, herpes and pyorrhea. Externally it is useful for conjunctivitis, bedsores, bleeding hemorrhoids, ringworm and athlete's foot.

Dosage: root tea - 1-2 tsp/8 oz. water, decoct 10 minutes, steep 1 hour. 2 cups per day. Extract: 20-30 drops, 2-3 times per day.

To the Cherokee, the use of herbs is only one tool of many necessary for regaining health. Traditionally it was (and still is) believed that it is crucial to not only heal the body, mind and spirit, but to reintegrate the ill person within the family, the community and with the earth itself. This is a holistic perspective beyond our culture's limited understanding. None of us can truly be well unless we recognize our connection to the rest of the Great Life.

Forgotten and Neglected American Medicinal Plants

DAVID LYTLE

In my work, I have the good fortune to deal with 180 different plants from many places throughout the country and the world—including their handling, processing and collecting. My main interest is a personal list of 64 plants native to North America.

I have a strong prejudice for native plants. I believe their particular value resides in the fact that we are here together. Not only are they useful as food and medicine, but hopefully we will gain from them a better understanding and respect for what really sustains us—our natural environment. It is my hope that many people of differing paths will use their skills to this end. I believe that change comes to individuals only as we are moved and motivated by direct experience. Our native plants provide us with ample opportunity for this experience.

I want to discuss four native medicinal plants that at one time were both widely used and highly valued. These plants have become more or less obscure and unjustly so. They are: *Stillingia sylvatica* (Queen's root), *Baptisia tinctoria* (Wild indigo), *Leptandra virginica* (Culver's root) and *Dicentra canadensis* (Cordydalis).

Stillingia sylvatic, or Queen's root, is becoming one of my favorite plants and I am using it more frequently. It is named in honor of Dr. Benjamin Stillingfleet (1702–1771), an English botanist and naturalist. It is also known commonly as Queen's delight, silver leaf and yaw root.

Stillingia is a member of the Euphoriaceae or Spurge family. The genus *Stillingia* consists of about 15 species native to tropical America and some Pacific islands. This is a perennial plant, rather woody and bushy, growing two to four feet tall. Queen's root has leathery, finely toothed leaves and exudes a milky sap when broken. This plant has distinctive glands at the base of the flower and blooms from March through October. Queen's root grows all along the southern Atlantic and Gulf coastal plains, from Virginia to Florida, west to Texas and as far north as Kansas. It grows in dry sandy soil and dry woods.

The root is the part of the plant that is used. These roots can get very large and woody but are preferred when of medium size and age. This root is decidedly most active when fresh or freshly dried—herbal practitioners of the last century declared the long-dried root worthless. The fresh roots have light tan exterior and are red and juicy when the bark is peeled back. The color and odor of the fresh root is such that one experience in handling it leaves a permanent impression. It has a distinctive unpleasant acrid odor and when ground assumes a beautiful pink color. A small piece of fresh root, when chewed for a few minutes, leaves the tongue and throat rough and raspy. Large amounts can cause vomiting and burning of the throat and stomach. This is most likely due to the presence of calcium oxalate in addition to its resin and acrid oil.

Queen's root acquired its reputation for being effective against syphilis. The Cherokee are reported to have used it for this condition. It is classified by the Eclectics, a large group of herb doctors of the last century and early 20th century, as an alterative unsurpassed by few if any other herbs. It seems to strongly influence the lymph glands.

It is most useful in throat and upper respiratory conditions where there is much mucus and congestion. I have recently seen a case where chronic ear congestion and one-sided sore throat were relieved by the use of a special form of Queen's root known as Compound Stillingia Liniment. Queen's root was a key ingredient for many of the old alterative, or blood purifying, compounds of the past. Some of these alterative formulas are still with us today, such as the famous Hoxey formula and its counterparts.

There are two reasons why I believe that Queen's root fell into a state of neglect. The first is that good quality material was not always used. As stated earlier, the fresh root is most active. If used in the dry state, the roots need to be replaced annually. Second, I believe that Queen's root became so associated with the alterative formulas that it ceased to be considered individually. When properly prepared and applied, Queen's root does exhibit its medicinal benefits. My own limited usage of this native plant leads me to believe that when clinically evaluated, its historical use will be validated.

The second neglected native plant I wish to discuss is *Baptisia tinctoria,* or Wild indigo. Wild indigo is a perennial of the Fabaceae, Legume or pea family. It consists of about 24 species. Baptisia is named after the Greek word meaning "to dye." The dried leaves of this plant and its related species were used as a coloring agent and substitute for indigo dye. Thus we get the common names wild or false indigo. Other common names are rattleweed, the dried pods being used as such by children, and shoofly or horsefly weed, since the flowering branches repel insects. Wild indigo grows two or three feet tall, bushy, with black spotted yellowish-green stems. It has the characteristic pods of the pea family plants. The leaves of most of the species turn bluish black or black when dried. Wild indigo has the smallest leaves of the Baptisia species. It grows on poor, dry, and often acidic soil in most of our eastern states. Baptisia has bright yellow flowers which bloom between June and September.

Although the leaves were used, the root and root bark were preferred by the Eclectics. This is another plant which was touted highly by them. Wild indigo was proclaimed to be an antiseptic of great power for both internal and external use. Foul ulcers, wounds, and putrid sore throats where the tissues appear deep red, blue or purple and seemed to be stagnant or dying were its indications for use. It seemed to these practitioners to be a specific for typhus. In fact, articles in the *Eclectic Medical Journal* proclaimed it to be a remedy for epidemics with success against cholera, Asian flu, diphtheria, measles and malaria. This is significant because we are talking about a time before the development of most of our modern pharmaceutical drugs for these diseases. I feel certain that the development of improved antiseptics, vaccines, and later, antibiotics were the reasons that wild indigo went from being widely used to a relatively obscure remedy.

My own experience with this medicinal plant is limited and less glamorous than the Eclectics. I have seen a few cases of Strep throat successfully treated with tincture of *Echinacea angustifolia* 80% and wild indigo 20%. In all of these cases, no antibiotics were being used and echinacea alone was not making much progress. This formula taken internally, and also used dilute in warm water as a gargle, was successful. In using this plant, I have ignored the warning not to use it in the acute inflammatory stage of illness because I have always combined it with echinacea, which is a good anti-inflammatory herb. I suspect that the Eclectic's indications for *Baptista* are too narrow.

It must be remembered that this plant is also irritating and possesses some degree of toxicity. Inappropriate use and dosage can cause dizziness and vomiting and blurred vision. Some Indian tribes made use of this action. The Cherokee are known to have used it as an emetic. Wild indigo and related species were reported to be used by at least a dozen other tribes including the Fox, Iroquois and Creek Indians. Their uses include a snake bite remedy, kidney trouble and spring tonic among others. From all of this information, it can be readily seen that Wild indigo deserves to be reconsidered as a medicinal plant of wide therapeutic range.

The third neglected native medicinal plant I wish to discuss is *Leptandra virginica*, or Culver's root. Leptandra is referred to scientifically as *Veronica virginica* but more accurately as *Veronicastrum virginicum*. It is commonly known as Culver's root, black root, Bowman's root and tall speedwell. I call it leptandra by force of habit. Leptandra belongs to the Scrophulariaceae or figwort family. It is the only species of its genus, although I have seen a reference to *Veronicastrum sibirica*, a plant of Siberia.

This is a beautiful perennial plant and can grow up to seven feet tall. The leaves are in whorls of four and seven and arise from a rhizome with a single tall stem. The fuzzy, white flowers appear as several spikes at the top of the stem, are fuzzy and white, and bloom between June and September. Leptandra seems to prefer alkaline soil and the plants growing in limestone areas are preferred medicinally. Growth occurs in moist, rich woods and meadows from Wisconsin to Vermont, south to Tennessee, the Carolinas and Georgia, and west through Alabama and eastern Texas.

The rhizome collected in the fall of its second year is preferred. It is best used when well dried. The fresh root is a drastic laxative and has been reported to have caused bloody stools and even abortion. This is in stark contrast to its action when dried, which is quite safe and mild. It is used as a mild laxative, cholagogue and liver tonic. This is well documented in the older botanical references. For use as a mild laxative, larger than normal single doses of the tincture are needed, or regular doses over a period of a few days. In my experience, the most effective dose of tincture is 2 drams, or 1/4 ounce, mixed with an equal part of neutralizing cordial. Stools are softened without watery discharge and no cramps or discomfort is produced. This is quite different than the case with *Cascara sagrada* or Senna, even when combined with carminatives like licorice root or fennel.

I believe that the word tonic is often abused as a term for describing herbs. However, leptandra is a true tonic and I believe its mild and beneficial effects on the liver, gall bladder and intestines cannot go unnoticed. Six Native American tribes are reported to have made medicinal use of this native plant. It had many uses for the Cherokee, Fox and Iroquois tribes. There are Iroquois references to Leptandra which suggest that it was a shamanic medicine and a panacea for all ailments.

The reasons why leptandra became so neglected seem much clearer than the other native plants discussed. Leptandra was for many years associated with what is known as the "Eclectic resinoid craze." This refers to a time in the middle of the last century when active isolated and concentrated components of plants were being sought (sound familiar?). One of the fathers of Eclecticism, Dr. John King, had successfully isolated the resin of *Podophyllum peltatum,* commonly known as American mandrake or mayapple. This powerful agent, which is in use even today, led the way for many other herbs to be made in this form. The process was simple enough; a high alcohol extract was mixed with cold water and the precipitate, or sediment, that formed was collected, dried and powdered. For years these preparations were sold until all but the few effective ones became discredited.

Leptandra was one of the plants to which resin isolation did not do justice. It seems that the benefit of leptandra resides not in its resin, but in a bitter principle which is washed out in solution. It was also shown that the resin content of leptandra significantly increases with the plant's age, which is why the rhizone of two-year-old plants is preferred because it has a more balanced set of components. Leptandra also suffered from neglect because faster acting and more powerful laxatives became preferred.

The fourth forgotten and neglected native medicinal plant I wish to discuss is *Dicentra canadensis,* known to the Eclectics as Corydalis and commonly known as turkey corn and squirrel corn. This name refers to the medicinal part, a small corn or tuber, a little larger than a pea. *Dicentra cucullaria,* or Dutchman's breeches, and *Dicentra exemia,* or bleeding heart, were collected indiscriminately during the time when this plant was available on the commercial market. This plant is listed in some of the oldest botany texts as *Bicuculla* species. It is classified in either the Papaveraceae (poppy) or Fumoriaceae (fumitory) family. Corydalis is now used to describe a genus of related plants that have only one spur on each flower. Dicentras, from the Greek word signifying two spurs, have two spurs on each flower. By habit, I will refer to *Dicentra canadensis* by the Eclectic designation, Corydalis.

Corydalis is a beautiful plant. It has smooth, finely divided light blue green leaves and many heart-shaped flowers. The tips of these look as if they were dipped in pink paint. The flowers hang down from arching stalks. It blooms in early spring until May or June. Corydalis grows in rich soil in woods from Quebec to Minnesota, east to parts of New England, south to North Carolina, and west through Tennessee and Missouri. Corydalis stands about a foot tall and has yellow tubers. *Dicentra cucullaria,* or Dutchman's breeches, is somewhat different. It needs to be discussed because commercial samples of the past usually contained more of this plant than *Dicentra canadensis.* The two spurs of Dutchman's breeches are angular and pointed, much like an upside-down pair of baggy pants, hence the common name. The flowers are white with yellow tips and it grows in a wider range to the south and west than Corydalis, also appearing in Washington and Oregon. The tubers of this plant are white and form a tighter cluster.

Corydalis is another herb that was used to remove syphilis and its conditions from the body. It was considered to be alterative and tonic, good for skin diseases and weak digestion. The use of this plant, like most native plants, was probably learned from Native Americans. The Iroquois are also reported to have used Dutchman's breeches leaves as a liniment for runners.

The tubers have a most interesting taste dynamic. Freeze-dried samples are light and crunchy like corn puffs and of the same color. The initial taste is bittersweet, somewhat like ginseng, with a strong, bitter aftertaste which is milder than, but not unlike, goldenseal or Oregon grape root. A slight numbing of the tongue is noticeable afterwards. The color and taste suggest to me the alkaloid berberine, a well-known active constituent of barberry root bark, Oregon grape root and goldenseal. I believe the main alkaloidal body has been designated as corydaline. The pharmacology of Asian and East Indian species of corydalis have been well studied. Constituents of some of these plants have been shown to relieve pain. Others contain components similar to our famous goldenseal. I read of one species, *Corydalis govaniana,* a native of the western Himalayas, which is used by the locals for exactly the same conditions as our Corydalis; syphilis, glandular, and skin conditions.

Corydalis was also, like stillingia, a key ingredient in some of the alterative formulas of the past. I am less clear about the reasons why this plant faded into obscurity. The factors I listed under Queen's root, in addition to the preference for other herbs such as goldenseal when treating like conditions, are probable reasons. Other factors affecting its collection may have come into play such as a low yield weight of tubers and a more limited range and local abundance. I have not had the opportunity to apply this herb medicinally, but I do think the high praise it received from the early Eclectic doctors and the results of study on related plants indicate that it deserves our consideration.

In conclusion, I would like to say that our heritage of native medicinal plant use, its folklore and traditions have provided us with more than enough information to give us a great foundation. Our Thomsonian,

Physio-medicalist, Eclectic and Naturopathic systems are well-founded but certainly underdeveloped. Our Native American herbal heritage, while having the advantage of antiquity, is nonetheless only partly known to us. Much more work in these disciplines will be required before the value of medicinal plants is fully known and appreciated by the society at large. I believe the primary impetus will come from the enthusiasts, gardeners, practitioners and the public itself. We rely too heavily on our sciences to bear out truths for us, as if what we gain from practical experience is not valid without scientific data. I think the proper role of science in this regard is one of a secondary supportive role to clinical discoveries.

The greatest task facing the herb enthusiast everywhere is the condition of our global environment in general and specifically the preservation of our native plant habitats. Inevitably we must learn to cultivate our medicinal plants if we do not manage our resources. However useful a plant is, it is nevertheless "bad medicine" to carelessly harvest wild plants. Check with botanists in your area to learn about any plant you intend to harvest. Talk with herbalists and wildcrafters about ethical and conscious methods. A plant may be abundant in one area and rare in another. Even if you see a whole hillside of an endangered species, it doesn't mean it is any less endangered. In the meantime, I would encourage everyone to take time out to stop and smell the flowers!

David Lytle is a well-respected herbalist and herb enthusiast who has been an herb product manufacturer for three years and presently manages the herb laboratory at the Eclectic Institute in Portland, Oregon, a leading research and manufacturing center for quality botanical medicines.

REFERENCES:

Britton, N.L. and Brown, A. *An Illustrated Flora of the Northern United States, Canada and the British Possessions.* Second edition. New York: Scribner & Sons, 1913, Vol. II, pp. 204, 345, 461.

Duke, J.A. *CRC Handbook of Medicinal Plants.* Boca Raton, Florida: CRC Press, Inc., 1985, p. 460.

Felter, H.W. and Lloyd, J.U. *King's American Dispensatory,* Volume I and II. Portland, Oregon: Eclectic Medical Publications, reprint 1983, pp. 323, 610, 1126, 1836.

Grey's Manual of Botany, 8th edition. New York: American Book Company, 1950, pp. 682–683, 887,1280.

Hussain, S.F., et al. "Two Spirobenzylisoquinoline Alkaloids from Corydalis Stevartii." *Journal of Natural Products,* Vol. 51, No. 6 (Nov.–Dec. 1988), pp. 1136-

1139.

Lloyd, John Uri. "Corydalis, Turkey Corn or Turkey Pea." *American Druggist and Pharmaceutical Record,* Nov. 1915.

"On the Resin of Leptandra." *American Journal of Pharmacy,* Oct. 1880, p. 489.

Moerman, Daniel E. *Medicinal Plants of Native America.* University of Michigan Museum of Anthropology, Technical Reports #19, Vol. I, pp. 89, 152, 470, 509–510.

Mukhopad Hyay, S., et al. "Alkaloids of Corydalis govaniana." *Journal of Natural Products,* Vol. 50, No. 2 (Mar.–Apr. 1987), pp. 270–272.

Rickett, Harold William. *Wildflowers of the United States,* Vols. I and II. New York: McGraw-Hill, 1967.

Scudder, J.M., Ed., et al. *Eclectic Medical Journal.* Cincinnati: J.M. Scudder Publishers, various volumes, 1960–1929.

Small, J.K. *Manual of the Southeastern Flora.* Chapel Hill: University of North Carolina Press, 1933, pp. 550, 674, 788, 1209.

The Benefits of Bian Zheng: More Precious Than Any Herb

DR. ROBERT FLAWS

All medical systems are either rational, empirical or some combination of the two. Rational systems are based on theoretical concepts of human physiology and pathophysiology and an individualized differential diagnosis. Empirical systems are based upon clinical experience and a mere cataloguing of symptoms and diseases. Traditional Chinese Medicine (TCM) as it is practiced today is a balanced blend of both rational and empirical methodologies. TCM practitioners primarily treat by administering polypharmacy, herbal formulas based on a combination of what are called *bian bing* and *bian zheng* diagnoses. *Bian bing* means to differentiate various named diseases and recognized pathological signs and symptoms. *Bian zheng*, on the other hand, means to discriminate various professional recognized patterns of disharmony. *Bing* and *zheng* are not the same. In Chinese medicine it is said,

> *Tong bing yi zhi,*
> *Yi bing tong zhi*
> One disease, different treatments;
> Different diseases, same treatment.

What this means is that a single disease may manifest various individualized patterns in different patients depending upon their varying constitutions. Therefore, although a number of the patients may be diagnosed as suffering from the same disease, they may each be given a different treatment since they may each manifest the disease in a unique and individualized way. Similarly, although diseases may differ, different diseases may manifest in two patients with the same pattern of signs and symptoms. In this case, they may both be treated in the same or similar way since their individual response to differing diseases is the same. It is diagnosis by *bian zheng* which is the definition and hallmark of TCM methodology and it is diagnosis by *bian zheng* which makes TCM the holistic and noniatrogenic medicine it is.

In comparison, practitioners of Western herbal medicine prescribe almost entirely on the basis of a disease diagnosis alone. Western herbal pharmacopeias list their indications entirely on the basis of a *bian bing* diagnosis. These indications may be individuals signs and symptoms or they may be modern Western disease categories. For instance, David Hoffman in *The Holistic Herbal* lists the indications of cramp bark as muscular tension and spasm, uterine muscular cramps, threatened miscarriage, excessive blood loss during menstruation, and bleeding associated with menopause.[1] Hoffman does not give any further differentiation as to why a particular woman may have menorrhagia and for what types of menorrhagia cramp bark is most effective. Although Hoffman calls his book holistic, this is no different from a modern Western medical diagnosis and provides no holistic understanding of the totality of an individual patient's constitution or pattern.

Although Western herbalists may have centuries and even millennia of experience behind them regarding the empirical indications of the medicinals they employ, without a *bian zheng* diagnosis further individualizing a patient, their methodology is liable to be as iatrogenic as a Western physician's. Western herbal medicine is often touted as being safer than modern Western pharmaceuticals. To the extent that this is true, this is a function of Western herbal medicine's less powerful and extreme pharmacodynamics. The physiologically active ingredients in herbs are typically not as concentrated as in Western pharmaceuticals and, therefore, their iatrogenesis tends to be less pronounced for that reason. However, as an American practitioner of TCM practicing in a city where Western herbal medicine is quite popular, I see a steady stream of patients whose symptoms have been worsened by taking the wrong Western herbs. In my experience, when this occurs, it is always due to a lack of individualized *bian zheng* diagnosis corroborated with a sophisticated understanding of the energetic nature and functions of the herbal medicinal.

It is my belief that the simplistic and naive opinion that somehow herbs are natural and therefore safe is erroneous and counterproductive. Although TCM is often described as an herbal medicine, in fact it is not. TCM uses medicinal ingredients from all three kingdoms—animal, vegetable and mineral. Because of this, I prefer to use the word medicinal instead of herbs and this has led me to examine what, if any, the differences are between herbs and other medicinals. It is true that vegetable medicinals tend to be more buffered, round and mild in their therapeutic action on the body and this point should not be overlooked. But, until all medicines are prescribed on the basis of both a disease and an individualized pattern diagnosis, the likelihood of iatrogenesis still exists.

Recently there has been a furor over the FDA's allowed Enkaid and Tambocor, two Western pharmaceuticals for heart arrhythmias, to be sold even though they have caused a number of deaths. Obviously, these two medicines help some people and harm others. Heart arrythmias are a symptom or a disease category. When such medicines are prescribed on this basis alone, they are bound to benefit some patients and harm others since there are a number of different energetic dyscrasias or imbalances which can give rise to heart arrhythmia.

In TCM, such arrhythmias may be due to insufficient heart blood or yin nourishing the heart, flaring of empty fire, insufficient heart *qi* or energy, liver fire flaring upward disturbing heart spirit, stomach fire flaring upward accumulating in the heart, phlegm blocking the orifices of the heart, stagnant liver *qi* obstructing the smooth flow of energy in the chest, stagnant blood obstructing the smooth flow of *qi* and blood in the chest or any of several combinations of these. Depending upon which of these patterns the patient exhibits evidenced by the total constellation of their constitutional signs and symptoms, different treatment principles are indicated. According to TCM theory, some of these causes of heart arrhythmia are diametrically opposite in their disease mechanism and therefore would be treated by opposite methodologies. In the case of stagnant *qi* and phlegm obstructing the heart, the treatment principles are to activate the *qi*, broaden the chest, transform the phlegm and open the orifices of the heart. Medicinals known to achieve these functions *and* which are empirically known to treat heart arrythmia are then indicated. However, if the patient actually is suffering from blood and yin insufficiency and medicinals with the above functions are employed on the basis of their being known to empirically treat heart arrythmia alone, they will further weaken and injure such a patient and could very well cause their demise. This is so whether those medicinals be made from vegetable, animal, mineral or synthetic sources.

There may not be anything wrong *per se* with Enkaid or Tambocor. The problem is that, in all probability, a sophisticated diagnosis similar to TCM's which would allow for a more precise prescription of these medicines is lacking. This is *the* main problem with Western medicine. Similarly, without such a diagnostic system, Western herbal medicine is in no way superior to modern Western medicine. It is only weaker.

That is not to say that Western herbal medicine has always lacked such a sophisticated system of pattern discrimination. It has not. There are two main traditions of Western herbal medicine. One is the Wise Woman tradition. This was a folk tradition and was primarily empirical. The other was the Galenic or Scholastic tradition. This was based on Greek and Roman vitalistic, humoral and elemental theories enriched by cross pollination from Chinese sources. Like TCM, this was a literate and professional system of medicine primarily relying on herbal medicinals but also using minerals and animal parts. It used a similarly sophisticated system of both *bian bing* and *bian zheng* diagnoses and dominated Western medical practice up until the middle of the 19th Century. Western Scholastic treatises on the cause of disease and differential pattern diagnosis are, by and large, understandable to TCM practitioners, and Galenic polypharmacy formulas are also familiar in their composition and rationale.

Galenic Scholasticism died out, however, because it became too rational and too conceptual. It lost touch with empirical reality and clinical practice and lent itself to charlatanism. Eventually, so-called modern Western medicine discredited Galenic Scholasticism and supplanted it. This same thing happened to Chinese medicine in Asia at exactly the same time. However, Western medicine in Asia did not become the monopoly it has become in the West, in part because there were too few practitioners and its medicines were too expensive. Traditional practitioners continued to carry on their practice amongst the people and continued to train their successors. In the last fifty years in China, TCM has been resurrected and promoted by the state, both for its efficiency and noniatrogenesis and for its cost-effectiveness. In this renaissance, great stress has been laid on developing TCM's system of dual diagnosis, not letting the mind create castles in the sky nor promoting merely symptomatic treatment. In modern TCM, rationality is tempered by and grounded in empirical, clinical experience thus achieving the superior middle way or the union of yin and yang.

Although Western Galenic medicine exists in books and is a living tradition in India where it has become the foundation of *Unani* (i.e., Ionian) or Islamic medicine, it is a dead tradition in the West. Its living lineage here has been cut and its concepts so discredited by seven generations of Western physicians that attempts to resurrect and employ this system here in the West again seem futile and counterproductive. On the other hand, TCM is a living, flourishing and mature medical system which has been endorsed by the World Health Organization for worldwide propagation and is legally practicable (under the aegis of acupuncture licensure) in almost half the states in the Union. TCM theory and methodology differ from Galenic Scholasticism in only minor, technical ways. Therefore, although the words are different, the concepts are not alien to traditional Western culture. For instance, when we say colloquially that we have caught a cold, this concept is derived from Galenic medicine and is based on the idea of a cold pathogen invading the body. This idea is essentially the same as the TCM etiology for this same disease. In the same way, the Galenic etiologies and disease mechanisms for migraines, gallstones, apoplexy and a host of other diseases are the same as in TCM.

TCM has proven its efficacy in over two thousand years of continuous clinical experience and this clinical experience has been recorded throughout this same two thousand years in not less than 10,000 extant medical books and manuscripts. Furthermore, Chinese medicine was developed in a vast country with a widely diverse genetic pool, varying social customs and mores, and a geographic environment stretching from sea level to the Himalayas and from the tropics to the arctic tundra with every other climate in between. In the last twenty years, TCM has been exported to Africa, Southwest Asia, Australia, North, Central and South America, and Europe where its practitioners have demonstrated its universal efficacy amongst all races and social classes and in virtually every climate, environment and social setting. Other traditional, rational medicines, such as traditional Tibetan medicine, are either no longer extant as living practices, lack an extensive professional literature or evolved to address the problems of a limited gene pool living in an extreme and unique environment. Therefore, TCM is unique in the world today as the oldest, most literate and most universal, rational alternative to modern Western medicine.

In suggesting that practitioners of Western herbal medicine adopt TCM theory and diagnosis, I am not suggesting that they must necessarily give up using the medicinals to which they have grown accustomed. Rather I am suggesting that it is TCM *bian zheng* diagnosis that they adopt and the methodology of prescription which is based on that differential diagnosis. AT least 20% of the standard TCM repertoire of single ingredients originally derived from non-Chinese sources. Medicinal ingredients entered China from Indochina, the Spice Islands, India, Tibet, Mongolia, Siberia, Turkestan, Persia, Greece, Rome and even America. For instance, American ginseng became a part of Chinese medicine in the 19th century filling a therapeutic niche not covered by Asian ginseng.

Sarsaparilla from the Caribbean was incorporated into Chinese medicine sometime in the 18th or 19th centuries. And *Cheli-donium* or greater celandine has been incorporated into TCM in the 20th century. However, when foreign medicinals have been incorporated into TCM, they have been prescribed both on the basis of *bian zheng* and *bian bing* diagnoses.

In order for practitioners of Western herbal medicines to begin using *bian zheng* diagnosis in their prescriptive methodology, two things must be done. First, Western herbal medicinals' TCM descriptions need to be worked out. A medicinal's TCM description must include not less than ten categories of information. These include:

1) Pharmacological information (i.e., species & part used)
2) Flavor (as categorized by the six flavors: pungent, sweet, bitter, salty, sour and bland or some combination thereof)
3) Temperature (as categorized by the five temperatures: cold, cool, neutral, warm and hot)
4) Channel concentration (i.e., what TCM organ or organs are most affected physiologically by the medicinal)
5) TCM functions (These functions are described in terms of TCM therapeutic principles logically juxtaposed to TCM patterns of disharmony.)
6) Disease, sign, and symptom indications
7) Empirically efficacious combinations
8) Contraindications (both *bing* & *zheng*)
9) Incompatibilities (with other medicinals, foods, preparation methods, etc.)
10) Dosages

Various parts of a given plant may have different medicinal uses in TCM. Therefore, it is important to specify in the name exactly what part of the herb is being discussed. In TCM pharmacopeias, or *ben cao*, different parts of a single plant having different medicinal usages are listed as separate ingredients. For instance, *Herba ephedrae* is pungent and warm and relieves the surface, thus causing sweating; while *Radix ephedrae* is sweet and neutral and astringes the surface, thus stopping sweating.

Flavor in TCM helps to explain a medicinal's functions and also its tropism for certain organs. For instance, the sweet flavor is nourishing and supplementing but is also heavy and promotes the secretion of body fluids. According to Five Phase theory, it is the flavor which tends to accumulate or gather in the TCM spleen. Therefore, a spleen supplement such as *Radix codonopsis pilosulae* is understandably sweet. However, if there is prominent dampness, *codonopsis* should not be used. Many medicinals are a combination of two or more tastes. Some medicinals, such as *Fructus schizandrae chinensis* contain all five flavors.

Temperature describes a medicinal's effect on the body's warmth, either local or systemic. This is a very important discrimination since the methodology of TCM says that a warm disease should be cooled and a cold disease heated up. Hot medicinals are contraindicated in hot diseases. However, because the body's inherent energy is warm and because digestion is essentially a process of warm transformation, even in pathologically hot conditions one must be careful not to overdose with cool and cold medicinals.

Channel concentration is *jung gui* in Chinese. Although the term channel or meridian is used, the medicinal's effect is not on the channel *per se* but on the organ. *Gui* means to gather, assemble or reunite. This term describes a medicinal's tropism for one or more organs or body tissues. It should be reiterated though that the organ named is the TCM organ, not the Western biological organ of that same name. The definition of a TCM organ may have little to do with Western morphology and physiology. Each TCM organ has its own description and functions and these must not be confused with those of the Western biological organs.

TCM functions are the rational conceptualization of a medicinal's therapeutic actions. Within TCM, there are a finite number of therapeutic functions regarded as appropriate for remedying a TCM imbalance or dyscrasia. These are technical terms with fairly precise TCM definitions and implications. For instance, if the *zheng* or pattern diagnosis is damp heat accumulating in the bladder causing pain and difficult urination, the TCM therapeutic principles are to clear heat and drain dampness, to stop pain and disinhibit urination. In this case, disinhibit means to promote the flow of body fluids. Dampness may also be perfused, transformed, eliminated, or purged depending upon the type of dampness and its location in the body. In the case of damp heat of the urinary bladder, anything but draining and disinhibiting is a categorically wrong approach to therapy. Therefore, in choosing medicinals to treat this condition, one must choose those which clear heat, drain dampness, disinhibit urination, and stop pain. It is these TCM functional or rational, theoretical descriptions which are the bridge between a TCM *bian zheng* diagnosis and holistic, individualized prescription.

Disease and symptom indications are those medically recognized signs and symptoms and disease categories for which a given medicinal has shown empirical efficacy. Two medicinals might each clear heat and eliminate dampness, but one may be particularly effective for the treatment of cholecystitis while the other may be especially effective in treating urinary cystitis. In addition, some medicinals have special empirical effects which are not accounted for by their energetic descriptions and are employed primarily due to their symptomatic efficacy. When such are used in TCM, they are employed as branch, rather than root treatments. A root treatment always seeks to rebalance the underlying terrain of disharmony or dyscrasia. Western herbal medicine is rich in its empirical experience and has well tabulated most of its medicinals' signs, symptoms and disease indications.

Efficacious combinations are those combinations of medicinals which have proven themselves to be especially empirically effective in clinical practice. Certain medicinals are synergistic and their combined effect achieves a larger, fuller therapeutic response. An example of this in TCM is the combination of *Rhizoma atractylodis macrocephalae* and *Sclerotium poriae cocos*. Atractylodes is a *qi* supplement which gathers in the spleen and aids in the aromatic perfusion and transformation of dampness. Poria is a damp draining medicinal which secondarily strengthens the spleen and harmonizes the middle burner. Since dampness is the most common, major impediment to proper spleen function, combining these two medicinals with slightly different functions together achieves a fuller, rounder effect than either would alone.

If the first rule of all medical practice is to do no harm, then contraindications are just as important as indications. In TCM, a medicinal may be contraindicated in the case of a particular symptom, for instance honey in the case of diarrhea, or may be contraindicated in certain *zheng* patterns. If a patient is suffering from emptiness of yin with night sweats, pungent, warm, surface relieving medicinals are contraindicated since they would exhaust yin fluids even further and thus worsen the patient's overall condition. When medicinals cause side effects, it is almost always because of a lack of precise *bian zheng* diagnosis and prescription. When one has such a diagnosis, one can then rationally predict a given medicinal's effect on a given individual.

Certain medicinals may react antagonistically to various foods, methods of preparation or other medicinals. These are technically called aversions in TCM. For instance, ginseng has an aversion to tannic acid and foods containing tannic acid. Some medicinals must be decocted and others merely infused in order to bring out their therapeutic efficacy. It is little use to spend one's time and money taking some medicine only to negate its effects by eating the wrong foods or preparing the medicinal in some inappropriate way, and it's even worse to take two medicinals together which both seemed appropriate when judged alone only to find that they cause some adverse reactions.

And finally, correct dosage is a very important part of prescribing. Too much of a medicinal may cause adverse reactions and too little may not achieve the desired healing effect. Dosage levels are typically determined through empirical experience. However, in TCM, knowing a person's TCM pattern diagnosis and the properties and functions of a particular medicinal ingredient, one can rationally determine if that patient needs more or less of that medicinal. Dosages in TCM are usually stated as a range from minimum to maximum dosages. Deciding which dosage to employ is a function of both empirical experience and rational deduction based on the *bian zheng* diagnosis.

Several Western practitioners of TCM, including myself, have tentatively begun the description of Western herbal medicinals according to the TCM categories above. I say tentative because such an endeavor requires a very high degree of proficiency in TCM theory and practice. This is not an exercise for beginners. It requires empirical experience with the medicinal, literary research, and a great deal of logical deduction using the premises and terminology of TCM in a very rigorous way. One first formulates a working hypothesis and then tests that hypothesis against all clinical information available on that medicinal. One often finds that, over a period of time, the initial impression about a medicinal's TCM functions was not quite right and has to be revised in the light of further clinical experience, research and insight. Discussions are under way amongst a number of Western practitioners concerning a cooperative effect extending over years to slowly develop the TCM descriptions of a core group of Western herbal medicinals. In *Something Old, Something New*, I present my methodology for working out any new medicinal's TCM description and the tentative TCM descriptions of a number of Western herbs as examples of this process.[2]

The second step in incorporating the insights of TCM *bian zheng* diagnosis into Western herbal medicine is for practitioners of Western herbal medicine to learn TCM theory and diagnosis. This may sound simple but it is not. TCM education sufficient to do internal medicine, i.e., the prescription of medicine taken internally, requires at least three years or more of study and clinical practice, preferably under supervision. Unlike acupuncture which can be learned in two years and which is relatively safe, the level of TCM diagnostic expertise required to do internal medicine safely and effectively is much greater since the possibility for iatrogenesis is also greater. This means that one cannot just learn a little TCM and make it work for them. TCM is a system of thought and not a bag of tricks. One must learn it systematically and this requires dedication, perseverance and the willingness to discipline oneself until one has plumbed the depths and closed the circle.

In China, doctors studying internal, albeit herbal, medicine spend four to six years in school. They are then posted to a clinic where they work as the amanuensis of a senior practitioner or *lao yi sheng*, literally "old doctor." This clinical apprenticeship may last from two to eight years during which time the old doctor diagnoses the patient and composes the prescription while the young doctor watches and writes the prescription down.

Although this level of training does not yet exist in the United States, still there are schools and colleges of TCM which offer three year courses of instruction which do include at least some clinical training. Without such professional training in terminology, diagnostics and conceptual and prescriptive methodology of TCM, it is not realistic to speak of adding a little TCM as some sort of learning to the practice of Western herbal medicine.

At the present time, there is a certain fascination among Western herbalists to include certain Chinese medicinals in their practice. These include ginseng, dang gui, shou wu aka fo ti, gingko, astragalus and Artemesia annua. However, the efficacy of these Chinese medicinals is to a large extent dependent upon their use as determined by *bian zheng* diagnosis. For instance, astragalus is popular in the West as a so-called tonic for the immune system. In TCM, astragalus is a *qi* supplement which specifically boosts the *wei* or defensive *qi*. *Wei qi* defends the body against invasion by external evils. Although this includes a part of Western immune function, astragalus consolidates the surface and controls excessive sweating when due to emptiness of defensive *qi*. It is possible for a patient to have immune deficiency as diagnosed and defined by Western medicine who suffers from a TCM pattern of empty yin with flaring of empty fire. In this case, astragalus might very well make this patient worse by closing the *qi men* or pores and trapping the heat inside. In such a case, the empty heat would consume body fluids and yin all the more making the patient worse, not better.

Similarly, Artemesia annua, or *Qing Hao* in Chinese, is widely touted as an anti-giardia herb. In TCM, this medicinal is indicated for summer heat diseases and for bone-steaming heat due to emptiness of yin. It is my clinical experience that this medicinal is not effective for treating giardiasis in patients who do not also present the TCM patterns for which Artemesia annua is traditionally indicated. I have had a number of patients referred to me by progressive Western MDs who have been treated for giardiasis with various Artemesia annua preparations whose stool samples are still positive for giardia. When this medicinal is applied solely on the basis of a Western *bian bing* diagnosis, it fails to achieve remarkable therapeutic effect within the human body even though *in vitro* its antiprotozoal effect is pronounced.

Therefore, I believe that the most valuable thing from Chinese herbal medicine practitioners of Western herbal medicine can incorporate into their practice is not exotic Chinese medicinals prescribed based on symptomatic usage or Western disease categories but rather TCM's *bian zheng* diagnosis and its theoretical and prescriptive methodology. Certainly there is no reason not to use herbal medicinals from around the world if they achieve a unique and superior effect. However, to merely add Chinese herbs to one's repertoire of materia medica and prescribe these on the basis of a *bian bing* diagnosis alone is like trading the crown to a kingdom for a bowl of mush.

TCM theory and diagnosis by *bian zheng* can supply the unifying ground theory for describing and utilizing, in a rational and discriminating way, potentially any medicinal, whether naturally occurring or human-made. TCM theory and diagnosis are so universally applicable that they can and I believe will provide the conceptual foundation for a new medical model for the 21st century. Through the amalgamation of *bian bing* and *bian zheng* diagnosis, one can make discriminating and inclusive use of both traditional humoral, elemental and vitalistic concepts and the scientific knowledge discovered in experimental laboratories. TCM excels at describing the holistic terrain. Western science excels at describing the smallest bits of individualized information. When both views are used in tandem, as they are in contemporary TCM, one sees both the field and the pattern, the forest and the trees.

That is not to say that an empirical folk tradition of herbal medicine did not exist in China nor that one cannot employ herbal medicinals here in the West on a purely empirical basis with a modicum of success. However, when compared to TCM's combination of rationality *cum* empiricism, such folk approaches lack the insight, sophistication and efficacy without iatrogenesis of such a high healing art. Empiricism without rational, individualized, holistic diagnosis is a stab in the dark. Those who are content to rely upon symptomatic treatment and intuition alone may be satisfied with this. But when logic and reason combine with experience and intuition, one practices as safe a medicine as fallible humans can.

ENDNOTES:

1. Hoffman, David, *The Holistic Herbal*, Element Books, Longnead, U.K., 1988, p. 188.

2. Flaws, Bob, *Something Old, Something New*, Blue Poppy Press, Boulder, Co., 1991.

Herbalists Using Herbs

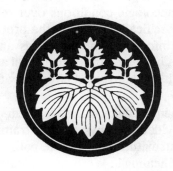

Botanical Treatment of Chronic Gynecological Conditions:
Infertility, Endometriosis, and Symptoms of Menopause*

SILENA HERON, R.N., N.D.

My goal is to present the general treatment strategy that has worked for a variety of chronic gynecologic conditions over several years of clinical practice. I will then specifically delineate the protocols that are derived from this model for infertility, endometriosis and menopause. These gynecologic conditions have structural, hormonal and psychological components, each of which can be treated effectively through botanical prescribing.

My clinical experience began with seven years of practice as a registered nurse. That provided the physiological training and exposure to a wide variety of patients with demonstrable pathology. I became disillusioned with the lack of healing in Western medicine so I dropped out for a while and studied alternative approaches.

After studying herbal medicine with a number of teachers, including Western, Chinese and Native Americans, I embarked upon a clinical practice of lay herbalism in 1973. Approximately two-thirds of my patients were women and a good percentage of those had gynecological complaints. Like any alternative practitioner, many of my patients sought my help because they were not satisfied with the treatments recommended by allopaths. I had enough success to consistently expand my practice each year.

I entered naturopathic medical school because I wanted to be able to explain why I was so successful as an herbal practitioner. I have certainly

*Presented at American Association of Naturopathic Physicians Convention, November 3, 1989

expanded my scope of practice, and refined my knowledge since that time. Yet, the foundation of my patient care still appears to be empirical and based on a deep appreciation of natural science. I have documented the majority of this presentation with current research and noted carefully when it could not be found. I can see that the greatest benefit is derived from the marriage of pharmacological analysis and clinical results. Each can point the direction for the other to follow, i.e., clinical experience can provide the wisest pharmacological hypothesis to explore while analysis of research can open new directions for successful clinical practice.

I have found that the best results in treating all chronic gynecological conditions are obtained when the follicular and luteal phases of the menstrual cycle are addressed. These are often simply called estrogenic and progesteronic formulas. I would like to clarify this approach by specifically addressing both infertility and endometriosis, as these two conditions are less frequently discussed by clinicians. These same standard formulas can be adapted to the treatment of other problems such as ovarian cysts, fibroids, menorrhagia, and metrorrhagia, by substituting other specific botanicals. I would like to discuss why each herb is added to the protocols for infertility, endometriosis and also menopause, to serve as a foundation upon which other individualized formulas can be developed.

Over the years, I have treated a number of women for infertility, but due to inconsistent compliance or followup I can only verify four cases of women who were infertile or chronic aborters who believe their healthy children were a result of my program. My approach is founded upon more than a decade's worth of observation of clinical outcome, and I believe this deserves wider exposure and trials.

Of the nine patients who got significant symptom relief with their endometriosis, three had confirmatory diagnoses with laparoscopy and four more had probable endometriosis found on ultrasound. Many others without confirmed diagnoses felt better and had decreased dysmenorrhea, premenstrual symptoms, ovarian pain and dypareunia. None of the patients had followup laparoscopies to determine that their transplanted tissue had disappeared or even diminished in size. Yet, the improved quality of life so many experienced needs to be passed on.

It is difficult to say how many menopausal women have obtained symptom relief under my care. This is a much more frequently encountered condition with a number of approaches that work. Yet, of the practitioners who have studied with me, many use my treatment protocol and report having a great deal of success.

Due to the many modalities used by naturopaths, it appears to me that not many have developed a broad base of understanding of a large number of botanical remedies. I rely more on whole plants than substances extracted from them, e.g., quercetin, catechin, other active constituents, or even vitamins and minerals that are also widely available in good quality botanical medicines. I am not comfortable with giving patients a large number of pills or capsules. Because liquid preparations are already in solution, they are typically easier to absorb. Tinctures and other extractions can be easily compounded, making a complex formula easy for a patient to take. In my practice I rarely use specific protocols, preferring to individualize my prescriptions. But here I have created these protocols for the purpose of sharing my knowledge with practitioners who have less direct experience with botanicals. My clinical experience over fifteen years leads me to believe that they would work synergistically in the formulas and standardized prescriptions facilitate the evaluation of results.

I will explain which botanicals appear to be hormonal balancers, have a more direct effect on the uterus, and other additional herbs which address the multi-leveled nature of these conditions. All of the formulas I present are given in substantial dosage to be sure that the physiological effect is accomplished with the large number of botanicals in each formula. The approach taken, called polypharmacy, is much in the manner of Chinese herbal prescribing, with a number of herbs working together to achieve a desired clinical effect. In order to simplify the prescription, I have recommended that each formula be calculated in parts, and that the total dose be 5 ml T.I.D. (3x a day) for each. The herbs are best absorbed on an empty stomach, and taken throughout the day to maintain blood levels. Therefore, the herbs should be given upon arising, one half hour before or two hours after lunch, and before bed.

INFERTILITY

Here I give two formulas: the estrogenic formula (A) is taken from the onset of menses through ovulation, and then the progesteronic formula (B) is substituted until the onset of the new cycle. While it is best to switch at ovulation, these botanicals contain precursors which do not act like drugs and thus no harm is done if ovulation is not clearly observed and the formulas are changed a few days early or late.

Vitex agnus castus (chaste tree) is found in each formula as it has such a significant hormone balancing effect. It is a Mediterranean shrub of the

Verbenaceae family that was once used to lower libido, as its name implies. It is also known as monk's pepper. More recently, it is described as either enhancing or suppressing sex drive, whatever is appropriate.[1] Current research clarifies its site of action on the diencephalo-hypophyseal system. It causes increased leutinizing hormone (LH) and inhibits the release of follicle stimulating hormone (FSH)[2], the promoting progesterone and the corpus luteum.[3] In balancing this hormonal effect, numerous symptoms including irregular cycles, premenstrual fluid retention, acne, etc. are relieved and fertility is enhanced. It must, however, be taken daily for at least a month and is usually recommended for at least three–six months.

The next herb, *Cimicifuga racemosa* (black cohosh), is a member of the Ranunculaceae family. Current research points to hormonal action, mainly estrogenic, which helps explain many of its traditional uses in gynecological conditions.[4,5] It is also a good spasmolytic and thus relieves dysmenorrhea. It has an excellent reputation in rheumatic complaints, neurologic and muscular pain, and has been shown to have an anti-inflammatory effect.[6] It is considered the specific herb/remedy when musculo-skeletal symptoms accompany gynecological imbalances.

Medicago sativa (alfalfa), a member of the Leguminoseae family, contains phytoestrogens[7] which can act either as an estrogen enhancer or balancer when there is too much production, by competition with estrogen for binding sites. When estrogen levels are low, they exert some estrogenic activity and if there is too much estrogen, they occupy estrogen receptor sites and thereby reduce overall estrogenic activity.[8,9] In a laboratory experiment where rats where fed massive doses of estradiol, those that were concurrently fed *Medicago* were protected from ovarian inhibition.[10] *Medicago sativa* also acts as a restorative tonic and blood builder because it is high in vitamins A, C, riboflavin and niacin, protein and chlorophyll, while also containing folic acid, biotin and flavonoids.[11-15]

Chamaelirium luteum (false unicorn root), previously called *Helonias dioica*, is a member of the Liliaceae family. It is tonic and strengthening to the reproductive tract.[16,17] It contains steroidal saponins that are primarily estrogenic[18], but also acts amphoterically, when menstrual cycles are irregular. A specific, along with *Vibernum prunifolium* for threatened abortion[16], it is also helpful when there is digestive or liver deficiency.[19]

Glycyrrhiza glabra (licorice root), a well recognized phytoestrogen[18,20], is a member of the Leguminaceae family and is another amphoteric (acts in both directions) like *Medicago sativa* on estrogen metabolism. When estrogen levels are high, it inhibits is action, and when estrogen is deficient, its activity is potentiated.[21] In a recent Japanese study, it was shown to induce normal ovulation in hyper-androgenic and oligomenorrheic women.[22] While its pseudoaldosterone activity is well documented[23], in a mixed botanical formula, used only in the first half of the menstrual month, it rarely causes fluid retention (I have never seen a case of increased blood pressure) and can usually be included in full or half dosage. It can, however, be left out of the formula in isolated cases where fluid retention is a persistent problem, though I personally have not seen a case where this small dose was contraindicated. When it is used, the additional benefits include cortisol-like anti-inflammatory, immunostimulatory and antihepatotoxic effects, via inhibition of the breakdown of cortisol in the liver.[24]

Leonurus cardiaca (motherwort), a labiatae, is specifically indicated when uterine pain or atony is associated with anxiety and tension. Its genus name—*cardiaca*—reminds us of its use in palpitations that are associated with anxiety, rather than founded in an organic cause. Laboratory experiments have demonstrated hypotensive, antispasmodic and sedative effects.[25] In addition to its uterine spasmolytic effect, like so many plant remedies that act in both directions and therefore have a balanced effect clinically, *L. cardiaca* has also been shown to have a very slight stimulating effect on the uterus and intestines.[26] As a relaxing emmenagogue, it is recommended for afterpains[19] and is a good galactagogue. One can see how it was bestowed its common name, motherwort.

Taraxacum officinalis radix (dandelion root) and/or *Berberis aquifolium* (Oregon grape root) is added to assist the liver in both its hormone metabolizing and eliminative function. Taraxacum is both nutritive[27] and choleretic, and therefore cleansing[28-30], while Berberis has a more stimulating effect on the hepatobiliary system.[1,17] Because Berberis can also be a uterine stimulant[20], it is left out of the progesteronic formula to prevent disruption of implantation of the potentially fertilized ovum.

Angelica sinsensis, the Chinese herb tang kuei (dong quai) has been applied for all female reproductive imbalances and now has a large body of literature to substantiate its benefits in infertility[31] and other female problems[32]. Hormonally, it is primarily estrogenic, so it is included in the follicular phase, but is best left out of the primary formula and then added to the formula from the end of menses until ovulation. When used during menstrual bleeding, it can increase the blood loss, so it needs to be used with care during menses until the practitioner knows how to carefully evaluate its effects. When it is added after menstrual bleeding is complete, it will tonify and, as the Chinese say, replace what has been lost in the menstrual blood. *Angelica acutiloba* (the Japanese species) has been demonstrated to cause an initial increase in uterine contraction followed by relaxation.[33,34] Thus, the reported emmenagogic and uterine tonifying effects are both present, which sheds light on the seemingly contradictory actions as abortifacient *and* tonic during pregnancy (often prescribed in the first trimester).

Several *Angelica* species have been demonstrated to relax smooth muscles throughout the body and so perhaps this is an explanation for its hypotensive (vascular smooth muscle), bronchial and intestinal spasmolytic effects in addition to its uterine antispasmodic effects.[33,34] Also, current research has demonstrated anti-allergic[35,36], immune enhancing anti-tumor[37] and some antibacterial effects of several species.[33]

While the European *Angelica archangelica* has been used primarily for its digestive and respiratory benefits[1], many native perennial woodland species of *Angelica* can be substituted for *A. sinensis*. Roots appear to increase their hormonal potency the longer they remain in the ground (i.e., the reverence for old *Panax* —ginseng roots). The European species is *A. archangelica*, a biennial, which only persists for 2 years instead of 3–30 years and therefore does not have as dynamic a hormonal effect.

Punica granatum (pomegranate seeds), from a fruit that is widely available in the autumn, are an ancient symbol of fertility. Recent investigation has revealed that they contain estrone[38], identical with the hormone. Heftmann et al measured 1.7 mg estrone per 100 g pomegranate seeds, which are thus an excellent source of plant estrone.[39] Here we have an opportunity to literally make medicine of our food.

After ovulation, the formulas are changed, but the same dose (5 ml T.I.D.) of the new progesteronic formula (B) is taken during the luteal phase, until the onset of menses.

Once again *Vitex agnus castus* is given and often in a higher dose than during the follicular phase. Then *Dioscorea* spp. (wild yam) is added, as it contains progesterone precursors (diosgenin and pregnenolone)[40], and is therefore the basis of contraceptive and steroidal hormone manufacture. It has the added benefit of being a spasmolytic and has been successfully employed in treating dysmenorrhea, ovarian neuralgia and afterpains.[1] Its anti-inflammatory effect is probably a combination of hormonal precursors to cortisone and beneficial effects on the liver[40].

Smilax ornata and *S. officinalis* (sarsaparilla) are members of the Liliaceae family. In this formula, it is necessary to use those species which grow in a tropical climate, not the ones from the Southeastern United

States as they are not considered strong enough. It is included in the progesteronic formula, as it also contains hormonal precursors. Its reputation as an alterative in rheumatic and skin conditions is probably in part associated with its ability to bind endotoxins in the gut, thus reducing the metabolic stress on the eliminative organs.[21] In China, other species are used in mercury poisoning and acute bacterial dysentery. In primary syphilis it is reportedly 90% effective (negative blood tests).[20]

Verbena officinalis (vervain) and other *Verbena* species have primarily been considered nerve remedies for relaxing tension, depression and stress[17], especially when due to some illness.[41] They are also smooth muscle relaxants with a slight favor for the uterus[42] and thus are specific for chronic uterine problems related to stress. The addition of a gentle hepatic stimulant rounds *Verbena* out to be an important addition to an infertility formula, especially in the premenstrual phase.

Eleuthrococcus senticosus (Siberian ginseng), is a member of the Araliaceae family and has been extensively tested in Russia for its excellent adaptogenic or non-specific immune enhancing effects.[43] As it helps the body to deal with stress on a cellular level, it has a broad range of applicability including preventing viral illness, improving performance and improving health during physiologic, climatic and pathological stress.[44] It is included here as the premenstrual phase more often requires this additional assistance, but it can be included in all parts of these protocols. Because *Eleuthrococcus* is suspected of working on the hypothalamus[44] and as a regulator of hormone release, it is specifically helpful in reproductive health.[45]

Alchemilla vulgaris (lady's mantle) is a much touted remedy in Europe, especially for female reproductive problems and revered by the alchemists for its ability to crystalize light in the dew upon its round leaves. Despite its reputation as a progesteronic herb that assists in balancing hormones[45], I could find no hard research supporting this fact. Like all members of the Rosaceae family, it contains tannins and it appears that its clearly documented uses can be attributed to its astringent and antihemorrhagic effect. In the treatment of 341 young women, ages eleven to seventeen with meno-metrorrhagia, it demonstrated an antihemorrhagic effect within three to five days. Given ten to fifteen days before the menstrual cycle, it showed a prophylactic effect and was considered effective orally and non-toxic.[46] It is reported to contain salicylates and to increase circulation to the reproductive area.[42] This herb clearly warrants further investigation to see if its reputation can be borne out in both laboratory research and clinical practice.

Mitchella repens (partridge berry squaw vine) is a Rubiaceae which is native to Southeast America. It was much revered as a woman's remedy among the Native Americans and was eagerly adopted into prominent and respected clinical use among botanical practitioners including the Eclectics. An important ingredient in "Mother's Cordial" (an old respected woman's formula consisting of *Mitchella, Helonias, Vibernum opulus,* and *Caulophyllium*), *Mitchella* is considered specific for pregnancy preparation, maintenance and successful outcome.[41]

It is reported to be a regulator in uterine and ovarian dysfunction, increasing circulation, allaying congestion and irritation of the organs, and relaxing the nervous system.[19] In addition, it is a diuretic and has been used topically on the nipples of nursing mothers.[16] Here is an American herb, greatly respected and widely used with consistently reported favorable results. It is included here because my own experience in clinical practice has usually confirmed traditional claims. While this plant apparently has not been seriously investigated in the laboratory, it is clearly a good candidate for thorough research. It is also important not to wait until technological documentation substantiates many years of clinical success.

Vibernum prunifolium (black haw bark) and *Vibernum opulus* (cramp bark) are often used interchangeably, but *V. prunifolium* is considered more specific for the female reproductive tract, while *V. opulus* has a more generalized effect. Both are members of the Caprifoliaceae family and I suspect that a variety of different species of *Vibernums* are sold as *V. prunifolium* or *V. opulus* because the collectors did not know taxonomic differences. Their long tradition as antispasmodics have now been demonstrated in the laboratory, most notably on the uterus itself[47], and they are hypotensive and relaxing upon myocardial contractibility.[48] Thus, we can explain its use in dysmenorrhea, and perhaps understand why it has been considered specific in threatened abortion. In addition, it is considered appropriate for a variety of spastic conditions, including that of the fallopian tubes, and perhaps, thereby facilitates conception when hypertonicity is a complicating factor.

Taraxacum officinalis (dandelion) is a Compositae of universal recognition. While its root (radix) is widely used in all conditions that are benefited by its hepatobiliary choleretic and liver trophorestorative effects[27-29], I specifically recommend using its leaf (herba) here. An effective diuretic[49,50], it is important in a variety of premenstrual imbalances. *Taraxacum* herba is not only superior to all other herbal remedies to which it has been compared, it has also been found to be comparable to the commonly used synthetic drug, Furosemide (Lasix).[4] In addition, the usual problem of potassium depletion associated with diuretic use is more than avoided. *Taraxacum* herba is actually a potassium supplement, containing 4.25% potassium.[49,50]

Silybum marianum semen (milk thistle seeds), a Compositae, has a profound effect on the liver in detoxification and overall protection.[51] I prefer to have patients add them to food, 1 tablespoon per day, soaked and ground, for at least three weeks out of the month.

ENDOMETRIOSIS

This protocol requires the use of three formulae: (A), during menses for symptom relief and estrogen balancing; (B), an estrogenic formula similar to that used for infertility, for the duration of the follicular phase; and (C), a progesteronic formula, also similar to that used for infertility, to be used during the luteal phase. Again, all formulae are given in the dose of 5 ml T.I.D. and the formula during menses can be given at more frequent intervals.

The protocol must be followed for at least six months or longer as there is usually a fair amount of adhesions, circulatory stasis and hormonal imbalance to counteract. I usually tell patients that they shouldn't expect noticeable changes before three months, yet in all but one case, there was significant symptom relief in just one month.

The basic goal of the entire treatment is to increase circulation in the pelvis, thereby promoting drainage, discouraging adhesions and facilitating removal of metabolites that promote the inflammation. In addition, hormonal balance is re-established, thereby decreasing premenstrual syndrome, menorrhagia and metrorrhagia. This is accomplished via the use of hormonal precursors and balancers, but also by improving liver function and thereby facilitating the inactivation of hormones. Almost always, digestive function is implicated, with constipation the most common symptom, but occasionally constipation alternating with diarrhea is reported. Many of the herbs directed at the reproductive system also have a beneficial effect on the liver and on digestion (i.e., *Chamaelirium, Glycyrrhiza, Cimicifuga, Angelica, Leonurus, Verbena, Dioscosea* and *Smilax*). *Taraxacum* and *Berberis aquifolium* are again added and have specific benefit in stimulating the liver and digestive processes.

The result is usually symptom relief as a result of treating the underlying cause. Patients consistently report a marked decrease in dysmenorrhea, dyspareunia, digestive symptoms, menorrhagia, ovulation pain, along with an improvement in mental outlook and decrease of lassitude to varying degrees. Of the six patients treated over months, only one remained on oral contraceptives and she reported that she was still afraid to completely abandon Western medicine because of many years of working as a pharmacist.

I will once again explain the inclusion of each herb in the protocols, but this time only discuss those that are not previously mentioned, unless they have another property that makes them specifically applicable in endometriosis.

The first formula (A) is taken from the onset of menses until its completion. It assists in relieving dysmenorrhea while balancing estrogen, improving circulation and relaxing the pelvic organs.

Anemone pulsatilla (pulsatilla or pasque flower), a member of the Ranunculaceae family, is an herb that is currently more familiar to homeopathic practitioners as its species name *Pulsatilla*. In a study of homeopathic *Pulsatilla*, it was shown to exhibit progesterone-like properties.[52] It had broad clinical use among the Eclectics[16,19,41] and in England, among the members of the National Institute of Medical Herbalists, it is regarded as the most specific pelvic anodyne.[53] In a paper presenting a therapeutic approach to endometriosis, Janet Hicks, MNIMH describes *Anemone* as both stimulating and relaxing to pelvic organs when added to a constitutional formula, but also, when given separately for quick relief of pain. Most of its indications are related to nervous tension in the reproductive system, with depression and irritability often associated. The Eclectic materia medica read almost like the homeopathic ones, with indications like "easily inclined to weep and mind wanders," while adding "faulty nutrition of the nerve centers."

It must be noted that lower dosage is often effective (thus 1/2–1 part) and while gastrointestinal irritation is noted in the texts, I have not seen a case. It is so often helpful in the dysmenorrhea and ovarian pain associated with endometriosis that if gastrointestinal irritation does occur, it should be separated out of the formula and given with meals to prevent this side effect.

Achillea millefolium (yarrow), a Compositae, has a long and much praised reputation in a variety of conditions due to its being anti-inflammatory[54,55], a digestive stimulant and carminative[56], choleretic[57] and spasmolytic.[58,59] In the old herbal tradition, I have called it a balanced and amphoterically-acting emmenagogue because of both the laboratory research finding thujone[56], a known uterine stimulant, along with its antispasmodic properties. In addition, it is an active hemostatic agent[60] and a tonic to the arterioles and venules[56], so we can understand its use in

Europe for angina pectoris and varicosities. All these complementary actions make it an ideal female reproductive balancer for menstrual regulation as it will both stimulate and relax the uterus in deficient or excess flow, facilitate digestive and liver function to metabolize estrogens, reduce inflammation and relieve uterine spasms or increase tonus, thereby assisting in analgesic effect, while actively treating the pathological state.

Humulus lupulus (hops), a member of the Moraceae family, is primarily used as a mild sedative with sleep problems, and, most specifically, to allay male sexual excitement.[2] It was noted before hops were picked mechanically that young women picking the strobuli had early menstrual periods. We have now verified the presence of a substance that has active estrogenic activity[61], and further research is being done in hopes of finding other hormonal substances, perhaps anti-androgenic. Hops also acts as a digestive bitter tonic, resulting in overall improved digestion, assimilation and circulation to the entire abdomen.[41,42] In addition, they have mild anodyne properties. Thus, the hormonal properties are specific for the follicular (estrogenic) phase; the balanced discharge of menses is promoted via enhanced assimilation and circulation, and the mild sedative and anodyne properties help to relieve dysmenorrhea. Thus, we can see how this herb aids the entire constitution, while also helping to relieve the symptoms.

Vitex agnus castus is included here as it is best taken daily for several months to achieve its pituitary hormonal balancing effect. *Chamaelirium luteum* is added because it is reported to relieve pain, while tonifying structure and facilitating hormone balance. *Vibernum prunifolium* is an important spasmolytic, and *Cimicifuga racemosa* is both antispasmodic, anti-inflammatory and hormone-balancing. Both *Leonurus cardiaca* and *Verbena officinalis* are added here because they are useful in allaying the anxiety and tension that is often associated with painful menses and each also acts specifically on the reproductive organs.

Valeriana sitchensis or *V. officinalis* (valerian), while not specific to the reproductive tract, is such a reliable remedy whenever there is anxiety, stress or pain[42], that I have also included it here. I have never encountered a case of endometriosis in someone who is not under a good deal of stress, but if that were the case, this botanical is the least important in the formula. Aside from being a specific for nervous tension, it is a good antispasmodic[62], but so many of the herbs in this formula are also spasmolytic that it is primarily included for its benefit in mental stress.[42] In addition, *Valeriana* is hypotensive[63] which is helpful in certain cases. It is anti-inflammatory[62] and slightly anaesthetic[64], which enhances its benefit in all endometriosis cases.

All the research I could find was on *V. officinalis*. I have found the local Northwest species, *V. sitchensis* to be even stronger. It has been noted in M. Grieve's "A Modern Herbal," that the Russians also consider *V. sitchensis* to be the most potent medicinally[65], but I could not find this direct reference. Formula (B), taken from the end of menses through ovulation, is the same as that given in infertility, with the addition of *Leonurus cardiaca* and *Anemone pulsatilla* as they both assist with the emotional component and pain that can also occur during ovulation in cases of endometriosis.

Borago officinalis succus (fresh borage juice), is added to both estrogenic and progesteronic formulas, primarily for its nutritive functions. It is generally recognized that the *Borago* semen (seeds) are high in gamma linolenic acid[66] and therefore anti-inflammatory. The leaves of the Boraginaceae also contain this acid[67], and therefore the flowering tops, including leaves and seeds, are likely a good source. Succus or fresh juice is the best way to take a plant that is generally nutritive as you are getting a lot more than its oils and active constituents.

Borago has been considered a hormonally active plant, most often described as an adrenal restorative. David Hoffmann suggests using it for an adrenal tonic for stress and to renew the glands after steroid treatments.[1] Early herbals describe its use in dispelling melancholy, gladdening the heart and promoting courage.[65] I have heard its heart tonic properties attributed to its high content of calcium and potassium. It also has been recommended as a galactagogue.[1]

I could not find any specific article documenting its adrenal restorative reputation. Perhaps someone can lead me in the right direction. However, in 1955, an endocrinological research group did find it hormonally active. The results of an experiment in attempting to inactivate pituitary hormones disclosed *Borago*'s significant antigonadotropic activity.[68] Since many phytoestrogens also have demonstrated antihormonal activity, and the actual hormones provide feedback to inactivate their pituitary tropic hormones, I surmise that we are at the beginning of a potentially productive search. In any event, *Borago* succus has demonstrated its effectiveness clinically and I await the definitive research project to explain why.

Once again, we switch to a reportedly progesteronic formula after ovulation, with the same dosing schedule as described previously. The formula is the same as the luteal formula for infertility. The two differences here are that *Leonurus cardiaca* is added and *Mitchella repens* deleted, and *Berberis aquifolium* is always included, while it is optional in the infertility formula. *Leonurus cardiaca* replaces *Mitchella* because of its more marked effect on the nervous system (Weiss states on the autonomic nervous system).[2] *Mitchella* has a stronger reputation in preparing the uterus for pregnancy.

Berberis aquifolium is required here due to almost consistent liver and digestive atonicity associated with endometriosis. *Anemone pulsatilla* can also be added here for its pelvic decongestant and anodyne properties.

MENOPAUSE

After female monthly cycling is completed, hormonal enhancement can be encouraged with one formula taken throughout the month. While I often give substantial physiologically active doses of botanicals, the recommended dose here varies from 3–5 ml, again T.I.D., spaced throughout the day on an empty stomach. This is because menopause is not pathological and there is a wider variation of patients wishing assistance with menopausal complaints. Some are more sensitive to botanical substances and therefore require a smaller dose.

Many conditions occur concomitant with menopause and each person can benefit most from an individualized prescription. I offer my menopausal protocol because it has been so successful in relieving many of the discomforts associated with this transition. I so often hear of patients who just return to refill their prescription because they are so satisfied with the results of taking this formula.

Several of the herbs which were previously discussed are repeated and I will mention their specific applications in menopause. Then I will discuss the two herbs not found in previous formulae.

Vitex agnus castus is used here again for its hormone balancing effect, *Leonurus cardiaca* for its assistance in anxiety, *Chamaelirium luteum* for hormonal and digestive benefit, and *Angelica sinensis*, *Glycyrrhiza glabra*, and *Medicago sativa* all for estrogen enhancement. *Vibernum prunifolium* is included as it allays spasticity which can promote hot flashes. *Cimicifuga racemosa* is a spasmolytic and estrogen enhancer. In a recent clinical study, sixty patients reporting climacteric symptoms after hysterectomy, were divided into four groups using either a type of estrogen replacement or an extract of *Cimicifuga racemosa*. Therapy was controlled using serum FSH and LH measurements and the gonadotropins in all groups decreased similarly. In addition, the group on *Cimicifuga* had the same therapeutic success as that of the groups on synthetic hormones.[69]

Salvia officinalis (garden sage), is a Labiateae and must always be differentiated from *Artemesias* (of the Compositae family) which are also commonly called sage. I suggest calling *Artemesias*, sagebrush, to avoid confusion. One important effect of *Salvia* is that it will decrease secretions[70], which has given this herb a reputation for stopping the flow of mother's milk.[70,71] This same property makes it specific for decreasing sweat[17] and thus helps to diminish hot flashes. It was reported in early journal research (1939) to contain 6,000 I.U. of estrogenic substance[71], thus making it doubly useful in menopause. This estrogenic effect might be the basis of its Eclectic use in spermatorrhea and as a general antiaphrodesiac.[41] *Salvia* extracts also have strong antioxidant properties.[20] They have been employed to preserve meats and suppress the odor of fish, and we can see their clinical application both in preventing and in treating specific conditions associated with aging.

Salvia, like all culinary herbs, is carminative and antispasmodic and stimulates the production of digestive fluids.[41,20,15] Here again, where digestion and assimilation is facilitated, almost all pathology improves and thus another reason for its inclusion in this formula. In addition, its volatile oil is antimicrobial and it contains a high concentration of zinc (5.9mg/100 gm).[15]

Hypericum perforatum (St. John's wort) and most other wild *Hypericum* species (but not the cultivated ground cover of the family, Hypericaeae) has had a long reputation in herbal and homeopathic use. It has come into the limelight recently because of its strong anti-retroviral activity.[72]

Its inclusion in this formula is primarily for two reasons. The first is its well documented and clinically proven antidepressive effect.[73,74] This is now thought to be a result of its function as a MAO inhibitor.[75] The best results are obtained when the herb is used for two–three months, though some effects can be seen in a few weeks. While not normally used for endogenous depression, it is considered effective for lightening moods and producing some euphoria.[2] I would like to point out that it is recognized in England that the mention in the British Herbal Pharmacopoeia (1983) of *Hypericum* being contraindicated in depressive states is an error that will be changed in the next edition.[42]

The second reason for its inclusion here is both empirical and hard to explain or document. *Hypericum* appears to benefit a variety of chronic pelvic conditions, especially those with a nervous component. Its reputation in the treatment of enuresis in Europe[2] and in the suppression of urine and chronic urinary infections points in this direction.[41] I see it as specifically applicable in many chronic female reproductive conditions and would like to quote Gibson from his homeopathic studies describing "a tight sensation felt in the pelvis," or in cases of delayed menses.[76] Its Eclectic recommendation for spinal cord injury or irritation is perhaps also related.[7] In the British Herbal Pharmacopoeia of 1983, the only specific indication of *Hypericum* is "menopausal neurosis."[17]

It's a well known homeopathic and herbal indication as the 'Arnica of the nerves'[41], and is worth mentioning here, especially in light of new research showing strong antiviral activity against HIV 1 and HIV 2, influenza and other viruses[77] and also EBV.[78] So we should use *Hypericum* in these commonly seen viruses and now have documentation of benefits that were alluded to long ago. In addition to antiviral effect, *Hypericum* has also shown antimicrobial activity against a broad spectrum of Gram-negative and Gram-positive bacteria.[79] The flurry of recent interest in *Hypericum perforatum* also revealed that its oil extract inhibits the growth of tumors and increases the body weight in rats.[80]

So we can see the potential for our time-honored gentle and effective herbal remedies of the past now standing up to current laboratory evaluation and testing. I see this as just another reminder to adhere to our empirical traditions and to trust the botanicals that have been widely used and respected over time. We don't need to make the same mistake the allopaths have made in revering our laboratory results more than our traditions. And yet, it is refreshing to find again the marriage of these apparently divergent and actually polar approaches to evaluation of true healing.

In ending with *Hypericum*, a famous old herbal remedy which is also becoming widely sought-after today for treatment of AIDS, herpes and EBV, you have a good model for my personal philosophy of planetary unity and hope. Not only has its traditional use been borne out in the laboratory of contemporary science, but its application is both clearly definable and also quite etheric. I believe that when we live closely to the cycles of nature as do all traditional cultures and observe with intense scrutiny her workings, then the secrets will be revealed. It doesn't matter if we look from a purely analytical Western scientific mind or a harmonious, intuitive, insightful, and empowered nature. The wisdom of the universe is available to us who seek it wholly.

I offer this paper as one small part of my personal study towards this end. I see the plant medicines as teachers and healers. I hope you will try these protocols in your clinical practice and report back to me your results.

INFERTILITY PROTOCOL

Both formulas are given as 5 ml T.I.D. (upon arising, 1/2 hr ac or 2 hr pc lunch and H.S.)

A. *Menses through ovulation (estrogenic) formula*
1 *Vitex agnus castus*
1–2 *Cimicifuga racemosa*
1-2 *Medicago sativa*
1 *Chamaelirium luteum* (= *Helonias dioica*)
1 *Glycyrrhiza glabra* (or 1/2 pt. in women who retain fluid readily—not just premenstrually)
1 *Leonurus cardiaca*
1 *Taraxacum officinalis radix* (add *Berberis aquifolium* when sluggish liver and/or digestive function is concomitant)

Angelica sinensis 1 ml T. I. D. is added to formula from end of menses through ovulation
Punica granatum semen (ad lib when available)

B. *Ovulation through menses (progesteronic) formula*
2 *Vitex agnus castus*
1 Dioscorea villosa or other *Dioscorea* spp.
1 *Smilax ornata*
1 *Verbena officinalis*
1 *eleutherococcus senticosus*
1 *Alchemilla vulgaris*
1 *Mitchella repens*
1 *Vibernum prunifolium*
2 *Taraxacum officinalis herba*

Silybum marianum semen (1 Tbl., soaked and ground, added to food for at least 3 weeks out of the month, whenever liver trophoestoration appropriate)

ENDOMETRIOSIS PROTOCOL

All 3 formulas are given as 5 ml. T.I.D. and the first formula A. can be given at more frequent intervals

A. *Day 1 through end of menses—formula for symptom relief and estrogen balancing*
1/2–1 *Anemone pulsatilla*
1 *Achillea millefolium*
1/2-1 *Humulus lupus*
1 *Vitex agnus castus*
1 *Chamaelirium luteum* (= *Helonias dioica*)
1 *Vibernum prunifolium*
1 *Cimicifuga racemosa*
1 *Leonurus cardiaca*
1 *Verena officinalis*
1 *Valeriana sitchensis* or *V. officinalis*

B. *End of menses through ovulation (estrogenic) formula*
1 *Vitex agnus castus*
1–2 *Cimicifuga racemosa*
1 *Medicago sativa*
1 *Chamaelirium luteum* (= *Helonias dioica*)
1 *Glycyrrhiza glabra* (or 1/2 pt. in women who retain fluid readily)
1–2 *Angelica sinensis*
1 *Leonurus cardiaca*
1 *Taraxacum officinalis radix*
1 *Berberis aquifolium*
Can add 1/2 *Anemone pulsatilla*
1 *Borago officinalis succus*

C. *Ovulation through menses (progesteronic) formula*
1 *Vitex agnus castus*
1 *Dioscorea villosa* or other *D.* spp.
1 *Smilax ornata*
1 *Verbena officinalis*
1–2 *Eleuthrococcus senticosus*
1 *Alchemilla vulgaris*
1 *Vibernum prunifolium*
2 *Taraxacum officinalis herba*
1/2–1 *Berberis aquifolium*

1 *Leonurus cardiaca*
Can add 1/2 *Anemone pulsatilla*
1 *Borago officinalis succus*

Silybum marianum semen (1 Tbl., soaked and ground, added to food for at least 3 weeks out of the month)

MENOPAUSE PROTOCOL

Formula given as 3–5 ml T.I.D. (upon arising, 1/2 hr ac or 2 hr pc lunch and H.S.)

2 *Vitex agnus castus*
1 *Leonurus cardiaca*
1 *Chamaelirium luteum* (= *Helonia dioica*)
1 *Angelica sinensis*
1–2 *Salvia officinalis*
1 *Hypericum perforatum*
1–2 *Cimicifuga racemosa*
1/2–1 *Glycyrrhiza glabra*
1/2–1 *Vibernum prunifolium*
1/2–1 *Medicago sativa*
Can add:
Taraxacum officinalis herba or radix
Berberis aquifolium
Silybum marianum semen (1 tbl./day)
Punica granatum semen (ad lib when available)

REFERENCES

1. Hoffmann, D. *The Holistic Herbal.* Dorset, England: Element Books. 1988.

2. Weiss, R. F. *Herbal Medicine.* Translated from the 6th German edition. England: Beaconsfield Pub. 1988.

3. De Capite, L. Histology, Anatomy and Antibiotic Properties of Vitex Agnus Castus." Ann Fac Agr Univ Studi Perugia 1967;22:109–26.

4. Jarry, H., Harnischfeger, G., Duker, E. Untersuchungen zur endokrinen wirksamdeit von inhaltssoffen aus Cimicifuga racemosa. Planta Medica 1985 (Aug.);(4):316–319.

5. Jarry, H., Harnischfeger, G., Duker, E. Untersuchungen zur endokrinen wirksamdeit von inhaltssoffen aus Cimicifuga racemosa. Planta Medica 1984 (Oct.);45–49.

6. Benoit, P. S., Fong, H. H. S., Svoboda, G. H., Farnsworth, N. R. Biological

and phytochemical evaluation of plants. XIV. Anti-inflammatory evaluation of 163 species of plant. Lloydia 1976;39(2–3):160–161.

7. Verdeal, K., Ryan, D. Naturally occurring estrogens in plant foodstuffs. A review. J Food Protection 1979;42(7):577–83.

8. Shemesh, M., Lindner, H. R., Ayalon, N. Affinity of rabbit uterine oestradiol receptor for phyto-estrogens and its use in competitive protein-binding radioassay for plasma coumestrol. J Reprod Fert 1972;29:1–9.

9. Martin, P., Horowitz, K., Ryan, D., McGuire, W. Phytoestrogen interaction with estrogen receptors in human breast cancer cells. Endocrinol 1979: p. 1560–66.

10. Ershoff, R. H., Hernandez, H. J., Matthews, J. H. Beneficial effects of alfalfa on the ovarian development of immature rats fed massive doses of alpha-estradiol. J Nutrition 1959;147–54.

11. Allen, O. N., Allen, E. K. *The Leguminoseae.* Madison, Wisconsin: University of Wisconsin Press. 1981: p. 424.

12. Hansen, C. (ed). *Alfalfa Science and Technology.* Madison, Wisconsin: American Society of Agrimony, Inc. 1972: pp. 1, 5, 6, 247–59, 253–77.

13. Lapedes, D. (ed). *Food, Agriculture and Nutrition.* New York: McGraw-Hill. p. 91.

14. *MADIS Manual.* New Jersey: Dr. Madis Laboratories, Inc. 1983: p. 19.

15. Pedersen, M. *Nutritional Herbology.* Bountiful, Utah: Pedersen Pub. 1987: pp. 70–74, 225–29.

16. Felter, H. W. *The Eclectic Materia Medica, Pharmacology and Therapeutics.* Reprint by Eclectic Medical Pub., Portland, OR. 1983 of original 1922 edition.

17. British Herbal Pharmacopoeia. British Medical Association Scientific Committee. 1983.

18. Costello, C. H., Lynn, E. V. Estrogenic substances from plants. I. Glycyrrhiza. J Am Pharm Soc 1950;39:177–80.

19. Ellingwood, F. *American Materia Medica, Therapeutics and Pharmacognosy,* 11th ed. Reprint by Eclectic Medical Pub., Portland OR. 1983 of original 1919 edition.

20. Leung, A. *Encyclopedia of Common Natural Ingredients Used in Food, Drugs, and Cosmetics.* New York: John Wiley & Sons. 1980: pp. 290–91, 294.

21. Pizzorno, J., Murray, M. *A Textbook of Natural Medicine.* Seattle: John Bastyr College Pub. 1985.

22. Yaginuma, T., Izumi, R., Yasui, H., Arai, T., Kawabata, M. Effect of traditional herbal medicine on serum testosterone levels and induction of regular ovulation in hyper-androgenic, and oligomenorrheic women. Nippon Sanka Fujinka Gakkai Zasshi 1983;34(7):939–944.

23. Epstein, M., Espiner, E., Donald, R., Hughes, H. Effects of eating licorice on the renin-angiotensin aldosterone axis in normal subjects. Br Med J 1977;1:488–90.

24. Kumagai, A., Nishino, K., Shimomura, A., Kin, T., Yamumura, Y. Effect of glycyrrhizin on estrogen action. Endocrinol Japan 1967;14(1):34–38.

25. Isaev, L, Bojadzieva, M. Obtaining galenic and neogalenic preparations and experiments on the isolation of active substances from Leonurus cardiaca. Nauchni Tr Visshiya Med Inst Sofiya 1960;37(5)145–52.

26. Erspamer, L. V. Pharmacology of Leonurus cardiaca and Leonurus

marrubiastrum L. Arch Intern Pharmacodynamie 1948;76:132–52.

27. Hyde, F. F. *New Herbal Practitioner*. 1975;1:76.

28. Benign, R., et al. *Planta Medica* (In Ver Dell. Beffa) 1964;2:1593.

29. Coicu, E., Racz, G. *Planta Medica* (Bucuresti 55i)1962.

30. Bohm, F., Schwabe, W., Karlsruhe. *Choleretic action of* some medicinal plants. Arzneimittel-Forsch 1959;9:376–78.

31. Luolan, Z. Observation on the results of treatment of female infertility in 343 cases. J Tradit Chin Med 1986;6(3):175–77.

32. Zhiping, H., Dazeng, W., Lingyi, S., Zuqian, W. Treating amenorrhea in vital energy-deficient patients with Angelica sinensis—Astragalus membranaceus menstruation-regulating decoction. J Trad Chin Med 1986;6(3):187–90.

33. Yoshiro, K. The physiological actions of Tang-Kuei and Cnidium. Bull Oriental Healing Arts Inst USA 1985;10:269–78.

34. Harada, M. Suzuki, M., Ozaki, Y. Effect of Japanese Angelica root and Peony root in uterine contractions in the rabbit in situ. J Pharm Dyn 1984;7:304–11.

35. Hikino, H. Recent research on oriental medicinal plants. Economic Medical Plant Research 1985;1:53–85.

36. Sung, C. P., Baker, A. P., Holden, D. A. et al. Effects of Angelica polymorpha on reaginic antibody production. J Natural Products 1982;45:398–406.

37. Berkarda, B., Bouffard-Eyuboglu, H., Derman, U. The effects of coumarin derivatives on the immunological system of man. Agents Actions 1983;13:50–52.

38. Moneam, N. M. A., El Sharaky, A. S, Badreldin, M. M. Oestrone content of pomegranate seeds. J Chromotography 1988:438–442.

39. Heftmann, E., Ko, S. T., Bennet, R. D. Naturwissenschaften 1965;52:451.

40. Mowrey. *The Scientific Validation of Herbal Medicine*. pp. 107–115, 151–56.

41. Felter, H. W., Lloyd, J. U. *Kings American Dispensatory*, 18th ed., 3rd revision. 2 volumes. Reprint by Eclectic Medical Pub., Portland, OR. 1983 of original 1898 edition.

42. Zeylstra, H. Notes from lectures at PCNM, JBC, NCNM. San Rafael, Calif. and communications 1982–1989; Director of Education, School of Herbal Medicine of the National Institute of Medical Herbalists, UK.

43. Brekham, I. I., Dardymor, I. V., Bezdetko, G. N., Khasina, E. Molecular aspects in the mechanism of increasing nonspecific resistivity caused by an Eleuthrococcus preparation. 5th International Congress Pharmacy, San Francisco, 1972.

44. Fulder, S. *The Tao of Medicine*. New York: Destiny Books. 1982.

45. Dardymov, I. V. On the gonadotropic effect of Eleuthrococcus glycosides. Lek. Srd. Dal'nego Vostoka 1972;11:60–65.

46. Petcu, P., Andronescu, E., Gheorgheci, V., Cucu-Cabadaief, L, Zsimond, Z. Treatment of juvenile meno-metrorrhagia with Alchemilla vulgaris fluid extract. Clujul Med 1979;52(3);266–70.

47. Jarboe, C. H., Schmidt, C. M., Nicholson, J. A., Zirvi, K. A. Uterine relaxant properties of Viburnum. Nature 1966;212(5064):837.

48. Nicholson, J. A., Darby, T. D., Jarobe, C. H. Viopudial, a hypotensive and smooth muscle antispasmotic from Vibernum opulus (36479). Proc Soc Exp Biol Med 1972;140(2):457–461.

49. Racz-Kotilla, E., et al. The action of Taraxacum offinale extracts on the

body weight and diuresis of laboratory animals. *Planta Medica* 1974;26:212–217.

50. Hyde, F. F. The leaf of Taraxacum officinale. *New Herbal Practitioner*. 1975;1(3):82.

51. Vogel, G. A peculiarity among the flavonoids: Silymarin, a compound active on the liver. *Proceedings of the International Bioflavonoid Symposium*, Munich, 1981: pp. 461–478.

52. Prasad, S., Chandrasekhar, K. Effect of Pulsatilla administered pituitary extracts of ovariectomized donor rats. *Indian J of Exp Biol* 1978;16:289–93.

53. Hicks, J. A therapeutic approach to endometriosis. *New Herbal Practitioner* 1983;10(1):27–31.

54. Sticher, O. Plant mono-di and sesquiterpenoids with pharmacological activity. In: Wagner, H., Wolff, P. (eds). *New Natural Product and Plant Drugs with Pharmacological, Biological, or Therapeutic Activity*. New York: Springer-Verlag. 1977:pp.137–176.

55. Goldberg, A. S., Mueller, E. C., et al. Isolation of the antiinflammatory principles from Achillea millefolium. *J Pharm Sci* 1969;58:939–941.

56. Zeylstra, H. Yarrow. *New Herbal Practitioner*, vol. 11 (no.1). April 1984:pp.46–58.

57. Muller, H. *Planta Medica* 1955;3:39.

58. Hoerhammer, L. Flavone concentration of medicinal plants with regard to their spasmolytic action (Chem Abstr 61:3571d). 21st Congress of Sci. Farm. Conf. Comun. Pisa, 1961:pp.578–588.

59. Tewari, J. P., Srivastava, M. C., Bajpai, J. L. Pharmacologic studies of Achillea millefolium Linn. *Indian J Med Sci* 1974;28(8):331–36.

60. Miller, F. M., Chow, L. M. Alkaloids of Achillea millefolium. Isolation and characterization of Achillleine. *J Am Chem Soc* 1954;76:1353–1354.

61. Kumai, A., Okamoto, R. Extraction of the hormonal substance from Hops. *Toxocol Letters* 1984;21:203–207.

62. Thies, D. W. *Tetrahedron Letters* 1966;11:1155.

63. Arora, R. B., Arora, C. K. Proc. Int. Pharmacol 2 Meeting, Prague, 1963. Oxford: Pergamon Press. pp. 51–60.

64. Hendriks, H., Bos, R., Allersma, D. P., Malingre, T. M., Koster, A. *Planta Medica* 1981;42:62–68.

65. Grieve, M. *A Modern Herbal*. New York: Dover Pub. 1971: pp. 120, 825.

66. Jamieson. *J Sci Food Agric* 1968;19:628–31.

67. Hitchock. *Plant Lipid Biochem* 1971: p.68.

68. Grahm, R., Nobel, R. Comparison of in vitro activity of various species of Lithospermum and other plants to inactivate gonadotrophin. *Endocrinol* 1955;56: 239–47.

69. Lehmann-Willenbrock, E., Riedel, H. H. Clinical and endocrinologic studies of the treatment of ovarian insufficiency manifestations following hysterectomy with intact adenexa. *Zentralbl Gynakol* 1988;110(10):611–18.

70. Moore, M. *Medicinal Plants of the Mountain West*. Museum of New Mexico Press. 1978: pp. 142–43.

71. Kroszcyniski, S., Bychowska, M. *Estrogenic action of sage* (Salvia officinalis). Compt. Rend. Soc. Biol. 1939;130:570–71.

72. Meruelo, D., Laurie, G., Laurie, D. Therapeutic agents with dramatic

antiretroviral activity and little toxicity at effective doses: Aromatic polycyclic diones hypericin and pseudohypericin. Proceedings of the National Academy of Sciences, USA, July, 1988. Vol. 85: pp. 5230–34.

73. Hoffman, J. Therapie von depressiven zustanden mit hypericin (hypericin treatment of depressive states). *Allgemein Med* 1979;55(12): pp. 776–82. ⌐

74. Muldner, H., Zoller, M. Antidepressive effect of a hypericin extract standardized to an active hypericine complex: biochemistry and clinical studies. *Anzneimittelforschung* 1984;34(8):918–20.

75. Suzuki, O., Katasumata, Y., Oya, M., Bladt, S., Wagner, H. Inhibition of monoamine oxidase by hypericin. *Planta Medica* 1984: pp. 272–74.

76. Gibson, D. *Studies of Homeopathic Remedies.* Beaconsfield, England: Beaconsfield Pubs. 1987: p. 251.

77. Laurie, D. Antiviral pharmaceutical compositions containing hypericin and pseudohypericin. European Patent Application #87111467.4 filed 8/8/87. European Patent Office Publication #0256452A2.

78. Someya, H. Effect of a constituent of Hypericum erectum on infection and multiplication of Epstein-Barr virus. *J of Tokyo Med College* 1985;43(5):815–26.

79. Barbagallo, C., Chisari, G. Antimicrobial activity of 3 Hypericum species. *Fitoterapia* 1987;LVIII93):175–77.

80. Valavichyus, Y. M, Ifanauskas, V. P, Yaskonas, Y. A. Antitumor activity of medicinal plants of Lithuania SSR USSR 6. Common St. John's Wort and Chamomilla recutita. Inst. Biochem., Acad Sci. Lith. SSR. Vilnius USSR *Liet Tsr Mokslu Adad Darb Ser C Biol Mokalai* 1986;0(3):110–113.

Herbs and the Mind
DAVID FRAWLEY

All herbs have an affect upon the mind because the body and mind form an integral and interrelated energy system. While the physical effects of herbs are more evident and easier to classify, those on the mind can also be examined, though they may require a different approach. Modern allopathic medicine concentrates on physical symptoms and tends to ignore psychological factors on the part of the patient as being subjective. On the other hand, traditional systems of medicine, including homeopathy, give much weight to psychological or spiritual factors. These may include the emotional condition of the patient or how they respond to circumstances and impressions. Such factors may be decisive in choosing the correct remedy or in determining the ultimate cause of the disease. To reclaim a truly holistic herbal medicine we must again explore the subtle effects of herbs on the mind and create a system for understanding them. Once we have understood how herbs affect the mind, we can use them to treat the mental and emotional imbalances which are often behind the disease process or accompany it. We can also use them to improve our general mental functioning — to promote creativity and intelligence.

While this is a large and complicated subject and requires much study, I hope at least to bring out potentials for further examination. We will base our study mainly on traditional medical systems, particularly the Ayurvedic medicine of India and the Traditional Chinese Medicine, as these countries have better preserved both their herbal and meditational traditions than the Western world, which both have a bearing on this issue.

How herbs affect the mind also depends upon what one perceives the nature of the mind to be. In modern science, upon which modern medicine is based, there is no recognition of a mind apart from the brain and its biochemical processes. This reflects a materialistic preconception, a view of the world based upon external or measurable factors. In oriental medicine and other traditional systems, on the other hand, there is the recognition of a mind that is not simply physical, and of a spirit which is not material at all. This also reflects a spiritual view of the world that recognizes a sacred nature to all life which cannot be measured or understood through external experimentation. While such concepts of a spiritual or sacred science may be speculative from the standpoint of modern science, they can be experienced by various yogic and shamanistic practices. Such subtler realities cannot be described in gross physical or biochemical terms, we should note, otherwise they themselves would only be physical and not beyond it. Hence to approach the subtle qualities of herbs may require a different view of reality than that afforded by modern science. As modern science, particularly in quantum physics, is discovering that reality is more subtle and variable than what it was previously thought to be by the mechanical Newtonian model, the nature of the mind may also have to be reexamined in this light as well. Hence there may be a point of convergence in the future of these two world-views of modern and ancient science.

It is also important to remember that herbal medicines function as part of a holistic life-style. Apart from this their effectiveness can be greatly reduced. Herbs are part of nature and are most effective when one follows a life-style in harmony with one's nature. In a mechanized and artificial environment, such as many of us live in, the sensitivity of our syste... to herbal medicines can be greatly reduced. Just as a flower cannot grow in cement, so do artificial life-styles inhibit nature's healing processes, particularly those on the subtle level of the mind. Moreover, herbs function as whole organic substances and cannot be understood by merely chemical analysis. This is even more true relative to their effect upon the mind because for herbs to reach the mind requires several subtle nutritional processes in which their chemistry can be altered. It is also influenced by psychological and environmental factors, particularly the kinds of impressions we take in through the senses.

THE MIND AND NATURE

According to Ayurveda, the traditional medicine of India, there are three basic qualities at work in the universe, called *Gunas* in Sanskrit. First there is a quality of intelligence and harmony that creates balance, called *Sattva*. Second, there is a quality of energy and agitation that destroys equilibrium, called *Rajas*. Third, there is a factor of heaviness and inertia that resists both balance and change, called *Tamas*. These three qualities underlie all actions in the universe. Sattva brings about the awakening of intelligence and the evolution of consciousness. Rajas develops energy and life and furthers our outward seeking. Tamas sustains form and materiality and causes us to resist change and growth.

The mind itself is also called Sattva because it is only when the mind is clear and balanced that it can perceive things as they are. Right perception and correct judgement occur only when the mind is calm. This has been compared to a lake that has to be still to receive the reflection of the moon. When the mind is agitated or disturbed (dominated by Rajas), misperception or false imagination occurs. When the mind is dull (under the rule of Tamas), there is dullness or non-perception.

The food we take in is similarly divided into three portions: The gross portion, which has a Tamasic nature, becomes excrement. The middle portion, which is Rajasic, builds the flesh and sustains the life-energy or vital force. The subtle portion, which is Sattvic, serves to nourish the mind, senses and nervous system. Hence Ayurveda understands a subtler level of nutrition than the physical, yet one that is affected by physical substances.

Ayurveda has thereby classified all food types according to these three qualities. Old, devitalized, overcooked, overly greasy, sticky and sweet food, including all meat or dead food, has a Tamasic quality or is heavy and dulling to both the body and mind.

Food that is too hot, spicy, sour or salty, or foods that cause gas and bloating, like most beans and cabbage family plants, have a Rajasic effect and are both stimulating and irritating to the body and mind.

Food that is pleasant and mild in taste and organic like fruit, most vegetables, whole grains, nuts and dairy products are Sattvic. They are calming, clearing and nurturing to the body and mind.

Herbs similarly operate to increase either the Sattvic, Rajasic or Tamasic qualities of the mind. Most drugs, whether medical or recreational, have a Tamasic or dulling effect. This is particularly true of sedatives or downers. Yet even stimulants have this effect in the long run because whatever artificially stimulates us must eventually weaken us and result in depression. As drugs are inorganic, metallic and heavy they must serve to make the mind heavy and block the flow of nerve impulses. The same is true of the herbal usage of heavy metals, like that of cinnabar in Chinese medicine. Animal products and insects like deer horn, gecko lizards, sea horses or scorpions in Chinese medicine are also heavy and Tamasic. Herbs that have a toxic or narcotic effect like cannabis, datura, and aconite are also Tamasic. Some very pungent herbs like garlic, onions, asafoetida or valerian also have some mild Tamasic effects through their sedative or aphrodisiac properties. Excess use of astringents (herbs to stop sweating, diarrhea or bleeding) has a Tamasic effect as astringents serve to hold waste-materials in the body.

Ayurveda does not consider that Tamasic herbs are good nutritional supplements to the mind, yet it does consider them to be very useful. Their main usage relative to the mind is as sedatives (again owing to their heavy nature). Yet as strong sedatives their usage should only be short term. Some are also useful for pain relief, as their dulling effect helps reduce nervous sensitivity. Others, like garlic or meat, can be helpful tonics as their heavy nature serves to give more bulk and stability to the tissues. For countering Rajasic or agitated states of mind, they can be used to restore balance or Sattva. Yet they are thought to generally obstruct perception and the practice of meditation and hence are prescribed in Ayurveda with caution.

Most stimulant herbs have a Rajasic energy. This includes spicy and aromatic herbs like cayenne, ephedra, black pepper, cloves, wintergreen, camphor, musk and bayberry. Such herbs can serve to clear the mind and open the senses and may counter pain owing to cold or stagnation as they work to improve circulation both of the blood and of nerve impulses. While useful for depression they can be irritating and can aggravate conditions of hypersensitivity, like conditions of insomnia. In addition, they help counter the side-effects of Tamasic substances. Sour herbs like hawthorn berries or lemon also have a stimulating or Rajasic effect.

Herbs of Sattvic nature are mainly nutritive tonics, balanced nervines, or sweet spices and aromas. Most oriental tonics fall into this category such as licorice, ginseng, dang guai (*Angelica sinensis*), or lycium berries (*Lycium chinense*), and Ayurvedic ashwagandha (*Withania somnifera*), shatavari (*Asparagus racemosa*) and bala (*Sida cordifolia*). Additional Western herbs useful in this way are comfrey root, marshmallow and solomon's seal. Sweet spices include ginger, cinnamon, cardamom, fennel and coriander. Sweet aromas are mainly flowers like rose, jasmine and lotus and some woods like sandalwood. In addition, there are other herbs whose nature, largely through experience, has been found to be highly Sattvic. These include Ayurvedic nervines like gotu kola (*Centella asiatica*) and calamus (*Acorus calamus*). Chinese tonic nervines like zizyphus seeds (*Zizyphus jujuba*) and biota seeds (*Biota orientalis*) are probably Sattvic as well.

Sattvic substances are helpful for long term balance of body and mind. They are often useful as food supplements to increase nutrition to the brain and nervous system. Some aid in longevity and rejuvenation.

Many are useful aids for concentration and meditation.

However, we should remember that the qualities of herbs depend upon their dosage and application. Inappropriate usage can cause a Sattvic substance to become Rajasic or Tamasic. The quality of herbs is not entirely intrinsic but can be altered by dosage or preparation.

Using this model of the three qualities of Sattva, Rajas and Tamas we have a simple yet meaningful way of understanding the spiritual and mental effect of herbs. Tamasic herbs may be useful for hypersensitive states but have mainly short term application. Rajasic herbs can help counter depression or dullness but can overstimulate. Sattvic herbs are good for general usage and as tonics to the mind but may be too mild in their effects to treat acute (Rajasic) or resistant (Tamasic) conditions.

CLASSIFICATION OF HERBS AND THE MIND

WESTERN HERBALISM

Western herbalism recognizes a group of nervine herbs or herbs which improve nerve function. This is its closest classification to herbs that work on the mind. These nervines act to alleviate nerve pain, calm the emotions, promote sleep, and treat various nervous system disorders. Typical such herbs are scullcap, valerian, lady's slipper, hops and passion flower.

Nervines are generally lumped together with anti-spasmodics or herbs that relieve the pain of muscle spasms (mainly the smooth muscles). Yet not all herbs share both functions or do so to the same degree.

However, many of these so-called nervines have different natures and qualities. Scullcap is a cooling, slightly bitter and pungent herb, composed mainly of air and ether elements with a Sattvic quality. It is particularly good for an overheated nervous system (*Pitta* aggravation in Ayurvedic medicine). Valerian, on the other hand, is a warming, pungent herb, composed mainly of earth and fire elements with a Tamasic quality. It is good for many conditions of cold and ungroundedness (Ayurvedic *Vata* disorders).

Hence, Western herbalism needs a better energetic system of discriminating the properties of its so-called nervines. Otherwise, in clinical usage one will not know which herb to use. While there is a recognition of the difference between sedative and stimulant nervines, even this is not always presented clearly, as some herbs can function in both ways. Basic distinctions of heat or cold, dampness or dryness, and excess and deficiency in the nervous system should be considered to bring more clarity in this regard.

CHINESE HERBALISM

Chinese herbalism has a different approach. It distinguishes four categories of herbs that work specifically on the mind, called "Substances to Calm the Spirit." The first is "Substances that Settle and Calm the Spirit" or mind-calming sedatives, which are usually heavy minerals and metals, like dragon bone, oyster shell, magnetite and cinnabar. They are for extreme, acute or "excess" conditions of nervous upset, where both the patient and the disease symptoms are strong. Some of them are toxic. Their nature is generally cooling and they are somewhat astringent as well (stopping sweating or palpitations). They are Tamasic or have a long term dulling effect upon the mind according to Ayurvedic understanding. Still they are milder and safer than most pharmaceutical drugs and stronger than most herbs which, as plants, have a generally light nature.

The second is "Herbs that Nourish the Heart and Calm the Spirit" or nervine tonics. They are for weak types or deficient conditions like nervous exhaustion. These have nutritive properties for the mind, brain and nerves and include such herbs as zizyphus seeds, biota seeds, jujube dates (*Zizyphus sativa*) and licorice. They are for chronic or "deficient" conditions of nervous debility or nervous exhaustion. They are considered to be sweet and generally neutral in energy as their action is moderating or balancing. They would be largely Sattvic according to Ayurvedic understanding and hence useful as nutritional supplements for the brain and mind.

The third is "Substances that Extinguish Wind and Stop Tremors." These are more specifically anti-spasmodic and anti-convulsion medicines and include herbs like gastrodia (*Gastrodia elata*) and gambir (*Uncaria rhyncholphylla*), as well as animal and insects like scorpions and centipedes. Some of these are toxic as well and they are generally Tamasic. They are used specifically to treat convulsions and tremors, which they tend to block by their heavy or toxic nature.

The fourth Chinese category is "Aromatic Substances that Open the Orifices." These are often nervine stimulants like camphor or musk, but some are for delirium owing to fever like bezoar (cow's gall stones, *Calculus bovis*). These herbs mainly treat conditions of coma and are used to revive consciousness. Their quality is generally Rajasic or stimulating.

It is interesting to note that some herbs classified as nervines in Western herbalism may not fall into any of these categories in Chinese herbalism. For example, scullcap may not fall into any of them but would probably be considered a heat-clearing herb. The Chinese also consider that many other types of herbs have effects upon the mind. Herbs to move the chi or unblock energy, like bupleurum (*Bupleurum scorzoneraefollium*) and cyperus (*Cyperus rotundus*), are considered very good for countering depression or blocked emotions particularly from the region of the liver. Tonic herbs like ginseng are considered to be generally good for nerve weakness or deficiency. The same is true of a number of other herbal categories.

AYURVEDA

The approach of Ayurveda is yet more complex. It derives from its Tridosha concept, its threefold division of individual constitutional types according to the three biological humors. Vata, or the biological air humor, governs nerve function and the transmission of nerve impulses. Pitta, the biological fire humor, governs digestion, including perception or mental digestion. Kapha, the biological water humor, nourishes the nerves.

Each of these three humors has a subtle counterpart in the brain. Vata relates to *Prana Vayu* which is the guiding life-force or intelligence that governs the reception of energy and impressions through the mind, senses and breath. Pitta relates to *Sadhak Pitta*, which governs our ability to digest thoughts, emotions and impressions. Kapha relates to *Tarpak Kapha*, which allows us to find nourishment and sustenance through thoughts, feelings and sensations.

These three nervous system aspects of the biological humors similarly have their counterparts in the mind. Sadhak Pitta relates to the energy of *Tejas*, or the fire of intelligence governing the mind that allows us to ascertain reality from unreality, truth from illusion. Tarpak Kapha relates to *Ojas*, the subtle essence of our bodily fluids, which sustains the immune and hormonal functions. Prana Vayu relates to the *Prana* in the mind, or the basic life-force, which governs all mental and vital activities as the master intelligence of the psycho-physical system.

The key to mental health is considered to be the balance of the three factors of Prana, Tejas and Ojas. This brings us back to the Ayurvedic classification of herbs. Ayurveda recognizes six tastes found in herbs: sweet, sour, salty, pungent, bitter and astringent. These mirror the six emotions of love, envy, greed, hatred, grief and fear. Each taste is made up of a combination of two elements: sweet is composed of earth and water; sour of earth and fire; salty of water and fire; pungent of fire and air; bitter of air and ether; and astringent of earth and air. The tastes and elements help us understand the effect of herbs on all levels.

Bitter nervines, like gotu kola, increase Prana. They serve to clear and open the mind and senses by their predominance of air and ether elements. Pungent nervines, like calamus or camphor which are primarily pungent in taste, increase Tejas. They work to stimulate the mind and senses and improve cerebral circulation by their predominance of fire and air elements. Sweet or bland tasting nervines, like ashwagandha, increase Ojas. They work to calm and nourish the mind by their predominance of earth and water elements.

Like Traditional Chinese Medicine, Ayurveda also uses many metals and minerals to affect the mind. In Chinese medicine there are two very basic methods of taking minerals. The first is to merely boil the raw mineral and drink the water, which may have little or none of the actual mineral. This process is used for mineral shells like oyster shell as well as minerals like gypsum or magnetite. The second is to take the raw mineral internally, which may be toxic as in the case of cinnabar. In Ayurveda, on the other hand, elaborate purifications are done to render the minerals suitable for internal usage and to make their quality become Sattvic. Such factors include mixing or cooking metals with organic substances (herbs like aloe vera or dairy products), or incinerating the mineral numerous times under various forms of heat (that from special types of wood or from cow dung) until the mineral forms a white oxide ash (*bhasma*). Such purified or humanized metals or minerals are considered to be non-toxic in the appropriate low dosages and clinical studies confirm this. In this way Ayurveda uses herbs along with purified minerals including sulphur, mercury, gold, silver and gem ashes from coral to diamond. Ayurveda regards such medicines to have a stronger and more direct affect upon the mind. They produce a whole series of nervine medicines, useful for all variety of conditions. They also are powerful remedies to treat deep seated imbalances and difficult chronic diseases, which usually have a psychological foundation. Such Ayurvedic purified mineral preparations mainly are called "*Rasa* preparations" or "*Siddha* medicines" and have been used for at least two thousand years.

A typical Ayurvedic nervine stimulant and tonic based on such purified metals is a Rasa preparation called "Makaradhwaj." It consists of purified sulphur and mercury (some varieties also use gold), along with herbs like camphor, nutmeg, long pepper and calamus. It is useful for nervous and sexual debility owing to conditions of cold and deficiency (primarily Vata conditions). It is very heating in nature, however, and so contraindicated in conditions of fever whether chronic or acute. It is often taken in the late fall or early winter as a stimulant tonic.

Another important nervine medicine that combines purified minerals with herbs and resins is called "Mahayogaraj Guggul." It consists of purified guggul resin (*Commiphora mukul,* a relative of myrrh) with herbs and purified minerals like silver, iron, mica and lead. It is good for nerve pain, particularly that due to cold and deficiency.

Unfortunately such mineral preparations, even though purified, are unlikely to be allowed into this country because of F.D.A. restrictions. Yet the herbalism of the coming century will undoubtedly have to examine them again and will most likely bring them back into the field of herbal medicine. Minerals are important medicines, particularly for conditions of the mind and nerves. Yet they need to be purified properly. Otherwise, however useful they may be in acute conditions, as toxic substances their residues must cause further imbalances.

CLASSIFICATION OF NERVINE STIMULANTS AND SEDATIVES

On this background, we can create a simplified classification for these different herbal traditions. It is important first of all to discriminate between a nervine sedative and a nervine stimulant. The former lowers or reduces hyperfunction of the nerves, as in conditions of hysteria or insomnia; the latter raises or increases hypofunction of the nerves, as in conditions of depression. Yet because there are different constitutional types, herbs may not always function in the same way for different individuals.

Typical nervine stimulants are camphor, sage, bayberry, wintergreen, eucalyptus and calamus. They are often aromatic, pungent and have analgesic properties (as they function as counterirritants). Their nature is generally warm and counters conditions of cold or stagnation in the mind and nervous system and emotional conditions of fear and depression.

Typical nervine sedatives are scullcap, hops, passion flower and gotu kola. They are more typically bitter in taste and have anti-inflammatory properties. Their energy is usually cooling and they counter fever, irritability, anger and an overheated nervous system.

Valerian, however, is another type of nervine sedative. While the bitter nervines act by cooling the mind, valerian, through its earth energy, helps to ground the mind. It is also a good anti-spasmodic, particularly for lower abdominal muscle cramps. Garlic and asafoetida (*Ferula asafoetida*) have similar effects. An Indian relative of valerian called jatamansi (*Nardostachys jatamansi*) is also useful in this regard. Yet it has a cooling nature and can be used safely by all constitutional types.

This is not to say that both these types of herbs cannot be used together. Nervine stimulants clear blockages in the nerve channels, which is often behind many nervous disorders. Bitter nervine sedatives also help relieve blockage due to heat or heaviness in the system, as the nature of bitter taste is cooling and light. Bitter and pungent nervines together increase fire, air and ether elements and hence make the mind more subtle and alert. The combination of a bitter with an aromatic nervine is thus good for clearing the nervous system and for promoting general mental functioning.

Mineral sedatives function more by their heavy nature, as they predominate in the element of earth. Yet owing to their inorganic nature they do not have any tonic or nutritive properties. Ayurvedic purified minerals, however, have a deep nutritive effect upon brain and nerve tissue, as well as being useful as sedatives or stimulants depending upon their nature (ie., purified mercury is very stimulating but purified iron and lead have sedative effects as their natures are heavier).

NERVINE TONICS

It is also important to discriminate between herbs that correct nerve function, in which category both stimulants and sedatives fall, and those which serve to tonify or nourish the nervous system. The former adjust hyper or hypofunctioning of the mind and nerves. The latter provide added nutrition to the nerves. In this regard Western herbalism has not had such a strong a sense of nervine tonics as do the oriental systems. We should also note that the term tonic, which refers to a nutritive effect in oriental herbalism, may only refer to some corrective action in Western herbalism as with the use of bitter tonics to strengthen the digestive system.

Of the Chinese nervine tonics, zizyphus seeds are considered to be the best. They treat insomnia, weak nerve function, nervous debility and night sweats. They are useful for conditions of nerve weakness whether caused by heat or cold.

Of the Ayurvedic nervine tonic herbs, ashwagandha is considered to be superior. It strengthens and builds the deeper tissues of the body including muscle, bone, nerves and reproductive tissue. It counters nerve pain, calms the mind and promotes deep sleep and meditation. Specifically, it relieves anxiety and is good for nervous exhaustion. Shatavari (*Asparagus racemosa*) is considered to be good for nourishing the heart and emotions and for promoting love and affection. Chinese medicine uses a related plant (*Asparagus lucidus*) in a similar way.

Ayurveda also uses different preparations to bring out the tonic properties of herbs. Gotu kola prepared in ghee (clarified butter) or made into an herbal jelly with sugar, honey and ghee (called *Brahma Rasayan*) becomes a good tonic for the mind, whereas the herb itself is better for its sedative purposes. Some nervine sedatives may also possess mild nervine tonic properties. This is the case with gotu kola and bhringraj (*Eclipta alba*). It appears to also be the case with lady's slipper and gastrodia (Chinese *Tian ma*). This is also better brought out through the right preparation or by combination with herbs that are more primarily tonic in nature. For example, gotu kola with ashwagandha becomes a good nervine tonic, whereas by itself it is better for inflammation or irritability of the nerves.

Such nervine tonics in Ayurveda may be taken as foods, particularly along with other nervine foods like milk, ghee (clarified butter), or nuts like almonds. They may also be made into herbal wines (like *Ashwagandhasrishta*, an ashwagandha herbal wine), which aid in their tonic properties and allow for easier digestion. Western herbalists should consider using or preparing such nervine tonics, rather than relying so exclusively on herbs that correct nerve function.

According to Ayurvedic understanding, nervine stimulants are best for Kapha or watery types who tend to suffer from heaviness, depression and lethargy. Nervine sedatives, particularly those which are cooling and bitter, are better for Pitta or fiery types who suffer from anger or fever. Nervine tonics are better for Vata or airy types as they are most prone to nervous debility and hypersensitivity. This, however, is only a general rule. Nervine tonics are often helpful for Pitta people suffering from nervous burnout or weakness of the blood. Nervine stimulants are often helpful for Vata types by clearing the nerve channels and alleviating cold. In the practice of Yoga, nervine stimulants are used for opening the mind and senses. The Indian variety of bayberry is sacred to Shiva, the God of pure consciousness, as is camphor. Calamus is important for improving the power of speech and gives a greater ability to articulate ideas.

Nervine sedatives are used for clearing and calming emotions and for alleviating anger or excess willfulness. Gotu kola (Sanskrit *Brahmi*) is the most typical in this case. It is good for clearing negative emotions from the liver and heart. In this regard it is good to combine it with an herb like turmeric or coriander which helps clear liver energy, or with a bitter like bayberry which helps decongest the bile. Gotu kola helps promote calm and meditation as it promotes the element of ether which sustains the mind.

AROMATIC OILS

Apart from the regular use of herbs, there are other methods of treating the mind. Aromatic oils are specific in this regard. They were often used in China and India to revive patients from conditions of coma or convulsions. Their usage of incense is well known.

Sweet flower oils are better for calming the mind and heart. They are usually cooling, counter fever and are useful in conditions of debility, unhappiness and grief. Typical are rose, saffron, jasmine, gardenia and honeysuckle. Some sweet aromatic woods like sandalwood or agaru (*aquilaria*) are particularly good for calming the mind, as wood has a heavier and more supportive energy.

Pungent spicy oils are better for opening the mind and senses and serve as nervine stimulants. Typical are musk, camphor, basil, eucalyptus and calamus. Aromatic resins have a generally clearing and opening affect but also cleanse the blood and clear mucus and congestion. Typical are myrrh and frankincense or Ayurvedic guggul.

Such oils can be applied externally at special sites, like that of the third eye, the heart center or the navel. They can also be added to various massage oils. Each can be mixed with larger amounts of water or other herbal decoctions and taken in small amounts internally.

Incense is not just for a pleasant affect; it also serves to cleanse the air of negative energies. This can work on a physical level to purify the atmosphere from bacteria and viruses or on a more subtle level to counter emotional disturbances. Aromas have an immediate effect upon the brain and mind and work to improve circulation in the subtle channels. They communicate with the Prana or master intelligence of the life-force and can thereby change the emotional structure directly through it.

OILS

Fatty oils like sesame oil are also very good for the mind and the nervous system. The skin can absorb these oils and take them into the nerve tissue via the bones. Sesame oil has the greatest penetrating power into the body. Herbs can be prepared in it and will be taken by it into the nerve tissue. Ayurveda has many such medicated sesame oils like Narayan Tail, Dashamula Tail, Nirgundi Tail and Prasarani Tail which are good for alleviating nerve and joint pain.

Regular use of oil massage helps keep the nerves nourished and in balance. It is good to apply small amounts of such oils to the orifices of the body including the eye lids, ear drums, nostrils, lips, gums, rectum and urethra. Brahmi oil (gotu kola prepared in a coconut oil base) is particularly good for this purpose. Ghee, particularly Triphala ghee (clarified butter prepared with the three herbs of haritaki, bibhitaki and amalaki or *Terminalia chebula, Terminalia belerica* and *Emblica officinalis*) is best for the eyes. Oil massage to the head is very good for calming the mind, particularly an oil drip on the forehead (*Shirodhara*).

These same oils work well taken in the form of enemas. In Ayurvedic medicine the membrane of the colon is the site where nutrients are absorbed to feed the nervous system. Oil enemas can thereby help treat many nervous system and mental disorders. Tonic herbs can be taken in this way also, as can milk decoctions, particularly of tonic herbs (like ashwagandha).

Western herbalists should also consider these different mediums for preparing herbs and different sites for their application.

TOXIC AND NARCOTIC HERBS

There is also a whole usage of toxic and narcotic herbs. Many toxic herbs in small dosages, like many of the nightshades (datura, henbane, belladonna, etc.), have excellent analgesic and antispasmodic properties. Many plant poisons that in higher dosages cause paralysis, in lower dosages relieve pain by blocking nerve impulses. Such toxic plants are used both in Ayurvedic and Chinese medicine in the appropriate dosage. Cannabis is excellent as a general analgesic and can be used for nerve pain and muscle pain, including intestinal pain. Several daturas have similar properties. Without being able to use such plants the herbalist is hampered particularly in providing pain relief. This does not mean that such herbs are without side-effects or that they can be used by the uninformed general public, but qualified herbalists should not be deprived of their power. They are herbs and are part of nature's herbal treasure that should be accessible to the herbalist.

Lastly, there is the use of psychotropic plants for various subtle effects upon the mind, including various forms of spiritual healing. This, though an interesting and controversial topic, is outside the scope of this article. While such things may be useful if done by a person with experience, according to Ayurveda they aggravate Vata, the biological air humor, and have a long term Tamasic effect. They should not be used on a recreational basis. Only an occasional sacramental usage may be safe. Yet while glimpses of subtle realities can be gotten through psychotropic drugs the only way to achieve these states is through yogic or related practices. For achieving these states, more subtle and less dramatic herbs may be more helpful through their functioning as long term nutritive or harmonizing agents for the mind.

CONCLUSION

Herbal usages based upon traditional energetic classifications and the result of thousands of years of clinical experience cannot be ignored. They may not be entirely provable by modern scientific methods but this may be because they are working on a different level. Just as modern science cannot necessarily prove that one painting is more beautiful than another, so too, the effects of herbs on the psyche is outside of the realm of simple measurement. Yet it can be observed and measured via clinical studies. A great deal more research must be done in this area before any final conclusions can be drawn. Tremendous resources as well as a great deal of knowledge and experience exists to be explored. Fortunately countries like India and China are able to continue such herbal usages and study them with modern scientific methods as well as clinical trials. The coming century should see a renaissance in this area and with the encounter between modern psychology and oriental yoga systems the psychological usage of herbs will be very important.

Our Eyes — Mirrors of Health

BRIGITTE MARS

The precious gift of sight, which brings light and color into our lives, is worth all the attention we can focus toward achieving and maintaining healthy vision. In Oriental Medicine, the liver governs the eyes and many eye disorders have their roots in liver disharmonies. For example, insufficient blood supply in the liver can be a cause of eyes that feel dry. Eyes that are often irritated and bloodshot may be due to the liver being irritated by coffee, alcohol and chemicals. Eyes that have a discharge of mucous may be aggravated by a diet too rich in congesting fats. In contrast, healthy organs give their purest energy to the eyes, creating brightness and awareness.

Besides eating a wholesome diet, foods that are known to be particularly beneficial to the eyes include sunflower and sesame seeds, carrots, green leafy vegetables, leeks, barley and blueberries. During World War II, Air Force pilots were given bilberry (*Vaccinium myrtillus*) jelly to improve their night vision. Bilberry extract is even available in capsule form these days. Also helpful are lycii berries (*Lycium chinense*), available in Oriental markets and some natural food stores. These sweet, reddish dried berries are considered to be a special liver tonic and helpful for blurred and poor vision. In our home, we use lycii berries like raisins — cooked into oatmeal, mixed into yoghurt or added to trail mix.

Some people may want to make a tasty beverage in their blender, rich in many nutrients for visual health:

2 cups raw carrot juice
1 teaspoon rose hip powder
1/4 cup raw, unsalted sunflower seeds
3 tablespoons of wheat germ (Buy it refrigerated to help prevent rancidity.

The herb eyebright (*Euphrasia officinalis*), a member of the Scrophularaceae family, has a long history of use in treating eye disorders. The French often refer to this herb as *casses lunettes* which means "break your glasses." Ancient peoples found this herb to slightly resemble an eye, and used it for poor sight. Eyebright has a cool, acrid, slightly bitter taste that stimulates the liver function, thus improving blood supply to the eyes. Eyebright can be taken internally as a tea, capsules and extract. To make tea, boil 1 cup of pure water, remove from heat, add 1 heaping teaspoon of herb, cover and let steep 10 minutes. Then strain and enjoy. Many people have found that using the strained tea as an eyewash helps to reduce eye inflammation.

A Chinese herbal tea blend is made with equal parts of lycii berries, fo ti (*Polygonum multiflorum*- a whole body tonic via the liver), red jujube dates (*Zizyphi jujubae* — a delicious liver tonic) and chrysanthemum flowers (*Chrysanthemum moriflolium* — clears the liver and brightens the eyes). Simmer 1 heaping teaspoon of each herb in 1 quart of water at a low boil while covered for 20 minutes. Strain and drink throughout the day.

Keep in mind that eye problems are usually a long time in the making and consistency is needed to make natural remedies show their full benefits. Research shows that certain vitamins and minerals help to maintain healthy eyes. Vitamin A is manufactured in the liver from carotene. The rod cells in our eyes contain a substance known as visual purple or rhodopsin. If the body is deficient in Vitamin A, the cells' ability to make visual purple is impaired and night blindness, dry eyes and loss of color vision may result. People who work in bright lights, sunlight, snow, face car headlights, as well as folks having to see in the dark may benefit from this nutrient.

Vitamin B1 deficiency may lead to dimness of sight. Riboflavin, or Vitamin B2, is also essential. A deficiency in this nutrient can manifest in blood shot eyes that burn, itch, water frequently or are extremely light sensitive (photophobia). People deficient in B2 may rub their eyes a lot. It is thought that light enters the eyes through a screen of riboflavin before reaching the visual purple.

The lenses of our eyes contain more Vitamin C than any other body part, except some endocrine glands. Vitamin C and E may both help prevent cataract formation by preventing oxidative damage. In cases of cataracts, Vitamin C is usually deficient. Vitamin E is necessary for good circulation and muscle strength. Consult with a nutritionally trained health professional for recommendations on appropriate dosages.

Nutritional therapy for poor eyesight is a good place to begin, but it is also necessary to distribute these valuable elements throughout the body with proper exercises. Eye exercises can increase circulation to the eye area. Attached to our eyeballs are six little muscles that can be tonified. When reading or focusing for long periods, squeeze eyes shut for a few seconds to increase blood flow to the area. If you spend your days looking close up at objects, take a break and gaze off into the distance every once in awhile.

Here is an exercise that has greatly improved my vision as well as that of many of my clients.

1. Keeping the head still, look up and down 7 times. Close eyes to rest 10 seconds.
2. Look from one side to the other 7 times. Close and rest 10 seconds.
3. Look diagonally from one direction to the other 7 times. Close and rest 10 seconds.
4. Look diagonally from the opposite direction to the other 7 times. Close and rest 10 seconds.
5. Roll the eyes in an upper half circle and back 7 times. Close and rest 10 seconds.
6. Roll eyes in a lower half circle and back 7 times. Close and rest 10 seconds.
7. Place the backs of both hands over closed eyes and rest for a full minute.

Many of us spend time exercising other parts of our bodies. It truly is worth improving circulation and strengthening the muscles attached to the eyes to keep them in working order. If your eyes need some extra help, you may want to massage the correlating reflex points at the base of the bottoms of the second and third toes in a firm circular motion. Deep massage at the base of the neck may help to relieve tension that impairs vision.

Glasses can help us see clearly but they don't improve actual vision. If you always wear glasses or contact lenses consider that we may be blocking Nature's full spectrum lighting. Light enters the eyes and affects the pineal gland. When it is safe and can be done without strain, try to spend a little time each day without anything covering your eyes. This is best done outside, preferably when surrounded by the calm, cooling green colors of Nature. Consider that cheap sunglasses filter only some rays, but allow other rays, to come through that may be harmful. Another beneficial eye strengthening technique is called "sunning." It is done by standing or sitting with closed eyes (though no glasses or contacts), then turning one's head gently from the left to the right, allowing the sun's rays to gently cross over closed eyes.

When your eyes feel tired, irritated and swollen, rather than resorting to synthetic eye drops, which give only temporary relief and can lead to more irritation later, try these gentler approaches. My grandmother taught me to lay down with a fresh slice of cucumber over each closed eye. Grated raw potato also gives blessed relief. If your eyes are begging for attention, it makes sense to take a few moments out to give them some genuine nurturing. There are some Swiss homeopathic eyedrops on the market which work very well. Remember that when our eyes are giving us trouble, we should look to the cause of the problem and do our best to remedy that. Please consult with a competent, preferably holistic orientated optometrist or ophthalmologist for problems such as seeing colored rings around lights, blurred or double vision, seeing imaginary spots, lines or flashes of light, burning, watery or itchy eyes for a proper diagnosis.

May your eyes enjoy the wonders of the world and be a reflection of your inner health and beauty.

SOME EXCELLENT BOOKS ON EYE HEALTH INCLUDE:
Natural Vision Improvement by Janet Goodrich
Better Eyesight Without Glasses by Doctor Bates
Better Eyesight by Patricia Bragg

Natural Remedies for Ear Ailments

BRIGITTE MARS

As a child, I suffered from frequent earaches and well remember the excruciating pain. My parents had the best of intentions, taking me frequently to the ear, nose and throat doctor, who was appropriately named Dr. Kaufman. As a result, I repeatedly took antibiotics for ten days of almost every month. Since that time I have learned, used and recommended many effective and natural methods for preventing and treating common earaches.

Recently, I spoke with the young mother of a four year old boy. Matthew had suffered the agony of five ear infections within a year. Each time he had been given antibiotics. Now a date had been set to surgically put tubes in his ears. Matthew's young mother, who was also a nurse, despaired over her child's sleepless nights and frequent pain. She wanted to do what was best for him. One of her neighbors suggested she try some alternative methods before doing surgery. The mother agreed to give it a try. She removed dairy products from his diet, used drops of echinacea extract when the pain and redness of an infection was apparent and used an herbal ear oil. So successful were these gentler approaches that the mom cancelled the impending surgery. It's been eight months since the child's last ear infection.

Our ears tune us in to the sounds of the world. They enable us to listen to the voices of our loved ones, the melodies of music and the orchestra of our natural (and unnatural environment). Because our sense of hearing is so essential, it is well worth understanding how to care for these wonderful receptors, our ears.

EAR INFECTIONS

Earaches are classified as *otitis externa* which is an infection and inflammation of the external ear and *otitis media* which pertains to the middle ear. The latter is where excess fluid and mucus impair ear drainage through the eustachian tubes. The ear, nose and throat are all connected through the eustachian tubes at the back of the throat.

Symptoms of ear infections include pain, throbbing, discharge and/or a feeling of fullness. Infants too young to talk may cry shrilly, pull and rub their ears, have low grade fever and/or diarrhea. They may still desire to eat food but refuse to nurse or take a bottle as this may cause increased ear pressure. Teething infants are often prone to earaches. Molars coming in may cause swelling in the maxilla bone plate.

There are a multitude of other possible causes of this malady, yet one of the most common is an allergy to cows' milk and other dairy products. A food sensitivity may cause an increase in mucus production and even swelling, thus creating blockage and pressure. Other common allergens to consider would include wheat, eggs, corn, soy, citrus and tomatoes. In hundreds of cases, I have seen children have less frequent occurences and often the disappearance of ear infections altogether with the elimination of dairy products (especially milk, cheese and ice cream). Naturopath Todd Nelson of Boulder, Colorado, finds that goats' milk is more easily tolerated and that its high flourine content actually helps to improve lymphatic drainage.For those with extreme sensitivities, even a tiny amount of the offending food may be a catalyst for an earache. For breast fed babies, the mother needs to be scrupulous in her avoidance of the offending substance, as it would be passed on to the baby through her milk.

Bottle fed babies have more frequent ear infections than those who are nursed. Not only is there more exposure to possible allergenic substances, but the baby given a bottle has to suck harder which creates more negative pressure in the eustachian tubes. Breast or bottle feeding while the baby is lying in a prone position may also contribute to more frequent ear infections as milk or fluid can drain into the ears. So it is best to hold the child slightly more upright. Children are more susceptible to earaches due to their eustachian tubes being shorter, straight and somewhat horizontal. This makes it easier for nasal secretions to enter the middle ear. The tubes enlarge as one grows, decreasing the frequency of ear troubles. Several other possible causes of ear infections may include complications of upper respiratory infections, forceful nose blowing that may push infected secretions into the middle ear, enlarged adenoids and bacteria from swimming water. Studies show there are more incidences of ear infections when parents smoke around their children. Dr. Julie Carpenter of Boulder, finds more frequent ear problems in children that attend day care centers. This may be due to diet or to exposure to more infections.

According to Louise Hay, author of *You Can Heal Your Life*, earaches can be the result of anger and not wanting to hear. If anger and turmoil fill one's household it certainly makes sense to do everything possible to create more harmony, so that children will feel less compelled to "tune out" the negativity by perhaps psychologically blocking the ears. Ms. Hay suggests that the person with the earaches, if old enough, frequently repeat the affirmation "Harmony surrounds me. I listen with love to the pleasant and the good. I am a center for love." Say it enough times and it may very likely make a difference not only with the ears, but with the lifestyle!

Earaches are responsible for about 8% of all pediatric visits. When visiting a medical doctor for ear problems, the ear will be examined with an otoscope, a funnel shaped flashlight. If a middle ear infection is present, the ear will look redder inside. However, a red or pink color does not necessarily mean an infection is present. Parents may want to buy their own otoscope to check the ears at home.

Ampicillin is one of the standard drugs recommended for children under four years old and Penicillin for those over four. Antibiotics destroy friendly bacteria in the intestines, can cause diarrhea, lead to the overgrowth of candida albicans and leave one even more prone to food and other allergies. A double blind study was done in the Netherlands in 1981, where 171 children had ear infections. One half of them were treated with antibiotics and the others were not. There was no difference in ear discharge, pain or recovery time in either group and none of the children had permanent hearing damage. Dr. Robert Mendelsohn, author of *How to Raise a Healthy Child in Spite of Your Doctor* would only prescribe antibiotics if pus was discharging from the ears, as he believed it would make the person more susceptible to another infection in four to six weeks. However, if one does take antibiotics, it is important to complete the entire series. To help bring the body back into balance a powdered supplement of lactobacillus acidophilus or lactobacillus bifidus (for very young children of nursing age) should be given for at least ten days following medication. Miso soup and unpasteurized sauerkraut would also be beneficial for the intestinal flora of older children. Many ear infections are now resistant to antibiotics, having become immune to them from overuse. One very resistant type of bacteria is the hardy *Branhamella catarrhalis*, which is often present in recurrent infections.

Everyday I talk to parents of young children and see that ear infections are one of the most common reasons that young children are being placed on antibiotics, which can create a vicious cycle. Frequent use of antibiotics greatly weakens the immune system. To help the body fight infection in a safer and more natural way, use the very effective herb echinacea (*Echinacea purpurea* or *angustifolia*). This herb has large polysaccharide molecules, which the body perceives as a bacteria, thus white blood cell production becomes activated, which actually makes the immune system stronger. One simple way to administer echinacea is in an extract or tincture form. Take the dosage size recommended on the bottle, but when fighting infection, it is necessary to use it more frequently - usually every one or two hours. (Except when sleeping, as rest is most healing). Dosages on the bottle will usually be for an adult. A general method for determining a child's dosage is as follows:

Take the child's weight and divide by the standard 150. For example, a weight of 50 pounds, divided by 150 would be one-third the adult dosage. Echinacea is available at natural food stores in a glycerite form which is alcohol free and may taste somewhat better to little ones. If one can only find the more commonly available alcohol extracts, it is easy to conceal a few drops in diluted juice or herb tea. To minimize alcohol consumption, add the drops of herbal extract to a small amount of just boiled water, allow the mixture to sit for ten minutes and you will have evaporated about 85% of the alcohol.

Other drugs often prescribed for ear infections include oral decongestants, often containing pseudoephedrine hydrochloride and chlorpheniramine. Alternatives would be to avoid congesting foods and consume plenty of warm fluids (tea and soups) to help thin secretions. Some herbs that are natural decongestants that could be included in tea would be Mormon tea (*Ephedra nevadensis*) for children as it is less stimulating, or its more powerful Chinese cousin ephedra (*Ephedra sinica*), for those with a hardier constitution. These herbs might be combined in teas with rose hips (for Vitamin C), elder flowers (to help reduce fevers), peppermint (as a mild decongestant) and licorice root (to sweeten the tea and for its anti-inflammatory properties).

In allopathic medicine, if one has frequent, recurring ear infections, a surgical technique called tympanotomy may be performed. This now replaces tonsilectomies as the most common childhood surgery. It involves puncturing the eardrum and inserting a polyethylene tube. This could, though rarely, lead to hearing loss and is best left to those cases where dietary changes and home remedies have not been effective. One mother told me that three of her children had tubes put in their ears and the doctor suggested doing the same for her fourth and youngest child "just in case," even though the child was perfectly healthy! "What is essential is to determine the cause of the ear problem and deal with it. A physician should help the parent or patient make an informed decision," says Dr. Bob Rowntree of Boulder, Colorado.

When an ear infection is present, gentle massage behind the ear, around the outer ear and ear opening, slight pulling on the earlobes, effleuraging down the neck to encourage lymphatic drainage and rubbing the temples all helps to increase blood flow to the area as well as to move toxins. Using some Tiger Balm or essential oils (two drops of either eucalyptus, lavender or wintergreen oil diluted in a teaspoon of sesame oil) for the massage will further help to relieve congestion and alleviate pain.

Few things in life feel as pleasant as a foot massage. When someone has an earache, help to take their mind off their ears with a firm yet gentle foot rub. While doing this, you can stimulate the reflex points to the ears by pressing deeply for about twenty seconds in a circular motion at the base of and between the fourth and fifth toes. These points may be tender yet often help give relief.

To treat the ears even more directly, I have had excellent results using herbal and oil drops found in health food stores, usually made with garlic, mullein flowers and olive oil. Before application, place the closed bottle in a glass of hot water to warm the oil. Have the person with the earache lie down on their stomach with the painful ear facing upward. Put two or three drops of oil in the ear. Pull down gently on the earlobe to facilitate the oil getting into the ear. The oil helps with the pain and to fight infection. It is best to treat both ears, even if only one seems afflicted, as infection may be present though not discernable.

I often make my own ear drops in the summer by gathering the fresh picked golden blossoms of mullein (*Verbascum thapsus*), layering them in a clean glass jar with slices of garlic and covering the mixture with olive oil. Cover the mixture with a piece of cheesecloth secured around the jar with a rubber band. This allows excess moisture to evaporate, while keeping dust and debris out. In two weeks, strain and rebottle the liquid portion into amber colored dropper bottles. These can be stored in the refrigerator for up to two years.

Once when travelling with my younger sister, she came down with a severe earache. There were no health food stores, herbal ear drops or mullein flowers in the area, so we made use of an even simpler folk remedy. I took the papery covering off a clove of garlic and gently inserted the whole clove into her ear (with most of the clove still showing, so it could be easily removed.) I covered her ear with a hot, wet wash cloth, which I kept rewarming. Every twenty minutes I removed the garlic, discarded it and added a fresh clove. Within an hour the earache had totally dissipated.

When someone is having a treatment done to their ears, whether it be with garlic, massage, or herbal oil drops, they should be encouraged to breathe deeply and visualize sending healing energy to their ears. A painful ear is an ear calling for attention! Deliberate yawning may also help to open blockages in the ear. For those familiar with yoga, the very simple Lion Pose also helps to open the ears. During the night, it is best to elevate the head slightly to promote better drainage of the ears.

Homeopathy has helped many people around the world deal with ear infections. The remedy depends upon the type of earache. Dosages are usually 3 pills every hour in 6x or 12x potency or as directed by your homeopath.

Aconite: Ear pain comes on suddenly. The ear is red and the face flushed. Often occurs after exposure to cold, dry weather.

Arsenicum: Burning discharge with a roaring sound in the ear. Hearing is impaired. The patient seems fearful and anxious.

Belladonna: Sudden, violent boring pains that seem to buzz through the ear. Pus and inflammation are present along with a hot, red ear. Usually the right ear is affected. Person may cry out during sleep. This is a remedy for the onset of such an earache.

Chamomilla: The patient has unbearable pain, is frantic and irritable. If a child, they want to be carried. One cheek may be pale, the other flushed. Often occurs during teething. Warm applications make the pain worse.

Dulcamara: For earaches that occur after cold, damp weather exposure. At night, the pain is worse.

Ferrum Phos: Use when gradual onset of an earache. The face will be flushed and the person will be very sensitive to noise.

Hepar Sulph: There is pain from the throat to the ear, with those areas being sore to touch.

Kali Mur: Use with mucus buildup in the eustachian tubes and diminished hearing. There may be cracking noises when the person swallows. This remedy is also used if there seems to be hearing impairment following an earache.

Mag Phos: Use when the ears hurt due to a cold wind, not from infection, right ear being the most affected. Warm pressure brings relief, where cold increases the pain.

Mercurius: Ears hurt more at night and are worse from damp weather conditions. The person perspires, has a sickly odor, much saliva, a swollen tongue with teeth impressions on the side.

Pulsatilla: Use when the outer ear is red, hot and swollen. Pain is worse at night, throbbing and darting, which may make hearing difficult. The patient feels cold and irritable and wants to be covered.

Homeopathy works best when coffee (even decaf), mint and camphor are avoided.

There are several vitamins to consider using, especially when one suffers from frequent ear infections. They include Vitamin A to strengthen the mucous membranes, Vitamin C to help prevent infections and zinc to boost the immune system. Calcium supplements are helpful for extreme hearing sensitivity. It may be worth giving a dairy free supplement to kids having to avoid milk products, particularily if they say "yuck" to other calcium rich foods such as sea vegetables, oatmeal, tahini and green leafy vegies.

If an earache persists for more than forty-eight hours, the person has a high fever or the earache is accompanied by a discharge of blood, green or yellow pus, it is time to consult with a health professional.

When an earache occurs there are many natural remedies to use that have been time tested for thousands of years by people around the globe. Our ears are such a valuable asset that it makes sense to do what will bring about true health.

AIRPLANE EARS

Also known as *barotitis*, this complaint occurs when a plane ascends or descends, the surrounding air pressure changes and vacuum pressure forms in the middle ear, causing pain. Simple remedies include swallowing, yawning and gum chewing. Infants can be nursed during takeoff and landing to help prevent a problem. For those with severe problems, look for an herbal decongestant at your natural food store. They will usually contain a form of the herb ephedra.

When flying back from L.A. with my two daughters, they requested some gum from the airport shop. I went to help them make a selection and was amazed by the number of sugarless gums that carried warnings that read: This product contains sacharrin, found to cause cancer in laboratory animals. I was well aware of the warnings on cigarettes, but many kids can consume two packs of chewing gum a day! Next time I fly with my kids, I'll look for maple or honey sweetened gum in the natural food store before the trip.

SWIMMERS' EAR

Swimming exposes the ears to a number of possible problem-causing bacteria. To prevent swimmers' ear, shake the head somewhat vigorously or jump up and down with the head tilted to one side after being in the water. If necessary, one can make a simple solution to put in the ears after swimming by adding 1 teaspoon of white vinegar to 4 tablespoons of freshly boiled water. Store in the refrigerator. After swimming, put 2 drops of the mixture in each ear.

BUG IN THE EAR

A buzzing bug in one's ear sounds extremely loud. For this annoyance, turn the ear toward the sun, as many bugs are attracted to the light. If it's nighttime, shine a flashlight in the ear to draw the pest out. If you have no results add 1 teaspoon of warm olive oil in the ear and let it sit with the ear turned upward for 1 to 2 minutes. The last resort is to gently fill the ear with warm water. These last two remedies are to drown the bug and get it to float to the top.

FOREIGN OBJECT IN THE EAR

Should you by accident get a foreign object in your ear, or happen to disobey your mother and put beans in your ears, remember that an imbedded object is best removed by a doctor who will have the tools to do so without puncturing the delicate membrane of the ears.

RINGING IN THE EARS

For this annoyance, it is important to determine the cause and attend to the source of the problem. Consider that ear ringing is sometimes caused by excess consumption of coffee or aspirin, high blood pressure, stress or a dying nerve. In Oriental medicine this is often considered to be a symptom of deficient kidney yang energy. A new book on the subject of tinnitus is called *Living with Tinnitus* by Richard Hallam. I have seen several cases where extracts of the herb, ginkgo (*Ginkgo biloba*) given orally has helped tinnitus by improving nerve signal transmission as well as increasing the brain's utilization of oxygen.

EAR WAX

Ear wax buildup is called ceruminosis. Its purpose is to lubricate and protect the ears. An excess of this substance may be due to overconsumption of fats and sugars in the diet. Dr. Mendelsohn would say that putting cotton swabs in the ears was akin to driving a tank across one's lawn. This treatment can end up pushing dirt and wax further into the ears. To safely remove earwax, add several drops of mullein flower oil into the ears every night for a week. Then one can use special ear wax candles, based on a tradition used by ancient Egyptians and Native Americans. These uniquely designed hollow candles are placed one at a time in a person's ear while they are lying down, a towel protecting their hair and face. An assisting person holds the candle and lights the top. When it burns down and feels warm to the person holding it, the candle is plunged into a nearby glass of water.

Upon examination of the candle, the bottom portion will be filled with one to several inches of wax. Amazing but true. I have found these candles beneficial in improving hearing when due to blockage and even in some cases of earaches. To order these, send $5 to Candles, 619 Oberlin, Glenwood Springs 81601

THE BETTER TO HEAR YOU WITH, MY DEAR

Helen Keller, who became blind and deaf early in childhood, considered hearing loss "a much worse misfortune." More than twelve million people in the U.S. are deaf and the number is increasing. Accumulations of fat and mucus in the inner ear can impair hearing, thus it may be helpful to eliminate foods like fatty meats and dairy products. The auditory nerve vibrates in response to sound and if it is coated it can lose its sensitivity. The cochlea contains a fluid that transmits sound vibration. Should this fluid become overly thick and sticky due to dietary imbalances sound transmission may also be impaired.

An eardrum that is overly loose (often due to excess use of sugary, cold foods and drugs) will not be able to conduct sound well. The food most likely to contribute to ear congestion would have to be ice cream, being dairy, cold and sugary. Foods that have a long tradition of being considered beneficial to the ears include azuki, kidney and black beans, green leafy vegetables like kale, collards and mustard greens, dark yellow vegetables such as pumpkin, acorn and butternut squashes, garlic and onions. One tablespoon of rice bran syrup taken daily improves circulation and may improve hearing. I am very fond of eating wild violet leaves (*Viola odorata*) in salads for strengthening the ears. Don't mow your lawn! Learn to eat it! In Oriental medicine, the ears are said to correlate to the kidneys. The kidneys are often treated with acupunture or moxibustion to help improve the ears. It is interesting that the ears and kidneys are similarily shaped.

Exercise benefits the ears by increasing lymph flow. Yoga postures that improve various ear disorders include The Palm Pose, The Lion, The Wheel, The Plow, The Shoulder Stand and The Neck Pose. An exercise to improve hearing is done by covering one ear at a time with the palm of one's hand. Tap firmly with two fingertips of the other hand 50 to 100 times every day. Also gently tap the sides of the head above the ears.

Massaging a few drops of cajeput oil in front of and behind the ears helps to improve hearing by increasing circulation. Applying a ginger compress over the ears and kidney area helps to break up accumulations of fat and mucus.

The herb ginkgo (*Ginkgo biloba*) has shown great potential in improving hearing loss, especially when due to nerve deafness. Ginkgo leaves increase cerebral and peripheral blood flow and improve nerve transmission. This herb may be used as a tea, extract or in capsule form.

Machinery is making the Western world noisier by one decibel a year. It is a blessing to retreat periodically into nature and really listen to the gentle sounds She makes. By focusing our awareness on the subtler sounds we learn another aspect of hearing. Humans can't hear frequencies below 16 cycles, which is truly a blessing, otherwise we would hear the sounds of air molecules colliding!

Our ears give us so much that we often take for granted. They are an asset worth learning how to nurture, keep clear and healthy and care for safely.

Listen to the sound of the Universe.

Herbs for Children

ROSEMARY GLADSTAR SLICK

A long time ago when I was just a child, my grandmother took me to her gardens and introduced me to her 'weeds.' When we would walk in the scented oak forest, she would rub my skin with fresh bay leaves assuring me it would prevent me from catching poison oak and the insects from swarming. When I fell in the nettle patches, she eased the painful welts with the fresh juice of the plant.

She taught me how to knit with chicken feathers and special games to play with the shiny, smooth bones she kept on the mantle. Her teachings were without fuss; strong and powerful like herself, they sank deep into the heart and there took root. That magic my grandmother taught me in the garden of my childhood has stayed with me throughout my life.

Herbalism instills in one a deep appreciation for the Mother Earth and a knowledge of natural healing and well being. Children learn this gift so quickly and what they learn stays with them throughout their lifetimes. I have taken many a group of small children out on herb walks. What a lively event. They scamper about in noisy excitement; their attention span lasts but a few moments. But in that precious time they learn and retain what most adults struggle for hours on an herb walk to learn.

Not only do herbs serve as wonderful teachers for our children, but they provide an effective, gentle system of healing for them. Children are so sensitive and respond naturally and quickly to the healing energy of herbs. Administered wisely, herbs do not upset the delicate ecological balance of their small bodies as does much of modern medicine, but rather work in harmony with their systems.

Though herbology as a healing art is recognized as the first of humanity's medicines and has been carried in the hearts of the people since time began, it is little understood today. In teaching our children how to use herbs as a way of life, we carry on the tradition of this beautiful, effective and ancient healing system.

HERBS FOR CHILDREN

Almost any herb that is safe for an adult is safe for a child's system and can be used in an herbal formula. However, there are some herbs that I consider "Children's Herbs." These herbs work with a gentle and sure action. Gentle here does not mean less effective; gentleness can be very strong, but there is a sweet presence to the gentle herbs, a soft beauty, the ability to be effective in a gentle, quiet way. It is reminiscent of feminine power. It is from these gentle herbs that I most often draw my botanics for children's formulas. If I must, or choose to, use stronger medicinals, I generally formulate them in a base of these gentle herbs. I find that a child's system is very sensitive and responsive. There is an inherent wisdom that is still very connected with the Mother Earth and her natural gifts. A child's body will often respond quickly to herbal medicine as if it innately understands it.

The following list of herbs will cover most children's health needs. Many are delicious and can be formulated with other less tasty herbs to make flavorful medicinal blends. Each of these herbs can safely be used over a long period of time with no harmful side effects. Though all are gentle and mild in their actions, they are also very effective. Remember, gentle does not mean less strong.

If you have small children in your household, I suggest having on hand one ounce of each of the following herbs. Store them in glass bottles with tight fitting lids. Be sure to label the jars for it is almost impossible to remember them all once they are neatly tucked away. Herbs will retain their properties best if stored in air tight glass jars out of direct light and in a cool storage area. It is important that you use *high quality* herbs and *store them properly* for them to be effective.

THE HERBS

Slippery Elm bark, *Ulmus fulva*
Marshmallow root and leaf, *Athea officinalis*
Comfrey leaf, *Symphytum officinalis*
Wild Cherry bark, *Prunus virginiana*
Fenugreek seeds, *Trigonella feonum-graecum*
Fennel seeds, *Foeniculum vulgare*
Chamomile flowers, *Anthemis nobillis* and related species
Catnip leaf and flowers, *Nepeta cataria*
Red Clover flowers, *Trifolium pratense*
Anise seed, *Pimpenella anisum*
Dill seed, *Anethum graveolens*

Borage flowers and leaves, *Borago officinalis*
Rosehips, *Rosa canina* and related species
Nettle leaf, *Urtica dioica*
Red Raspberry leaf and flower, *Rubis idaeus*
Oatstraw, *Avena fatva* and *sativa*
Hibiscus flowers, *Hibiscus sabdariffa* and related species
Spearmint, *Mentha spicata*
Peppermint, *Mentha piperata*
Licorice root, *Glycyrrhiza glabra*
Echinacea, *Augustafolia, Purpurea* and related species

People often express concern about using strong herbs such as gold-enseal, echinacea, valerian and yellow dock for children. I've found them to be extremely useful and effective and I don't hesitate to use them when necessary. But I do recommend they be used in conjunction with the milder herbs listed above. Follow the dosages recommended on the Dosage Chart as well. Do not make the common mistake of thinking that what is stronger is always what is most effective. In herbal medicine, some of the most gentle herbs have the ability to produce the surest results and long-term benefits.

CHILDREN'S HERBAL TEA FORMULAS FOR GENERAL HEALTH

I've included here some of my favorite tea recipes for children's good health. Each of the following recipes taste delicious and can be drunk either by itself or mixed with fruit juice to sweeten. If there is a particular tea recipe your child enjoys and/or needs, I suggest mixing up a quart of the blend so it is on hand. Always keep a teapot full and warm on the stove, and in the warmer months, keep a bottle of iced herbal tea in the refrigerator.

High Calcium Tea

An excellent blend of herbs that adds high quality bio-chelated calcium and other important minerals to the diet. Good for children before and during teething, and during growth spurts. This is an excellent tea to administer if there is any bone or musculature injury.

1 part nettle
1 part oatstraw
1 part raspberry leaf
1 part comfrey leaf
2 parts lemon grass

2 parts spearmint and/or peppermint
3 parts rosehips
6 parts fennel seed
1/2 part cinnamon
*Optional: 1/8 part stevia (sweet herb)

Calming/Relaxing Tea

This blend is especially useful for calming a fussy child. It is gently soothing and can be used over a period of time as a tonic for the nervous system. This blend is also helpful during crisis such as colic, fevers, teething and other stressful situations.

1/2 part oatstraw
1/2 part comfrey leaf
1/2 part catnip
1/2 part passion flower
1 part licorice root
1 part slippery elm bark
1 part rose petals
2 parts chamomile
2 parts chrysanthemum flower
2 parts spearmint or peppermint
*Optional: 1/8 part stevia (sweet herb)

High C Tea

A wonderfully refreshing blend, High C Tea provides the bioflavinoids and vitamin C in an organic, naturally bio-chelated base so that all the nutrients are readily available for assimilation. We are so used to seeing ridiculously high dosages of vitamins and minerals and are taught to think these high numbers mean more efficiency. In fact, our bodies are better able to assimilate vitamins and minerals in the dosages and balanced formulas that nature has provided for centuries.

1 part cinnamon chips
2 parts lemon grass
1 part hibiscus
1 part nettle
4 parts rosehips
1/2 part orange peel
1 part spearmint

3 parts wintergreen
*Optional: 1/8 part stevia (sweet herb)

Respiratory Tonic Tea

This blend is an effective and tasty tea for building strong, healthy lungs. It is especially helpful for children that have recurring respiratory problems such as colds, flus, hay fever, asthma, ear infections and general congestion. Used over a period of time, it will aid in creating a healthy respiratory system.

1 part red clover flower
1 part comfrey leaf
1 part mullein
1 part coltsfoot
2 parts lemon grass
4 parts rosehips
4 parts fennel
1 part calendula

HOW TO DETERMINE DOSAGE FOR CHILDREN

There are several different techniques used to determine the proper dosage for children. Most herbalists rely on years of experience and intuition. When I am suggesting herbs for small children, I take into account the size of the child, general constitution, the illness and the herbs being used. Then I pray and let the old herb spirit guide me. The following charts will help provide sound guidelines for prescribing the proper amount of herbs. It is important, however, to consider the size, weight and general constitution of the child. Also consider the nature of the illness and the quality and strength of the herbs being used. These are all important considerations, especially when you're using the stronger, more potent herbs in the child's formula.

A. Young's Rule: Child's age divided by twelve plus the age.
   i.e. Dosage for a 4-year-old: $4/(12+4) = 4/16 = 1/4$ of adult
B. Cowling's Rule: Year number of next birthday is divided by 24.
   i.e. 3 turning 4 years old: $4/24 = 1/6$ of adult.
C. Dosage Chart
1. When Adult Dose is One Teacupful
Children 1- year old or less   2 teaspoonfuls
Children 2 to 4 years old   3 teaspoonfuls

| Children 4 to 7 years old | 1 tablespoon |
| Children 7 to 11 years old | 2 tablespoons |

2. When Adult Dose is One Teaspoonful, or Sixty Grains/Drops

Children 3 months old or less	2 grains
Children 3 to 6 months	3 grains
Children 6 to 9 months	4 grains
Children 9 to 12 months	5 grains
Children 12 to 18 months	7 grains
Children 18 to 24 months	8 grains
Children 2 to 3 years	10 grains
Children 3 to 4 years	12 grains
Children 4 to 6 years	15 grains
Children 6 to 9 years	24 grains
Children 9 to 12 years	30 grains

HOW TO ADMINISTER HERBS TO CHILDREN

One has to be innovative when administering herbs to children. Often times the herbs taste unfamiliar or bitter and children are not always willing to try them. Since consistency, both when treating adults and children, is the key to the herbs' effectiveness, it is necessary to develop preparations and recipes that are pleasant and easy to take. I'd like to share some of my favorite ways to administer herbs to children. These suggestions come from years of observing what children will and will not accept. Each child, of course is unique, and what is acceptable for one may or may not work for another. Each age group brings with it a different set of challenges. Be innovative and creative with a willingness to work with the individual nature of each child. The following suggestions are offered as gentle guidelines.

HERB TEAS

There are many delicious and naturally sweet herbs that can be used to flavor the bitter and less familiar flavors of some of the medicinal herbs. With a little creativity you can make good-tasting medicinal blends that both you and your children will enjoy. For instance, try mixing herbs like stevia (sweet herb), marshmallow root, licorice root, fennel seed, anise seed, Chinese star anise, mints, hibiscus, cinnamon, ginger, etc. in for flavor and effect. Teas can also be sweetened by mixing with fruit juice. Warm apple juice mixed with most teas is very good, especially if you add a stick of cinnamon. For a medicinal tea to be effective, it must be administered several times daily. Use the Dosage Chart as a guideline.

HERB CANDY

I call these "Jump for Joy Balls." They are a favorite way to administer herbs to children (and adults) both because they taste delicious and are very effective. The herbs are powdered, then mixed into a paste made with ground fruits and nuts and/or nut butters and honey. You can flavor these in so many ways.

The basic recipe is:

1. Grind raisins, dates, apricots and walnuts in a food processor or grinder.
2. Stir in coconut and carob powder. Mix the herb powders in well.
3. A variation on this recipe is to mix nut butter with honey, about equal portions. Stir in powdered herbs, coconut, carob chips, and other goodies.
4. Roll into balls and roll again in powdered carob or coconut. Store in refrigerator.
5. To determine the daily dosage, it is necessary to know how much powdered herb you included in the total recipe and how many herb balls this amount made. Determine the dosage of herb by using charts provided below. Divide the candy into daily dosages.

SYRUPS

Syrups are delicious, concentrated extracts of the herbs cooked into a sweet medicine with the addition of honey and/or fruit juice. Glycerin may be substituted for honey. It is an excellent medium for the herbs and is very nutritious for children. (For recipe for syrup see my pamphlet *Medicinal Herbal Preparations.*)

HERBAL BATHS

Soothing and calming, an herbal bath can work wonders on a child's nervous system (and the parents, as well). Herbal baths are also an excellent way to get the essence of the herbs into the child's system. The warm water opens the pores of the skin, the largest organ of elimination and assimilation, and the herbal nutrients flow in. The various temperatures of the water will affect the healing quality of the bath. Cool to tepid water is excellent when trying to lower the temperature of fevers. A warm bath relaxes the child and is soothing to the nervous system. There are many herbs that can be used in the baby's bath. My favorites are chamomile, lavender, roses, comfrey, and calendula.

HERB POWDERS

Herbs can be powdered and used directly in food and drinks. This is an excellent way to administer herbs to children because it is simple, effective, and the flavors of the bitter herbs can usually be masked. It is also easy to regulate the dosage of the herbs being used.

TINCTURES

Tinctures are concentrated extracts of herbs. They are taken simply by diluting a few drops of the tincture in warm water/juice. The flavor can usually be masked by the juice, so children readily take it. Most tinctures are made with alcohol as the primary solvent. Though the amount of alcohol is very small, many people choose not to use alcohol based tinctures for a variety of reasons. Tinctures can also be made by using either vegetable glycerin or apple cider vinegar as the solvent, both of which are very effective for children. The alcohol in alcohol based tinctures can also be removed quite easily by placing the tincture in boiling water for one to two minutes. The alcohol will quickly boil away, leaving just the herb residue. Since tinctures are quite concentrated, it is important to follow the recommended dosages on the individual bottle and/or the guidelines on the Dosage Chart provided.

MOTHER'S MILK

For infants this is the most effective and safest way to administer herbs. The mother drinks the herbal medicine in tea and/or tincture form. It quickly goes into the blood stream and then into the mother's milk making it readily available to the nursing child. It is necessary for the mother to drink at least 6-8 cups of the tea daily. Not only will the baby have the benefits of the gentle healing herbs, but mother will as well.

HERBAL POPS

These herbal popsicles are a fun and easy way to get a child to take their prescribed tea formula. Make a strong herbal tea and mix with equal amounts of fruit juice. Place in ice cube trays or popsicle molds. These herbal pops are refreshing in the summer time and provide the wonderful healing properties of the herbs in a delicious and fun form. Because they are so cold, I do not recommend them for cold types of imbalances such as flus, sore throats, colic, ear infections, etc.

HERBAL ENEMAS

Warm catnip enemas will bring down a child's fever and provide necessary fluid to the system when nothing else works. It is also an excellent way to administer the healing essences of the herbs into a sick and feverish body. Though unfamiliar to most people these days, enemas are a time-tested home remedy and quite painless for the recipient. To prepare an herbal enema for a child with a fever, cold or flu: Make 1/2 quart of catnip tea using 2 tablespoons of herb per 1/2 quart of water. Remove from heat and let cool to proper temperature; use a cool enema to lower fevers and to cleanse the lower bowels; use a warm (body temperature) enema to calm the nervous system and for colic, tension, etc. Strain well and pour liquid (about 1/2 quarter) into enema bag. Place enema bag at shoulder height so that liquid can flow smoothly. Lubricate the tip of enema with herbal salve or oil. *Slowly* release a gentle flow of liquid. You would be wise to have the child in a tub. The longer the child holds the liquid in the more effective the enema. It is helpful, after withdrawing the tip, to fold a towel and press slightly over the anus for a few minutes to aid in retention. But even if the child holds the enema in for just a couple of minutes, the enema will be effective.

HERBAL REMEDIES FOR CHILDREN'S HEALTH PROBLEMS

The following information is gathered from years of working with parents and their children and observing them going through the crises of growing up. Many of those children I met in the early days of my herbal work now bring children of their own to see me. It touches my heart with wonder.

This information is shared in the spirit that it may assist you in helping your child through the illnesses of childhood. It is not meant to replace the professional advice of your family doctor, but rather to complement and to assist it.

TEETHING

Unavoidable, teething happens to all children with varying degrees of discomfort. Though not an illness, it generally is a time of frustration for both parent and child; for parents because it seems no matter how hard they try they can't remove the pain and thus feel helpless; for the child because he/she is experiencing one of the early pains of life and it hurts!

There are certainly steps one can take to eliminate some of the discomfort:

1. Catnip tea is an old standby for both child and parent during the teething times. Catnip is soothing to the nervous system and helps to relieve acute pain. It is also helpful for teething-related fevers.

Administer as tea and/or tincture. Give in small dosages frequently. The tea itself is not tasty so you may wish to formulate with other gentle nervines such as chamomile, roses, passion flower, etc.

2. High Calcium Tea is very helpful to give to the child throughout the teething period. It is most effective if it is given several weeks/months before teething begins.

3. Teething symptoms can often be relieved by giving frequent doses of a high vitamin C syrup. Give 2 to 4 drops of rose hip syrup every hour for infants. For older children give 100 to 200 mg vitamin C in acerola tablets daily along with frequent doses of rose hip syrup.

4. Hyland's Homeopathic Pharmacy makes a wonderful herbal teething tablet for children. I've had several parents tell me that Hyland's Colic formula is even more effective for teething than the teething tablet. They both work well and are available in most natural food stores.

5. Iced Catnip/Chamomile Popsicles are excellent for the child to suck on. The cold helps numb the gums and relieves the pain.

*I do not recommend using clove oil on a child's gums. Though very effective for relieving toothaches in adults, the oil is far too strong for a child's mouth. Some people do dilute it in vegetable oil for teething children. However, I still caution about its use on children. *Never let children put clove oil on their own gums.*

COLIC

Colic, a term used to describe an infant's tummy ache, can be a heartwrenching experience both for the parents and infant. It is caused by painful spasmodic contractions of the infant's immature digestive tract and by air and gas being trapped in the intestines. The digestive tract of an infant is very sensitive at birth and generally takes about 3 months to mature. (Miraculously, this is the time period in which most colic clears up.) Depending on the degree of sensitivity, mealtimes can be a painful ordeal both for the parent and infant. The following suggestions are all gentle and effective and work in harmony with the sensitive nature of the infant child.

1. Often colicky children are extremely sensitive to their environment. Since you, the parent, *are* its primary environment and source of emotional and physical nourishment, your well-being can contribute to the presence or absence of colic. Quiet peaceful music during mealtimes is often helpful. Drink warm nervine teas

before nursing. Feeding time should, whenever possible, be a quiet restful sharing. Turn the TV off. If you are feeling stressed out and tense, the infant will often respond with similar energy. This does not mean that all colicky babies have stressed out parents, but it is important to note that the environment is conducive to creating peace and well-being for the child.

2. If nursing, mothers should avoid foods that are irritating to the infant's digestive tract. The brassica family which includes cabbage, broccoli, cauliflower, kale, collards, etc. are high in sulphur which creates gas in the intestines. Avoid hot spicy foods; an infant's system just isn't ready for them yet. And avoid chocolate, peanuts/peanut butter, and foods rich in sugar; these foods slow down the digestive action and will add to the spasms and contractions of colic. Though the amount of caffeine in your daily coffee may not seem to directly affect you anymore, it is nonetheless a powerful stimulant. Your child's young system will respond readily to this drug's stimulating properties and may become nervous and highly excitable. Coffee is also very acidic and will adversely affect the immature digestive system of the infant adding to the difficulties of colic.

3. Acidophilus is highly recommended for infant colic. It helps to build up a healthy intestinal flora and supports the growth of digestive enzymes. There are special preparations of acidophilus for children available in most natural food stores. Be sure you get an active, viable form of acidophilus. Double the amount suggested on the label for treating colic. A standard dose would be 1/4 teaspoon 4–5 times daily for relieving the symptoms of colic.

4. If the child is eating solid foods, include daily servings of yogurt, kefir and buttermilk. These foods aid in the development of healthy intestinal flora. If nursing, the mother should eat several servings a day of these foods.

5. The herbs most helpful for the acute symptoms of colic are slippery elm, fennel, anise, dill and catnip. The following teas are ones we've successfully used for the acute symptoms of colic.

Slippery Elm Gruel
1 part Slippery Elm bark
1 part Marshmallow root
1/2 part Cinnamon bark chips
Sweeten with maple syrup

Add 1 tablespoon of herb mixture to 1 cup of boiling water and simmer over *low* heat for 15 to 20 minutes. (Keep lid on the pan.) Straining the gruel will be the hardest part of making this tea. Both slippery elm and comfrey are extremely mucilaginous which, though very soothing and healing to the intestinal tract, is very difficult to strain. Line a large strainer with cheesecloth, pour the tea into it, and let it slowly drain through. When cool enough to handle, gather up the cheese cloth and squeeze the remaining gruel through. Sweeten with maple syrup. This gruel (thick tea) is wonderfully soothing and healing. It is also extremely nourishing. Store the liquid in the refrigerator and warm to use. The infant may drink as much of this tea as he/she wishes. If nursing, the mother should drink 3–4 cups daily.

Seed Tea
Dill and anise were at one time such favorite herbs for colic that English nursery rhymes were written in honor of them. The following tea helps to expel gas and relieve the systems of colic.
1 part fennel
1 part Dill
3 parts Anise
3 parts Chamomile
1/4 part Catnip
1/8 part Stevia
Infuse 1 teaspoon in 1 cup boiled water and let sit, covered, for 45 minutes. Strain. Give the infant teaspoon dosages every few minutes until colic pain ceases. This tea may also be given effectively in small dosages before feeding time.

6. Hyland's Pharmacy has a homeopathic colic tablet that is very good. It is available in most natural food stores.
7. In the midst of a colic attack, there are a couple of old fashioned and effective techniques to try. One, place your baby in a warm herb bath. If bottle fed, the baby can enjoy his/her feeding from the comfort of a warm, soothing bath. Or, you may relax the stomach muscles by placing a towel that was soaked in hot herb tea such as chamomile and lavender (both nervines) over the stomach area. Be certain the towel is adequately warm but not hot. The combination of warm water and herbal essence will often be just what's needed to stop the muscle spasms. A drop or two of lavender and/

or chamomile essential oil dropped in either the bath water or on the towel will often work wonders.

8. And there is always the old reliable bounce-n-pat technique. Bounce the child on your knee and/or pat on your shoulder until he/she is hypnotized into forgetting the problem. It really seems to work.

CRADLE CAP

Neither a serious or contagious problem, a child will usually outgrow cradle cap in time. The sebaceous glands of most infants are not developed and may oversecrete causing a yellowish oily crust on the child's scalp. You can remove the "cap" and help regulate the activity of the sebaceous glands by gently massaging a mixture of herbs and olive oil (recipe below) into the scalp two or three times daily. Leave the herb/oil mixture on overnight. The next morning the crust can be easily removed by gently massaging. Shampoo with a mild baby shampoo.

Most children will just outgrow cradle cap but if it persists, give the infant a warm tea of the following herbs:

Tea for Cradle Cap
1 part Red Clover flower
1 part Burdock root
1 part Mullein leaf
To make: Steep 1 teaspoon of herb mixture in 1 cup boiled water for half an hour. Strain. To an infant, administer 2 teaspoons of the tea 3–4 times daily.

Oil/Herb Mixture for Cradle Cap
1 part dried Nettle
1 part Chamomile flowers
1 part Mullein leaf
To make: Put herbs in a double boiler and cover with olive oil. Cook over very low heat for about one hour. Strain and bottle. Store at room temperature for easier, warmer application.

DIAPER RASH

Most diaper rashes respond readily to natural therapy. Follow the suggestions listed with good faith; all have been used successfully by countless mothers. If the diaper rash is persistent and does not get better, it could be a herpes-related virus and/or yeast type fungus. Consult your family practitioner in such cases.

Diaper rashes are generally caused by:

1. Irritating, harsh detergents which leave a soap residue on the diapers. Simply change soaps. Use mild soap flakes such as Ivory or a liquid soap such as Heavenly Horsetail or Basic H. Do not use detergents, ammonia or bleach.
2. Foods that irritate the child's digestive system. Citrus and other high acid foods are major irritants and can affect the child both through the mother's milk or by eating these foods directly.
3. Teething, fever and other stress-related incidents.

What to do:

1. Administer 1/4 teaspoon acidophilus culture three times daily. Use a preparation prepared especially for children.
2. Diapers

   Leave diapers off as much as possible. The more exposure to air and sunlight the better. If sunlight is not in season and the diaper rash is persistent, a sunlamp will prove helpful. Expose baby's bottom for five minutes to it, 3–4 times daily.

   Use only 100% cotton diapers and change after every bowel movement. Rinse the baby's bottom frequently and dry thoroughly.

   If your child is prone to diaper rash, you may choose to do away with plastic panties, a prime contributor to rashes. Use instead, a natural wool soaker. These are nonirritating, are highly absorbent, and are available in places that supply baby products.
3. Use arrowroot powder and/or a special clay/herb mix for your baby powder and as a remedy for diaper rash. (Recipes follow.) Cornstarch, an old-fashioned powder used frequently on babies, is also very effective, but is not recommended for use on yeast-related diaper rashes as it may encourage the growth of certain yeast. Commercial baby powder is made with talc which is a known carcinogen. It also contains synthetic scents which can be irritating to an infant's sensitive skin. Make your own baby powder or buy those that are made with natural ingredients that are beneficial to your baby.
4. An herbal salve made with St. John's wort, comfrey leaf and root, and calendula is one of the best remedies I know of for diaper rash. (Recipe follows.) Wash and dry the baby's bottom, after each bowel movement, apply the herbal salve and light dust with clay/herb powder. This treatment plan used in conjunction with the other suggestions listed will generally clear up a diaper rash.

5. For a more serious rash, mix the clay/herb powder with water or a tea of comfrey to form a thin paste. Smooth over rash and leave on for half an hour to forty-five minutes. To remove, gently rinse with warm water or soak off in a warm tub.

INFANT DIARRHEA

There are probably few babies that have not had a bout of diarrhea, or its counterpart, constipation. Diarrhea can have a number of causes, the most common being: reactions to or excesses of certain food groups, reactions to bacteria and viruses, teething, fever, emotional upset, or as a complication of infection elsewhere in the body.

The primary concern with infant diarrhea is to be aware of dehydration. It can occur quickly if fluid intake is not being carefully monitored and can be fatal if severe. Be mindful that the infant's fluid intake is adequate. Monitor the amount of liquid the child drinks and give the child warm baths and/or enemas. These will help in the absorption of liquid.

Though liquid intake is essential, it is not necessary that the child eat solid food. It is actually best if they fast on liquids such as herb teas, vegetable broths and chicken soup. Eating solid food will make the already stressed digestive system work overtime. It also means more runny diapers as everything eaten will quickly come out. If the child wishes to eat, allow foods such as yogurt, kefir, buttermilk, cottage cheese, potato soup, mashed potatoes (no gravy or butter) and slippery elm gruel. These foods are easy to digest and will contribute to healing the digestive system.

Along with a high fluid intake, herbal baths, and a very simple diet as suggested above, the following suggestions should remedy the diarrhea:

1. **Blackberry Root Tincture.**
   Mix 1 teaspoon of tincture in 1/2 cup warm water and administer 1/4 teaspoon of this preparation every hour.

2. **Tea for Diarrhea**
   3 parts Blackberry root
   2 parts Slippery Elm bark
   To make: Simmer 1 teaspoon of the herb mixture in 1 cup water for 20 minutes. Strain and cool. Administer 2–4 tablespoons every hour or more often as needed.

3. Administer 1/8 teaspoon of acidophilus culture every hour until diarrhea stops.

CONSTIPATION

If your child develops constipation, the first step is to avoid all foods that could possibly contribute to the problem. Definitely eliminate dairy foods, cheese, wheat, eggs and refined, processed foods. If the child is nursing, the mother should avoid these foods in her diet until the constipation clears up. If the child is bottle fed on cow's milk, switch to goat's milk.

Include in the diet those foods which contribute to good elimination: fruits, vegetables, liquids, molasses, dried fruit and foods that supply bulk in the system. There are several herbs that should be included daily: carob powder, slippery elm, flax seed, psyllium seeds and Irish moss. None of these are laxative herbs per se, but provide necessary bulk in the diet.

The following suggestions combined with the dietary recommendations should help with your child's constipation:

1. 1/2 teaspoon acidophilus with meals.
2. Grind equal amounts of slippery elm powder, flax seed and psyllium seed together until finely powdered. Mix 1 teaspoon of the mixture in with food at each meal time.
3. Make a special "candy" by grinding prunes, figs, apricots and raisins together. Mix in powdered psyllium seed, slippery elm and fennel seed. To flavor, mix in carob powder, coconut and ground walnuts. Roll into balls and serve daily as a nourishing snack.
4. The following tea mixture will aid in curing constipation:
   1 part Slippery Elm
   1 part Irish Moss
   2 parts Psyllium seed
   4 parts Fennel seed
   2 parts Spearmint
   1/4 part Orange peel
   1/2 part Cinnamon
   To make: Simmer 1 teaspoon herb mixture in 1 cup boiling water for 20 minutes. Strain and cool. Administer 1/8 to 1/2 cup tea with meals and/or as often as needed.
5. For acute constipation administer a catnip enema. Follow directions as given on page 173.

EARACHES

Until a child is three or four years old, the ear canals are not fully formed and consequently do not drain well. When a child gets congested or has a cold, the ear canals get plugged up with excess mucus which cannot drain properly. Bacteria begins to grow in the extra moisture and infections occur. The use of antibiotics, though effective for acute situations, do not correct the cause of the problem. Antibiotics are also nondiscriminatory in what they destroy, so while doing their duty of destroying the infecting bacteria, they are also destroying the helpful bacteria needed to fight recurring infections. It is important when using antibiotics to follow the suggestions listed below.

Ear infections can be potentially serious. Treated improperly, they can leave a child with impaired hearing, or worse, permanently deaf. It is important to treat an ear infection at the first sign of the infection and to work conjointly with a holistic practitioner and/or your family pediatrician. If treated at the onset of the problem, ear infections can be avoided. Watch for the early signs of infection: congestion, colds, runny nose, fevers, excessive rubbing/pulling of the ear lobe combined with irritability and fussiness.

Ear infections can result from allergies. If your child has recurring ear infections despite your best efforts, check the possibility of allergies. Wheat, citrus and dairy products including milk, cheese and ice cream are the most common offenders.

What to do for Ear Infections

1. One of the best herbal remedies is garlic and/or mullein flower oil. Warm to the temperature of mother's milk and drop a couple of drops down each ear. It is important to treat both ears; the ear canals are connected and the infection can move back and forth. Administer the warm herb oil every half hour or as often as needed. It not only helps fight the infection, but relieves the pain as well.

   To make Garlic/Mullein Flower Oil:
   Chop fresh garlic. Mix with 1/2 ounce of fresh or dried mullein *flowers* (not the leaves). Place in double boiler and cover with olive oil. Over very low heat, warm for one hour. Strain well and bottle. To use, take a small amount of oil in a teaspoon and hold over candle or stove top to warm to the temperature of 'mother's milk.' Suction into dropper and apply into each ear.

2. Avoid all congesting type foods: eggs, dairy, wheat, sugar, orange juice and all refined, processed foods.

3. Administer 1/8 teaspoon of the following tincture diluted in warm water or juice three times daily:
   1 part Golden Seal root

1 part Myrrh
2 parts Slippery Elm bark
1 part Echinacea root
1 part Ginger root
*These herbs can also be powdered and capsulated to administer to older children.

4. Acidophilus culture, 1/2 teaspoon several times daily.
5. A tasty tea of fresh grated ginger, fresh squeezed lemons and honey or maple syrup is a refreshing, decongesting blend.
6. Be certain the child's kidneys are working well and he/she is taking in sufficient fluid. Warm packs placed over the lower back (the area of the kidneys) can help relieve ear infections.
7. It is imperative that the child gets plenty of rest and does not go out into the cold air prematurely. It is a common mistake to think a child has recovered from the ear infection and can be sent out to play. Ear infections should be treated for at least a week following the acute stage.
8. As prevention, hats with ear flaps should be worn by children prone to ear infections. Also, keep the area of the kidneys warm during cold weather.

FEVERS

Use the following techniques for lowering and/or controlling a child's fever. Fevers are a natural mechanism to rid the body of infection. It is only when the fever gets too high or lingers too long, that it can be debilitating. With small children, it is imperative to keep fluid intake high. Dehydration is the greatest danger of childhood fevers.

1. To lower a fever, bathe the child in a tepid bath. Mix 1/4 cup apple cider vinegar into the tub. Be certain there are no drafts in the room. After the bath, quickly wrap the child in a warm flannel sheet. Placing a drop or two of chamomile oil on the sheet is very helpful.
2. Wrap the child's feet in a cool cloth that has been dipped in a mixture of apple cider vinegar and water. Keep the child bundled warmly.
3. Administer a catnip enema in acute stages of fever. This will not only help to break the fever but insures fluid intake.
4. The following tea administered every 1/2 hour in small dosages is excellent for lowering fever:
2 parts Catnip
2 parts Elder

2 parts Peppermint
1 part Echinacea root
To make: Steep 1 teaspoon of the mixture in 1 cup boiled water for
one hour. Administer every 1/2 hour. See Dosage Chart.

RECIPES FOR CHILDREN'S PRODUCTS

I wanted to share some of my favorite recipes for baby products with
you. All are 100% natural and easy and fun to make.

Sleep Pillow

Create a very special sleep pillow to soothe your infant into a calm,
peaceful sleep. These herb pillows have proven helpful to children who
have trouble sleeping deeply and restfully.

To make: Mix equal amounts of chamomile, lavender, roses, and
hops together. Use about 4–6 ounces of herb per pillow and sew into an 8
x 8 inch cotton pillow. Use soft natural fabric for your pillow covering;
flannel is wonderful! Place near baby's head to help with a peaceful,
aromatic sleep.

Baby's Bath herbs

Use the following mixtures in the bath water. Place herbs in a cotton
cloth bag and allow to steep in the water. Use the fragrant herbal bag for
a wash cloth.

To make:
1 part Roses
2 parts Chamomile
2 parts Calendula
1 part Lavender
2 parts Comfrey

Mix together and use about 1 small handful for each bath.

Baby Salve

This is my very favorite salve recipe for diaper rash, cuts and scrapes,
and irritated skin.

1 part Comfrey leaf
1 part Comfrey root
1 part St. John's Wort flower
1 part Calendula flower

To make: Steep 2 ounces of herb mixture in 1 pint of olive oil for two
weeks. At the end of two weeks, place mixture in a double boiler and

slowly over *very* low heat, warm for 1 hour. Strain. To each cup of herbal oil, add 1/4 cup of beeswax. Grate the beeswax and add to warm oil. You may need to warm the oil a little longer to melt the beeswax. When the beeswax is melted, check for desired consistency by placing one table-spoon of the mixture in the refrigerator for a few minutes. If the salve is too hard, add a little more oil; if too soft, add a little more beeswax. Pour into a glass jar. This salve does not need to be refrigerated and will last for months (or years) if stored in a cool area.

Baby Powder

For an excellent daily baby powder mix the following ingredients together:

> 2 parts White Clay (Available in natural food stores and ceramic supply stores)
> 2 parts Arrowroot powder
> 1/4 part Slippery Elm powder
> 1/4 part Comfrey root powder

To make: Mix the powder together and place in a shaker bottle such as a spice jar. You may wish to lightly scent your baby powder but use only pure essential oils and be certain it is nonirritating to a child's sensitive skin. Orange oil is light and refreshing and often used as the scent for baby powders.

For diaper rash:

To the previous mixture, add 1/8 part golden seal powder, 1/8 part myrrh powder and 1/8 part echinacea. Apply as a powder, or mix into a thin paste and apply as a poultice to the rash.

Baby Oil

This is an excellent all-purpose oil and is wonderful to rub on baby after baths. It makes a great massage oil for babies also.

> 1 pint Apricot or Almond oil
> 1/2 ounce Roses
> 1 ounce Chamomile
> 1/2 ounce Comfrey

To make: Mix herbs and oil together and let sit in a glass jar with tight-fitting lid for two weeks. In a double boiler, slowly warm the mixture over very low heat for one hour. Strain and bottle. You may lightly scent with a pure essential oil such as chamomile or orange oil.

In Conclusion

I dearly hope the above information will help you in aiding your children through some of the problems of childhood. Many of the suggestions presented have been successfully used for years. This information combined with the advice of your family doctor and the inherent healing wisdom you possess, should enable you to make wise decisions about your child's health.

Rheumatoid Arthritis: A Case History

David Hoffman, B.S.C., M.N.I.M.H.

Name: E.J., Age: 42, Sex: Female, Marital Status: Married
Date of First Visit: June 1982
Address: Laugharne, Dyfed, Cymru (Wales)

Present Complaint: Rheumatoid Arthritis
Site of pain: Swelling, pain and increased temperature primarily in the knees, ankles, fingers. Generalized joint tenderness.
Duration of pain: Almost constant, with only slight diurnal changes.
Severity of pain: Confined to wheelchair most of the time. She described pain as "excruciating."
Timing of pain: Worse in the morning. Extreme fatigue in the afternoon and difficulty in sleeping.
Character: Constant deep ache, "excruciating" pain on movement.
Aggravating Factors: Heat and stress.
Relieving Factors: None other than medication.
Medical Treatment: Steroidal anti-inflammatories during flare-ups, aspirin regularly.
Previous History of Present Complaint: Rapid onset at age 23, initially in right knee.
Accompanying Symptoms: Gastric discomfort. Sleep disturbance because of pain. Depression. Obesity.
Medical History: Good health before onset of these symptoms.
Social History: Farmer. Little or no exercise. Does not smoke or drink alcohol. Typical Welsh diet (!).

SYSTEM REVIEW
Cardio-Vascular System: No cardio-vascular signs or symptoms. Blood pressure normal.
Respiratory System: Some dyspnea on exertion.

Gastro-Intestinal System: Appetite too good! Occasional constipation, with normal stools. Epigastric pain on empty stomach, triggered by non-steroidal anti-inflammatories.

Nervous System: Occasional headaches, diagnosed by Rheumatologist as early sign of arthritis in the cervical vertebrae. "Pins & Needles" and cramps regularly down both legs. Marked depression. Very disturbed sleep because of pain and worry.

Urinary System: No signs or symptoms.

Reproductive System: No signs or symptoms.

Musculo/Skeletal System: Pain in knees, ankles, fingers. Generalized joint tenderness, worse in morning. Generalized stiffness that is worse in the morning. Aggravated by heat, stress, sleeplessness. Patient not aware of any relieving factors other than medication. Generalized muscular fatigue.

Skin: No signs or symptoms.

The *Merck Manual* defines rheumatoid arthritis as "a chronic syndrome characterized by nonspecific, usually symmetric inflammation of the peripheral joints, potentially resulting in progressive destruction of articular and periarticular structures; generalized manifestations may also be present." It is a chronic inflammatory condition that involves not only the joints but other connective tissue as well, and being an auto-immune condition, it is identified by the presence of rheumatoid factor in the blood.

The joint destruction that can occur results from inflammation of the synovial membrane. As part of the auto-immune response, white blood cells and antibodies infiltrate the membranes causing them to proliferate. Persistent inflammation causes permanent damage to the joint cartilage, bones, ligaments and tendons, resulting in painful joints, loss of mobility, generalized soreness and depression.

ACTIONS INDICATED:

Immune System Support is essential for any fundamental change in this problem. However, what form this should take is problematic.

Anti-Rheumatics help but their selection must be based upon a rationale that relates to the individual.

Anti-Inflammatories are very important as much of the symptom picture is the direct result of the inflammatory process. The saponin-containing anti-inflammatories come into their own here, but the salicylate-containing herbs are still helpful, complementing each other well.

Alteratives are often the key to any attempt at transforming the systemic problem.

Anti-Spasmodics lessen the impact of physical friction by relaxing the muscular envelope around joints.

Circulatory Stimulants are not as important as in Osteo-Arthritis, but still must be considered. This difference reflects the role of the blood in both conditions.

Analgesics will ease both the pain and the stress response to this pain.

Nervines are especially relevant considering the acknowledged "psycho-somatic" component of this problem. Nervine relaxants also help as anti-spasmodics and nervine tonics help the person deal with the constant stress of the pain and discomfort. Hypnotics may help sleep in the face of pain. Tonics and anti-depressants will support the work of coping with this extremely tiring and debilitating condition.

Other actions such as bitters, diuretics or hepatics may be appropriate.

SPECIFIC REMEDIES:

There are no specific remedies for rheumatoid arthritis. This is only to be expected when the multifactorial nature of auto-immune conditions is taken into account. Of special relevance are the alterative anti-rheumatics, including *Menyanthes trifoliata* (bogbean), *Harpagophytum procumbens* (devil's claw), *Smilax* spp. (sarsaparilla) and *Arctium lappa* (burdock). *Guaiacum officinale* (Lignum vitae) and *Dioscorea villosa* (wild yam) are especially useful as anti-inflammatories. Beyond this it is down to the diagnostic skills of the practitioner combined with the patient's observance of dietary, lifestyle and dosage regime.

FIRST CONSULTATION

E.J. was in so much pain that she was unable to climb the stairs to my clinic, and so the first consultation took place in her car. I prioritized the treatment plan thus, giving medicine for 1 week:

- Alleviation of epigastric symptoms by reducing gastric inflammation, especially as the core remedies I wanted to give for the R.A. can irritate the mucosa, disrupting assimilation in a number of ways.
- Helping her sleep.

For epigastric symptoms (#1):

Symphytum officinale 25 ml. Liquid extract 1:1 in 25% alcohol (BHP[1])

Althaea officinalis 25 ml. Liquid extract 1:1 in 25% alcohol (BHP)

Filipendula ulmaria 25 ml. Tincture 1:5 in 45% alcohol (BHP)

Water 25 ml.

Total 100 ml.

for one week at a dosage of 5 ml. in total 3 times a day.

Infusion of *Matricaria recutita* or *Mellissa officinalis* sipped slowly throughout the day will help.

Note: Even though *F. ulmaria* is rich in salicylates, it not only does not cause inflammation, it can reverse many of the gastric symptoms caused by aspirin.

For sleep and pain relief (#2):

Valeriana officinalis 100 ml. Tincture 1:5 in 45% alcohol (BPC 1949)

Passiflora incarnata 50 ml. Tincture 1:8 in 45% alcohol (BHP)

Piscidia erythrina 25 ml. Liquid extract 1:1 in 60% alcohol (BPC 1939)

5–15 ml. of total 1/2 hour before retiring.

Note: Although few legal and effective analgesics are left for the phytotherapist, this combination often helps sleeplessness due to pain.

SECOND CONSULTATION

E.J. was in much better spirits, though still in extreme pain. She climbed the stairs with great difficulty, but was confident that the herbs would help. Her sleep had become easier and stomach problems had settled down. Medication was dispensed for 2 weeks. This consisted of:

- Repeat prescriptions of both #1 and #2 for symptomatic relief when necessary.
- Beginning treatment of the joint inflammation, but starting gently to avoid any potential irritation.

Prescription (#3):

Filipendula ulmaria 100 ml. Tincture 1:5 in 45% alcohol (BHP)

Salix alba 50 ml. Liquid extract 1:1 in 25% alcohol (BHP)

Valeriana officinalis 50 ml. Tincture 1:5 in 45% alcohol (BPC 1949)

Cimicifuga racemosa 50 ml. Tincture 1:10 in 60% alcohol (BPC 1934)

Apium graveolens 50 ml. Tincture 1:1 in 90% alcohol (BPC 1934)

Total 300 ml. for 2 weeks

First day 1/2 teaspoonful (2.5 ml.) 3 times a day with food.

Second day 1 teaspoonful (5 ml.) 3 times a day with food. If no gastric problems occur, increase to 1 teaspoonful 4 times a day with food.

Note: The focus is on anti-inflammatories and nervines, avoiding the stronger alteratives at this stage.

THIRD CONSULTATION

A slight subjective improvement in pain and stiffness, but observable brightening of demeanor. She told me that she felt "better in myself," a classic Welsh expression. There had been no epigastric or abdominal problems so I started the main treatment, dispensing enough for 1 month.

Long-term medication (#4):

> *Menyanthes trifoliata* 50 ml. Tincture 1:5 in 45% alcohol (BHP)
> *Filipendula ulmaria* 25 ml. Tincture 1:5 in 45% alcohol (BHP)
> *Dioscorea villosa* 25 ml. Tincture 1:5 in 45% alcohol (BHP)
> *Valeriana officinalis* 15 ml. Tincture 1:5 in 45% alcohol (BPC 1949)
> *Cimicifuga racemosa* 15 ml. Tincture 1:10 in 60% alcohol (BPC 1934)
> *Apium graveolens* 15 ml. Tincture 1:1 in 90% alcohol (BPC 1934)
> *Angelica archangelica* (folia) 15 ml. Tincture 1:5 in 45% alcohol (BHP)
> *Achillea millefolium* 15 ml. Tincture 1:5 in 45% alcohol (BHP)
> *Hypericum perforatum* 15 ml. Tincture 1:10 in 45% alcohol (BHP)
> *Guaiacum officinale* 10 ml. Tincture 1:5 in 90% alcohol (BPC 1934)
> Total 200 ml. For 2 weeks

First and second day 1/2 teaspoonful (2.5 ml.) 3 times a day with food.

If no gastric problems occur, increase to 1 teaspoonful (5 ml.) 3 times a day with food.

The digestive system must be working well so treat any stomach irritation as a priority. This combination does not take such problems into account. If there had been epigastric tenderness due to the *Menyanthes* or *Guaiacum*, I would have added *Althaea*. This combination provides a range of actions:

- alterative remedies—*Menyanthes, Guaiacum* and *Cimicifuga*
- salicylate anti-inflammatory—*Filipendula*
- saponin containing anti-inflammatory—*Dioscorea*
- general anti-inflammatories—*Angelica, Menyanthes, Guaiacum* and *Cimicifuga*
- nervine anti-spasmodics—*Valeriana, Cimicifuga* and *Apium*
- nervine tonic and anti-depressive—*Hypericum*
- diuretics—*Apium and Achillea*
- "stomachics," in this case carminatives and intestinal anti-inflmmatories—*Angelica, Valeriana* and *Apium*
- bitter tonics—*Menyanthes* and *Achillea*

BROADER CONTEXT OF TREATMENT

Nutritional factors are very important in the successful treatment of R.A., but unfortunately Wales is not a very nutritionally aware country! To ensure that my guidelines would be followed, I was forced to keep dietary constraints to a minimum. The focus was on avoiding foods that would aggravate her problems. The simple diet given to E.J. was:

- no coffee, whether decaf. or regular
- no red meat of any kind in any form
- no vinegar or anything based upon vinegar, such as pickles
- no vegetables that contain high levels of plant acids: e.g. tomatoes, rhubarb
- no berries rich in fruit acids such as gooseberries, red and black currants
- no red wine, port or sherry
- no carbonated drinks
- no shell fish
- no refined white sugar or products that contain it
- no refined white flour or its multitude of products
- no artificial additives, flavorings and preservatives
- no processed foods
- no food or beverage that causes the patient specific problems
- eat plenty of fresh green vegetables
- drink plenty of fresh spring water (from her own spring)
- eat whole grains whilst reducing potatoes.

Such diets produce the most dramatic results in the more acute stages, as happened with E.J. In the extreme of long-standing R.A., there is a balance that must be found between nutritional dogma that might not be too effective and eating habits that have a positive psychological effect on the patient.

Attention must be given to physical aids and support for the patient who is becoming disabled by this disease. There are a wealth of simple devices available that ease the simple daily tasks of life that have become taxing for the patient. These range from specially designed kitchen devices such as cutlery, can openers and faucet grips, to brushes with extended handles and adaptations to telephones. Using such Activities of Daily Living (A.D.L.) devices can ease the patient's experience of life enormously. These were supplied to E.J. by her National Health Service doctor.

Initially I had planned a stress management program for her, but when the pain and inflammation subsided it was no longer necessary.

OUTCOME

On her next consultation there was a measurable increase in movement of knees, and a further decrease in pain and stiffness. Treatment continued with visits every two months. There was a gradual improvement over the next six months leading to complete abandonment of the wheelchair. She still had arthritic pain but she considered it to be completely livable. A maintenance dose of a half teaspoonful (2.5) of prescription #4 twice a day was started. The following summer, during a rare Welsh heat wave, she had a bad flare-up, but it was quickly brought under control by increasing her maintenance dose temporarily.

Four years later, when I moved to America, she was still maintaining her much improved condition.

ENDNOTES

1. *British Herbal Pharmacopoeia,* 1983, pub. by The British Herbal Medicine Association.

HIV Positive:
A Case History

MICHAEL TIERRA, O.M.D.

Name: R.E., Age: 30, Sex: male,
Date of first consultation: July 1991
Address: Port Arthur, Texas
Primary Complaint: HIV Positive

Diagnosed with a T-cell count of 340 (normal may vary from 1400 to 2700 in children). His mother reported accompanying symptoms of repeated susceptibility to respiratory illness, mental haziness, weakness and diarrhea. He did not want to undergo conventional medical treatment using AZT and preferred using herbs.

DIAGNOSIS:

Deficient kidney and lung yin because of the generalized wasting syndrome characteristic of later stages of this disease, with deficient heat.

DISCUSSION:

AIDS and the related HIV syndromes are caused by a severe compromise of the immune system accompanied by degenerative wasting, inflammation and skin cancer. The root cause of the disease in Traditional Chinese medicine is centered around kidney yin deficiency with damage to the body's essence chi. A further extension of this is manifested with a deficiency of lung yin which results in respiratory illness and most dangerously, pneumonia. According to TCM, the lungs also govern the skin so that in advanced stages of AIDS there is the appearance of various lesions and cancers.

Treatment must focus on nourishing the yin with demulcent, nourishing tonic herbs such as American ginseng (*Panax quinquefolium*), marshmallow root (*Althea officinalis*), slippery elm (*Ulmus fulva*), Iceland moss (*cetraria islandica*), comfrey root (*Symphytum officinalis*), acorn gruel, oatmeal, raw eggs, Siberian ginseng (*Eleutherococcus senticosus*), *Schizandra chinensis, Rehmannia glutinosa,* lycii berries, ho shou wu (*Polygonum multiflorum*), privet berries (*Ligustrum lucidi*) and saw palmetto berries (*Serrenoa*).

While many of these have scientifically proven immune potentiating properties, two of the most important herbs, known to stimulate the deep immune system, increasing both T and B cells, are *Astragalus membranicus* (huang chi) and reishi mushroom (*Ganoderma lucidum*).

The advantage of using reishi mushroom over astragalus is that it is classified as having a spirit strengthening but neutral energy, strengthening all vital organs of the body, especially the lungs. Astragalus is classified as a chi tonic which focuses on strengthening the spleen-pancreas (deep assimilation) and lungs. It tonifies the "wei chi" or defensive immune system of the lungs which makes it very important to prevent respiratory illness and other externally contracted diseases. Having a mildly warm energy, however, alone it may be unsuitable especially for advanced cases of AIDS with severe inflammation. The extreme complication of this condition absolutely necessitates an approach combining both warming, tonifying and nourishing herbs and foods, with some cooling, anti-inflammatory herbs.

Some anti-inflammatory herbs appropriate for the treatment of this condition include: echinacea root (*Echinacea angustifolia, pallida* or *purpureum*), chaparral (*Larrea tridenta*), pau d'arco (*Tabebuia heptaphylla*), garlic (*Allium sativum*) and goldenseal (*Hydrastis canadensis*).

Other herbs to help regulate digestion and assimilation include tangerine peel (*chen pi*) and *Atractylodes alba*. Finally, herbs to help stabilize the spirit and calm the mind are useful because of the complication of the accompanied anxiety.

TREATMENT:

Because of the complex nature of this condition I prescribed herbal formulas which I use in my clinical practice:

Reishi Mushroom Supreme

Ganoderma (reishi) mushroom extract, polygala root (*Polygalae tenuifoliae*), which serves to both calm the spirit as well as help to expel phlegm from the lungs, *Zizyphus spinosa* seed which nourishes and calms the spirit, *Codonopsis pilosula* which tonifies chi and aids digestion and assimilation, *Atracylodes alba* and *Astragalus membranicus,* both of which tonify chi and help digestion, *Schizandra chinensis* berries which is an astringent herb that tonifies yin, nourishes essence, prevents leakage of energy, tangerine peel which helps assimilation, tang kuei (*Angelica sinensis*) which tonifies blood and promotes circulation, processes *Rehmannia glutinosa* which also tonifies blood and liver and kidney yin, *Poria cocos* which helps digestion.

Recommended dose per day of this formula was about 6 grams four times a day.

The next formula was the Yin Energetics Complex based on the famous Liu Wei di Huang formula from the sixth century. It consists of the following:

Yin tonics: lycii berries, ophiopogon root, *Rehmannia glutinosa, Schizandra chinensis*. These tonify the yin of kidney-adrenals, lung and heart.

Diuretics and herbs that direct the tonic action to the kidneys: *Fructus cornus, Radix alisma, Poria cocos*. Chi tonics: human placenta, *Dioscorea batatas*.

Anti-inflammatory: moutan peony.

Herbs which serve as catalysts to help balance the formula: achryanthes root, eucommia bark.

Recommended dose per day of this formula was 3 grams four times daily.

The next formula is Defense Force which consists of a number of the anti-inflammatory herbs together with immune tonic and yin nourishing herbs. It consists of the following: chaparral leaf, echinacea root, garlic, goldenseal, pau d'arco, ginger root, Siberian ginseng, suma (*Pfaffia paniculata*), astragalus root, *Ligustrum lucidum, Schizandra chinensis,* reishi mushroom.

Recommended dose per day of this formula was 3 grams three times daily.

Along with these formulas which were prescribed in tablet form, I recommended that the patient purchase a pound of good quality astragalus root and use approximately four slices per day boiled in a quart of water. This resultant tea is then used as stock to cook oatmeal and rice and/or make soup.

I did not have the opportunity during this first session to recommend the macrobiotic diet which is my usual procedure. This was done later after the patient experienced the following improvements.

After two weeks on the combined herbal program his T-cell count dramatically came up to 486. He then contracted a minor respiratory illness for which his doctor prescribed antibiotics. During this time he continued to take the herbs but his T-cell count dropped slightly. Two weeks after recovering from the illness his T-cell count went up to 514 with no further symptoms. After using the herbs for only ten weeks, his doctor feels that his condition is sufficiently stabilized. The patient is quite athletic, works out at the gym daily, has no further symptoms of diarrhea, weakness or unclear haziness.

Simpler Scents:
The Combined Uses of Herbs and Essential Oils

MINDY GREEN

Aromatherapy can be viewed as an extension of herbalism—a progression in learning more about the way plants can heal. Herbalism and aromatherapy have much to offer each other. In this chapter I will share with you the combined uses of plants in the form of herbs (phytotherapy) and plants in the form of essential oils (aromatherapy).

As herbalists most of us are aware that not all the plants in our materia medica contain essential oils. Many plant actions stem from the energy of alkaloids, saponins, mucilage, glycosides, etc. Essential oils are concentrated forms of powerful aromatic molecules that produce ketones, phenols, aldehydes, ethers and so forth. In many instances the synergy of whole plants used with essential oils provides a greater capacity for healing.

Essential oils are an extremely concentrated form of plant energy. They must be used with caution, respect and educated awareness of their power. Essential oils are approximately 70 times more powerful than the whole plants they come from. Consequently, their healing activity and their potential toxicity is increased. When you consider the amount of plant material it takes to produce even the smallest amount of essential oil you can see why this is so. One kilo of essential oil produced from one hundred kilos of herb is considered a high yield. It requires approximately a ton and a half of roses to produce one pound of rose oil or thirty roses to make one precious drop.

AROMATIC MOLECULE PRODUCTION

Aromatic molecules are the active principles of essential oils and the combination of several or even several hundred aromatic molecules can comprise a single essential oil. Briefly examining the dynamic process of essential oil synthesis within a plant we find that aromatic molecules are produced by a process of absorption of energy by photons within chlorophyll glands and secretory cells. Simply put, essential oils occur when energy from the sun is transformed into a complex of aromatic molecules. Genes and enzymes are responsible for deciding which of the aromatic molecules will be produced. The secretory cells or glands can be found in different parts of different plants. For example, with sage they appear on hairs of the leaf structure; with eucalyptus these glands appear within the leaf structure. In sandalwood and rosewood, glandular canals and pocket canals respectively produce these essential oil resins.

To extract essential oils from plants, the processes of distillation, expression, enfleurage, or solvents are used. The latter two processes are far less preferable to the health care practitioner than the two former as these involve synthetic and/or toxic chemicals.

THE HEALING POWER OF AROMATIC SUBSTANCES

The effectiveness of essential oils lies in several areas: their immediate effect on the olfactory sense, their power of penetration and their physiological action within the body.

Much can be said about the sense of smell and its role in health and immune response. It is our most primitive sense, our first sense to be developed and our most direct link from the outside world to the brain. Olfactory neurons are the only nerve cells in the body that replace themselves. Every 30–40 days these cells are completely renewed. Through the sense of smell essential oils are able to cross the blood/brain barrier, the lipid membrane that protects the brain. This is partly due to the extremely small size of aromatic molecules, and also because olfactory nerves evolved before the brain. Aromatherapy is truly the sensual approach to healing; scents affect our limbic brain, the seat of our emotions and memory. In turn, this affects everything from the hypothalamus, pituitary and endocrine system to appetite, body temperature and insulin and hormone levels. They affect us not only on the physical level but can be calming and centering on an emotional/psychological level as well. Psychological effect alone can have a big role in healing the body as evidence by recent studies done with the use of aromatics employed strictly through inhalation. Placebo studies show that our state of mind may have more to do with healing than any herb or other substance used.

From fighting infection to boosting the immune system and calming the nerves, essential oils are effective healing agents. The key here is the active principles of the aromatic molecules and their ability to penetrate the skin and mucous membranes, both internally and externally. When used externally they easily enter the bloodstream through the small blood capillaries in the skin (the ingestion of essential oils is not always necessary or advisable for the beginner). Their extremely small molecular size makes this possible along with the fact that they are also highly lipotrophic (attracted to the oils in the skin). Essential oils penetrate the skin 100 times faster than water. Their ability to affect the nervous system is quite remarkable and they can be used to stimulate or relax. They penetrate via the nerve extremities and are effective for treating depression, stress, anxiety, shock and insomnia.

Antimicrobial action within the cell is another way that essential oils work to maintain a balanced internal ecology. Their actions affect bacteria and infection in a very simple yet effective way. Being lipid soluble, essential oils enter the cell walls of bacteria and interrupt oxygenation (primary energy metabolism) and consequent formation of ATP. This impaired "breathing" efficiently interrupts reproduction of bacteria. Because this oxygenation process is such a basic function of survival, bacteria do not develop a resistance to the use of essential oils as they can with antibiotics. They also act indirectly to "correct the terrain"; many essential oils lower the pH of the blood, especially those with a high phenol or alcohol content. This creates a less hospitable environment for the presence of bacteria.

It is interesting to note that all essential oils have a positive/negative charge or polarity that can be measured. To my knowledge, little study has been done to incorporate this information as it would apply in the energetics of disease symptoms for those with experience in TCM or Ayurveda. This would be an interesting area of study that could result in the more effective use of the yin/yang properties of essential oils for specific diseases.

CAUTIONS

Essential oils should be diluted prior to application on the skin. There are a few exceptions but most oils will irritate and burn if applied neat (undiluted). This is especially true if a poor quality essential oil is used. When using oil blends externally it is important to rotate your use of oils every 4–7 days as many oils can be toxic to certain organs (especially the liver) when used over extended periods. They should never be taken orally without the supervision of a trained and experienced aromatherapist. They are safest when used as inhalants, massage oils and in the bath.

Dosage is a very important consideration and more is not better when it comes to aromatherapy. Often lower doses can be more effective than high doses, so start slowly and if you are a beginner choose only 2–4 oils when making blends.

APPLICATIONS

There are some easy ways to incorporate the use of essential oils into your practice or into a client's busy schedule.

Externally the use of essential oils applied in diluted form is very effective and has great therapeutic benefit especially when employed as anti-inflammatory, sedative and analgesic agents. A normal dilution ranges from 1% to 10%, but generally, for most purposes, 2% is sufficient, safe and effective. To make a 2% dilution combine 10–12 drops of a single or blend of essential oils with 1 oz. of vegetable oil (often referred to as a carrier oil) such as almond, hazelnut, olive, etc. Full body massage is most effective, but when used as an after bath/body oil or applied over an affected area, it can provide good results.

Inhalation is an effective method of application for various lung disorders. Depending on the essential oil employed, different results can be achieved such as expectorant, mucolytic and antispasmodic actions. Lower concentrations are often more effective for a secretion stimulating effect as high doses can become suppressant. The best method of application is by the use of an aromatic micro-diffusor, but a vaporiser or hot water method will also work. Inhale the fragrant steam for 5 to 10 minutes at a time, as needed. Oils used in a diffusor effectively disinfect a sick room because they destroy a wide range of airborne bacteria on contact.

Bathing with essential oils is highly beneficial, especially if relaxation and stress reduction is the goal. Begin cautiously as some oils can irritate the skin. A safe start is 2–5 drops of essential oil per tub. The floral oils are less irritating than the spice or citrus oils. For most people lavender and geranium are nonirritating, even at 15 drops per tub, though doses of more than 10 drops of a total blend are more of a waste than an added benefit. For those with very sensitive skin, essential oils can be diluted in a carrier oil first. Add the essential oils after the tub is full and swish the water around before entering. If irritation occurs from the bath, rinse with cold water and apply pure vegetable oil to the skin.

Oral use of essential oils can be an effective way of administration, but so much knowledge and caution is needed regarding toxicity, dosage and length of treatment that it is best to avoid this area of application in the context of this article.

Rectal or vaginal application of diluted essential oils in the form of suppositories, implants or douches is an option in the treatment of certain conditions. Consulting with an experienced practitioner is recommended as these forms of application require nearly as much caution and knowledge as the oral administration of essential oils.

THERAPEUTIC COMBINATIONS

USING ESSENTIAL OILS WITH HERBAL PREPARATIONS
HAYFEVER AND OTHER ALLERGIES

Alleviation of allergy symptoms is a typical example of the efficacy and the synergistic effect of herbs and essential oils. A traditional herbal remedy might employ several of the following herbs: ma huang, eyebright, nettle, goldenseal, yarrow, golden rod, horseradish and sage.

From an aromatherapy perspective an effective adjunct would be the combination of *Cupressus sempervirens* (cypress) for its astringent effect, *Matricaria chamomilla* (chamomile) or *Melissa officinalis* (melissa) as anti-allergenics and possibly *Lavandula vera* (lavender) for its general therapeutic and relaxing benefits. Also helpful is the mucolytic action of oils such as *Rosemary officinalis* (chemotype verbenon) and *Inula graveolens*. The aromatic hydrosol of rose or myrtle may be used as compresses on the eyes to relieve inflammation, redness and itching. A suggested method for incorporating these two therapies is as follows:

Combine these nonirritating essential oils (equal parts is fine) and use 4–8 drops daily in the bath. As a massage oil, dilute to 2% (10 drops in 1 oz. of carrier oil) and apply to the entire body. The mucolytic oils may be diluted to 5% and applied in the nostrils with a Q-tip as needed. The herbs can be used in any combination and taken as a tea (1 tsp. of the combined herbs per cup of water) 3–5 times per day.

ADRENAL INSUFFICIENCY

This malady can be the result of, or contributing factor to, a number of other problems such as allergies, severe infections, chronic fatigue and hormonal imbalances to name a few. While adaptogenic, alterative and tonic herbs such as Astragalus, Siberian ginseng, echinacea, yellow dock, licorice, red clover, etc. are indicated, an aromatherapy treatment can complement their actions. Essential oils of *Picea mariana* (black spruce) and *Pinus sylvestris* (sea pine) are the perfect choice. Apply externally directly over the adrenal area in a higher than normal dilution of 20%. To prepare this add 60 drops (approx. 2 ml.) of each essential oil to one ounce of vegetable oil. Apply daily as needed but not for more than one week.

The herbal treatment of herpes generally involves the use of nervines such as scullcap, wild oat and valerian along with anti-microbials such as calendula and myrrh, and immune modulators such as echinacea. As herpes is a viral infection, the use of essential oils is found to be very effective. There are many to choose from: several species of eucalyptus (*E. polybractea, E. radiata, E. globulus*) and melaleuca (*M. alternifolia, M. Quinquinervia*) are specific as well as lavender, myrrh, rose and bergamot. A fatty oil of *Caulophyllum inophyllum* is the carrier of choice but any vegetable oil will do. Dilute 3–5% by using 20–30 drops of an essential oil blend to one ounce of carrier oil. Apply as needed to outbreak.

While many acute infectious diseases require the ingestion of essential oils (a process too lengthy to go into here) there is one external therapy that can be employed with good results. According to leading researcher, Pierre Franchomme, the use of phenolic oils, normally too irritating to be applied to the skin, may be used on the soles of the feet with no damage or irritation. The oils are quickly absorbed into the bloodstream and work to fight the infection from within. Essential oils of *Oreganum compactum* (oregano), *Thymus vulgaris* (thyme), *Satureja montana* (savory) and *Cinnamomum zeylandicum* (cinnamon leaf) may be used in a 10% dilution (60 drops of EO to 1 oz. of carrier) on the soles several times a day for an acute condition. Use no longer than 3 days.

Estrogen replacement therapy is most effective when herbs and essential oils are combined. Herbal therapy may include herb combinations of vitex, dong quai, licorice, angelica, fennel and black or blue cohash. The essential oils that contain estrogen-like aromatic molecules of sclariol or the sesquiterpenic alcohol of viridiflorol are *Salvia sclaria* (clary sage), *Salvia officinalis* (sage) and *Melaleuca viridiflora* (niaouli). These oils may be combined in a 3–5% dilution and applied to the abdomen and lower back daily (or as a vaginal suppository used 4 to 5 days per week) to treat ammenorrhea or aid menopausal transition. These oils are also helpful for PMS but should be avoided if the client has estrogen-dependent breast cysts or uterine fibroids.

Because whole natural plant substances treat the body in its entirety, true healing can begin. But we mustn't forget to examine why these symptoms manifest. Determining and correcting the cause is always the primary objective in healing and this may require dietary and lifestyle changes.

The uses of plant medicines, biologically familiar to the body, act to correct diseased terrain and help eliminate pathogenic micro-organisms. Herbs and essential oils will tonify and boost the body's own immune process and response and are a wonderful and effective start on one's journey to good health!

Herbalists on
the Practice of
Herbalism

An Energetic Model for Western Herbology

LESLEY GUNSAULUS TIERRA, L.AC., DIP. AC.

Originally, herbs were used in the West according to a systematic approach, called the Humor system. Promoted by Hippocrates in Greece, this system categorized each person as one of several physiological types. It likewise classified herbs and applied them for healing in a corresponding fashion. In this system, like all traditional healing systems with a theoretical foundation, the individual was evaluated, taking into account any strengths and weaknesses causing the disease. Then the effect the herbal medicine had on the organs, the person and the disease was considered. It was next matched with the cause of the individual's condition.

With the advent of materialistic thinking in the 17th and 18th centuries, a mechanistic view of nature has occurred. This proclaims that only what can be substantiated materially is reality. Extending to the human body, this way of thought views the body as a machine governed by mechanical laws and comprised of chemical constituents. As a result, modern medicine has come to view and treat disease separately from the person who experiences it. The disease is identified and then the common treatment for it given. Thus, everyone who receives the same diagnosis gets the same cure.

In the same way Western herbology has turned from applying herbs according to the Humor system to using them mechanistically. Herbs are applied to treat diseases solely according to their therapeutic properties and chemical constituents. Again, the disease is separated from the individual and a plant's components are separated from the whole plant to treat the disease.

Such an approach is based on the fallacy of isolation. It sees that one aspect of a person can be isolated and treated separately regardless of the other aspects of the person, or that an herb can be used in isolation irrespective of the rest of the plant's components. It results in our simplified approach of asking, "What is in this herb and what is it good for?" and, "What herb can I use for my headache?" This simplistic method of using herbs isolates the disease from the person and the chemical aspects of an herbs from its overall individual therapeutic effect.

SYMPTOMATIC VERSUS ENERGETIC MEDICINE

This approach to using herbs applies herbs symptomatically. With this method, the disease is isolated from the person and herbs are given to treat the disease symptoms, just like modern medicine. For example, if we get a headache, we take willow bark. Sometimes we combine several herbs into a formula for this ailment, yet our approach is always the same: willow bark is good for headaches, therefore, if you have a headache, take willow bark. While this frequently works, it doesn't always. Not every headache is relieved by the same herb. Thus, it is a "hit or miss" approach: something is missing.

Many traditional cultures use herbs energetically. Chinese, East Indian Ayurveda, Tibetan, Middle Eastern Unani and Native American Cherokee medicines are all founded on an energetic basis, although each system is different. To use herbs energetically, we look beyond the symptoms of the disease to alleviating the underlying imbalance which caused the disease. This cause varies according to each individual because all aspects of a person are taken into account, not just the disease itself.

Likewise, each herb is evaluated energetically and according to all of its aspects, such as its hot or cold effects, tastes, properties, colors, growing conditions, chemical constituents and so on. The appropriate herbs are then selected which alleviate the underlying cause of the disease. Herbal energies are matched with that of the person, the disease and its cause.

Rather than making the headache the main treatment focus, it looks at the person to see what is occurring in the body to cause the headache. The cause for it is then treated instead of just the headache itself. In eliminating the cause, the headache goes, too.

Some causes of a headache may be: 1) liver congestion, 2) stomach upset, 3) tension, or 4) weakness in the body. Which cause it is varies according to each person's body and whatever health imbalances exist. Dandelion and feverfew help headaches due to liver congestion; catnip can relieve headaches due to stomach upset; valerian often eases tension headaches; and cinnamon can eliminate headaches due to weakness in the body. Each of these herbs is different, yet each relieves a headache in its own way. This is quite a different approach to simply giving willow bark for any one of these types of headache.

What is missing in the symptomatic method of giving herbs is that only the headache is looked at while the person who has the headache is completely ignored! We assume that every headache is the same and forget that because every one of us is different, each headache is due to a different cause. Thus, the symptomatic way of using herbs is to treat the disease, while the energetic method is to treat the person who has the disease.

A new model for healing is needed, one which renews our use of herbs wholistically. To learn how to use herbs for healing according to an energetic system, many factors are involved. We first learn how to determine an herb's energy, taking into account all of its various aspects. Then we determine the underlying factors causing the illness. Next, we match the appropriate herbs to the determined condition.

THE ENERGY OF HERBS

In order to apply Western herbology to a new energetic model of healing, it is first important to start looking at herbs according to their energy, rather than just their properties and chemical constituents. Herbs have a cold or hot energy and both affect the body differently. Therefore, we want to learn what the energy of each herb is before we use it so we know which effect it will have and if this is the effect we want to happen.

The energy of an herb is a natural inherent part of the herb and it has several different aspects. All of these work together in an herb to give a unique personality and use and determine the conditions for which it is effective. These aspects are: heating or cooling energy, the five tastes, the four directions, other energies and special properties. When using herbs according to their energies, perhaps the first and most important aspect is its heating or cooling energy. The effects of tastes, directions and other energies and special properties all contribute to this basic heating-cooling category.

When we use an herb that has a warm energy it causes warmth in the body and vice versa for cool-natured herbs. Another way of looking at it is the effect an herb has on the body's metabolism. When it causes the metabolism in the body to speed up, it is heating. When it causes the metabolism to slow down, it is cooling.

Warming and cooling energies are on a continuum. Some herbs are hot, some slightly warm, others cool, some very cold and others neutral. Each herb varies in energy, yet overall it is stated that the herb is either hot, warm, neutral, cool or cold. There are very few hot or cold herbs, and so warming or cooling energies are the most common.

If there is already heat in the body, then taking a warm-natured herb will create further heat. However, taking an herb with a cool energy will clear the heat, creating balance. Likewise, if there is coldness in the body, taking a cool-natured herb creates more coldness. Yet, taking a warm-natured herb will warm that coldness and create balance. This is very simplified, but it demonstrates how the warming and cooling energies of herbs can affect the body and how we feel.

Therefore, one of the best ways to tell the inner nature of an herb is to see how you feel after taking it. A further key to learning the energy of an herb is how it affects the body. Usually herbs which give us more energy and strength and activate our blood circulation have a warm energy. Herbs which cause us to go to the bathroom, sweat or to feel calm have a cool energy.

Overall, there are general qualities which give an herb its warming or cooling energy. In general, warming herbs include hard leaves, twigs, branches, seeds, barks and long roots which take a long time to grow and mature. They tend to have a spicy or complex sweet taste (made up of complex carbohydrates), with more minerals and protein. They strengthen the energy and have little or no volatile oils. Examples include fennel, elecampane, angelica, prickly ash, cinnamon, ginseng and astragalus.

Cooling herbs in general are softer leaves, flowers, juicy fruits, fast growing roots and tubers and have a sour, bitter or salty taste. They are more eliminating and contain an abundance of volatile oils. They tend to grow and mature quickly and have a detoxifying and cooling effect in the body. Examples include dandelion, goldenseal, red clover and peppermint.

The energy of an herb can be altered somewhat by external applications. To make an herb warmer in energy: 1) add heat or cook; 2) cook a long time; 3) use pressure (pressure cook or use weights, as in a pressed salad or for making pickles); 4) roast; 5) use dry. To make an herb cooler: 1) add liquid or make soupy; 2) prepare with vinegar; 3) add simple sweets such as sugar, fruit or fruit juice; 4) cook quickly; 5) use cool; 6) use raw.

Although this is very simplified for learning how to determine the energy of an herb, several books are available with more detailed information. What should be stressed here is that because each herb has a unique energy, then herbal properties have different energies, too. Most herbal properties can be differentiated as cold and hot.

For example, there are diaphoretics which have a cool energy and diaphoretics which have a warm energy. The same is true of expectorants, diuretics, nervines, antispasmodics and so forth. Which diaphoretics are cool and which are warm depends on the herbs and their energies. Some herbal properties do contain herbs of all the same energy, such as Yang tonics all being warm and Yin tonics all being cool. Yet, herbs should first be differentiated by their energies and then applied according to their herbal properties.

AN ENERGETIC MODEL: DIFFERENTIAL DIAGNOSIS

In looking at a new model for healing with herbs, traditional Chinese medicine offers a valuable approach for Western herbalists. Chinese diagnostics uses several systems of diagnoses that provide a system of viewing the same problem from several different perspectives. One model in particular is a useful system to adopt for incorporating Western herbalism into an energetic point of view.

Called Differential Diagnosis, this system is a method of evaluating all the characteristics of an illness and then seeing what pattern they form. The pattern is then treated, rather than the disease. This allows for the treatment of all problems a person is experiencing, not just the supposed "disease" that has been defined. Such an approach is important because it provides a method for understanding and healing the cause of "untreatable" complex conditions, such as cancer, arthritis, AIDS and chronic fatigue syndrome, for instance.

It also takes into account all aspects a person is experiencing. Some of us think we have a disease, like candida or chronic fatigue syndrome, but when we look deeper at the cause of the problem we learn we really don't have that disease. Further, many of us experience problems which can't be identified as a known disease. Instead, we are told to go home because there is nothing wrong with us, or else to seek psychiatric help. That is why it is important to treat the person, not the condition. In treating the person the imbalance can be discovered and corrected. When treating the condition, often a "cure" doesn't exist or our condition doesn't exist!

Differential Diagnosis classifies all diseases according to eight individual principles. Of the eight, there are two primary ones termed Yin and Yang. The remaining six are categorized under them and actually provide a further definition of them. These eight principles are:

Internal	External
Deficient	Excess
Cold	Hot
Yin	Yang

Internal and External define the location of the disease. Deficient and Excess describe the strength of the disease in relation to the strength of the patient. Cold and Hot refer to the energy of the disease, or its hypo-metabolic or hyper-metabolic state.

Yin and Yang represent a combination of all the six preceding principles. In general, diseases which are Internal, Deficient, Cold and Yin are chronic and hypo-metabolic (asthenic) in effect. Diseases which are External, Excess, Hot and Yang are acute and hyper-metabolic (sthenic) in effect.

Other combinations of these eight principles occur such as Internal, Deficient and Hot, or External, Excess and Cold. Each of these requires a different understanding and corresponding applications for herbal treatment. Yet, they each allow for paradoxical symptoms to co-exist and be treated.

Once the disease is categorized according to the appropriate combination of these eight principles, the herbal treatment approach is automatically determined. If a disease is Internal, Hot, Excess and Yang, for instance, then we know there is an excess amount of internal heat which needs to be cleared. To treat this, herbs which are internally cooling and eliminating in energy are used. This typically corresponds to the Western property of alteratives.

As a specific example, if a person has a cold with chills, low energy, little or no fever, runny white mucus and clear-colored urine, this person is experiencing an External Cold Deficient and thus, Yin condition. The treatment approach then, is to use warming, stimulating and strengthening herbs with an energy that flows to the surface or external part of the body. This corresponds to diaphoretics, expectorants and stimulants with a warm energy in Western Herbology.

Thus, the Western herbal approach of using herbs according to their properties can be incorporated into the Chinese model of determining and treating disease energetically. First, we evaluate the condition according to the Eight Principles. Then we determine the corresponding treatment approach and appropriate herbal energy. Next, we see which Western herbal properties match the treatment approach and herbal energy that is needed.

The following is a description of each of the eight principle categories and their combinations with assignments of the appropriate Western herbal properties for their proper therapeutic approach.

THE EIGHT PRINCIPLES

INTERNAL-EXTERNAL

Whether a disease is internal—in the body, or external—more on the surface of the body, defines the depth of the disease. Internal conditions affect the internal organs and bodily systems. Herbs whose energy is inward, downward and some with an upward energy are used, such as tonics, diuretics, laxatives, emmenagogues and some stimulants.

External conditions affect the skin, nose, throat and outer parts of the body. This includes chills, fever, sore throat, body aches, sinus conditions and skin eruptions. Herbs with an outward and upward energy are used, such as diaphoretics, expectorants and some stimulants and alteratives.

DEFICIENT-EXCESS

The strength of the disease in relation to the strength of the patient defines whether the illness is one of deficiency or excess. A deficient condition occurs when there is a lack of something, such as a lack of blood (anemia), energy or heat. An excess condition occurs when there is too much of something, such as too much heat or dampness. To determine which it is, we look at the root cause, not just the symptoms, and gauge that according to the capacity of the individual to maintain a continued resistance to the onslaught of disease. This is taken in a general sense and denotes the overall condition of the patient and/or the disease.

Deficient states are those which hang on, take a long time to develop and have a tendency to recur. There is a low symptomatic condition, weakness, lack of blood, fluids, energy or heat. This is a situation of chronic conditions and usually is accompanied by weakness and tiredness. Often there is not enough energy to throw off the disease.

Deficient states are an incapacity to find or produce what is necessary for the body to maintain its immunity to disease. It often takes a longer time to reach a deficient state and so treatment to restore the body can take longer, too. Here herbal tonics for the blood, energy, substance, heat or coolness of the body are given.

Excess states are characterized by the person having strength in either the acute or chronic condition, buoyancy of spirits and the condition itself is extreme in its manifestation. In these instances there is an abundance of whatever is occurring be it fever, phlegm, heat, coldness, dampness and so forth. Herbs which have an eliminating or dispersing quality are used, such as purgatives, alteratives, diuretics, expectorants or diaphoretics. The idea here is to eliminate the excess.

It is not unusual for western people, whose diets are high in meat protein, to experience excess diseases more frequently. Taken to extreme, however, they result in congestion and deficient states where the immunity of the body is so taxed that it can no longer deal with the excessive conditions created. All states eventually lead to deficiency when left untended over time.

If we look at the body as a container which holds energy, heat, blood and fluids, we can view deficient and excess conditions in a different way. In a deficient condition the container is porous. It allows the energy, heat, blood or fluids to leak out. Thus, a person with this type of container is weak in any of these qualities. This person is overly sensitive to everything. Strong nourishment is needed to plug the holes and build a strong container.

In an excess condition the container is over packed and bulging. There is no room so the energy, blood or fluids tend to stop moving and stagnate. Heat can increase until steam needs to be released, like a pressure cooker. If the excess continues, it eventually blows holes in the sides and weakness results. Thus, the excess needs to be eliminated to create a healthy container with its contents flowing easily and smoothly.

The following chart gives the characteristics of deficiency and excess states:

Deficiency	Excess
weak	strong
silent	talkative
odorless	strong smells
light sweating, breathing and discharges	heavy sweating, breathing and discharges
lack of blood, energy, fluids	too much dampness or heat
flaccidity	congestion and stagnation
low grade, even chronic fever	high fever

In treating deficient conditions, it may be necessary to combine both tonifying and eliminative treatment. This needs to be done to build the person's strength to aid the deficiency while giving eliminative treatment to cure the particular symptoms. Applying both may be done in a single herbal formula.

In treating excess conditions, especially acute ones, one should never tonify as this only feeds the disease rather than the body's normal energy. Elimination first needs to occur, even if there is a weakness. After the first stages of elimination are complete, some tonifying therapy can be given concurrently, if appropriate.

COLD–HOT

The energy of an illness refers to its cold–hot state. Conditions not as extreme are classified as cool or warm and most illnesses fall under this. Illnesses of cold are characterized by cold signs and illnesses of heat are characterized by heat signs. To determine if an illness is one of coldness or heat, at least three or more signs of coldness or heat will occur.

Coldness tends to congeal and contract like ice. It causes a person to hunch over or curl up in order to minimize body surface and maintain inner warmth. With lack of heat, activity in all forms slows down. Usually there is tiredness, lack of energy or weakness.

Heat causes extreme activity in the body with a tendency to rise up and out, like the heat from a fire. When it does this, it often moves other things with it, such as blood (high blood pressure or blood in the stools, phlegm and so forth) or the tongue (being talkative).

The following chart delineates the symptoms for each category. Remember that this represents a continuum. Thus, a person with a little coldness, for instance, will show only a few of the cold signs and these will not be very pronounced or will only occur occasionally. The same is true for someone with just a little heat.

Cold Symptoms	*Hot Symptoms*
watery stool; frequent; or diarrhea; little odor	hard, solid stool; dry; usually constipated; strong smelling
clear or white urine; usually frequent and copious	yellow and thick urine; interrupted or stopped urine
appears very depressed	appears very agitated
weak, tired, thin, quiet	strong, stout, muscular, restless, active, irritable
cold skin temperature, hands and feet, five senses are weak	warm skin temperature, hands and feet, five senses are strong
curled, lying posture	stretching posture in sleep, likes to stretch
soft voice, silent	loud voice, talkative
soft and shallow breathing	heavy, coarse breathing

wet mouth; poor taste and appetite; prefers warm food and drinks	thirst, dry mouth; prefers cold drinks and food, good appetite
prefers deep massage	dislikes pressure, massage
fat, pale, wet tongue; white or coat	red, solid tongue; cracks, yellow, thick coat

Sometimes there are mixed signs of both cold and hot, such as a hot disease manifesting in a cold body and vice versa. To determine which it truly is and how to treat it, combine information on the constitution with that of the illness.

For instance, a person who has a bladder infection but also feels cold, weak, tired, gets frequent colds and flus and eats a lot of salads and fruit in a vegetarian diet is a situation of a hot disease manifesting in a cold body. The infection itself is hot with burning, scanty or yellow or bloody urine. Yet, the body is cold with feelings of cold, lowered immunity, little energy and strength.

In this case there are signs of both heat and coldness. To treat this, the heat of infection needs to be cleared directly and gently, while the coldness of the body needs to be warmed. This can be done by using warming stimulants with slightly cool antibiotic herbs.

An example of a cold disease manifesting in a hot body is chronic asthma with clear to white phlegm, yet the body and breathing are strong, the person feels warm and perhaps the face is red. In this case, warming expectorants for the lungs are combined with alteratives to clear the excess condition in the body.

YIN–YANG

Yin and Yang represent an combination of all the six preceding factors. Yin diseases tend to be Internal, Deficient and Cold while Yang diseases tend to be External, Excess and Hot. Therefore, when one summarizes a person's condition as being Yin or Yang, what is meant is that there exists a state of Deficiency or Excess respectively.

Yet, Yin and Yang in the body are fundamental properties themselves. Yin includes blood and all other bodily fluids and is moistening and cooling in nature. Yang includes energy and heat and is drying, heating and moving in nature. Therefore, the Yin of the body refers to its blood, moistening and cooling properties, and the Yang of the body refers to its energy, moving and heating properties.

Yin and Yang are usually seen in various combinations with the other six principles such as Deficient Yin, Deficient Yang, Excess Yin or Excess Yang. The treatment for each varies accordingly, using herbs which tonify Yin or Yang, or herbs which eliminate dampness (Excess Yin), such as diaphoretics, expectorants and stimulants with a warm energy, or eliminate heat (Excess Yang), such as alteratives, febrifuges and cooling diaphoretics.

COMBINATIONS OF THE EIGHT PRINCIPLES

Disease is seen as a combination of the eight principles in various ways. To determine which category it is, there must be at least three or more signs from that category showing in the illness. The following outlines these various combinations with their particular signs. The treatment principle is then given which delineates which herbs to use according to their properties used in Western herbology.

INTERNAL COLD

Signs: feelings of coldness, no thirst, diarrhea or loose stools, no sweating, aversion to cold, slowness, craves warmth, sleeps a lot, pale moist tongue, white tongue coat, slow or deep pulse, pale, frigid appearance, lack of circulation, achy pain in joints and flesh, low blood pressure, cold extremities, poor appetite, poor digestion, clear discharges such as urine, nasal and mucus, tendency toward stagnation and contraction.

Treatment Principle: Warm the inside of the body and eliminate the cold, tonify Yang; use warming stimulants, emmenagogues, carminatives, antispasmodics, nervines and Yang tonics.

EXTERNAL COLD

Signs: sudden onset of illness, chills with slight fever, little sweating, no thirst, fear of cold, body aches, needs lots of covers, craves warm food and drinks.

Treatment Principle: Use surface relieving herbs with a spicy warm energy, warming diaphoretics, stimulants, antispasmodics and nervines.

INTERNAL HEAT

Signs: constipation, red face and/or eyes, thirst, aversion to heat, dark yellow or red urine, dark, scanty urination, craving of cold, hemorrhaging, bloody nose, stools or urine, irritability, yellow mucus, stools or urine, fast pulse, sweats easily, blood in any discharges, yellow coated tongue, red tongue body, strong appetite, burning digestion, preference for cold, fever, infections, inflammations, sticky, thick and hot-feeling excretions, dryness internally or externally.

Extreme heat causes a more severe condition which includes several of the heat signs above plus: delirium, coma, shortness of breath, heat stroke, restlessness, disturbed mind, depletion of fluids, exhaustion, sudden high fever, profuse sweating.

Heat in the body can result in *dryness*. Its signs include: dehydration, dry stools or cough, dry, rough, chapped or cracked skin or tongue and unusual thirst. Dryness is treated by moistening, lubricating and aiding the body to absorb the moisture it already contains. Demulcents, emollients and certain diuretics do this.

Treatment Principles: Clear the heat in its corresponding location, be it blood, toxicity, dampness and so forth. Use cooling diaphoretics, purgatives, alteratives, antipyretics, diuretics, refrigerants, laxatives, febrifuges, antispasmodics, nervines, analgesics, cholagogues, demulcents, hemostatics, expectorants and laxatives.

EXTERNAL HEAT

Signs: sudden onset of illness, high fever, slight chills, great thirst, profuse sweating, craves cool food and drinks, headaches, fear of heat, throws covers and clothes off, sore, swollen and possible red throat, carbuncles, boils, red skin eruptions.

Treatment Principle: Use herbs to relieve the surface with a spicy cool energy, cooling diaphoretics, expectorants, febrifuges, alteratives, antipyretics, antispasmodics, nervines, antibiotics, demulcents, emollients, analgesics, hemostatics, vulneraries and laxatives.

DEFICIENT COLD

With Deficiency Cold in the body there is a state of Deficiency and coldness. Here the Yang is Deficient and so is not strong enough to move, heat and transform the fluids which then congest and manifest in Cold Damp symptoms. This fits the Deficient Yang category below.

DEFICIENT HEAT

Deficient Heat is a state of heat arising out of a lack of bodily fluids, or Yin. Thus, the Yin is not strong enough to hold the Yang energy and so Yang symptoms of heat manifest. This fits the Deficient Yin category below and is called "false heat."

EXCESS COLD

Excess Cold is a condition of excessive coldness in the body. This is usually due to an Excess Yin or a Deficiency of Yang. Refer to those categories for their signs and treatment.

EXCESS HEAT

Excess Heat is a condition of Excess Yang in the body. Refer to the categories of Internal and External Heat for its signs and treatment.

DEFICIENT YIN

When there is a deficiency of Yin, there is a lack of body fluids. This results in dryness and heat signs. Yet, there is also an accompanying weakness and lack of strength. These causes often occur from burnout: overworking, thinking or doing which depletes the essential fluids of the body.

Signs: thinness and emaciation, agitated manner, warm palms and soles, insomnia, superficial red flush on cheeks and/or nose, night sweats, thirst, possible bleeding, red tongue with no coat, fast but thin pulse, dry skin or hair, possibly talkative, but in spurts with no underlying strength, nervous energy.

Treatment Principle: The heat needs to be gently cleared and the Yin substance of the body needs to be nourished and moistened by using: Yin tonics with cooling demulcents, alteratives, nervines, antispasmodics, hemostatics, laxatives, blood tonics, diaphoretics, vulneraries, emollients and plenty of rest.

EXCESS YIN

Yin in Excess creates dampness in the body. Because Yin is cold in energy, there is usually accompanying coldness. However, there is not the weakness that occurs in a person with true coldness. The face may be pale, voice soft, hands and feet cold, or a lack of sweat or appetite occur, but overall the person is strong, buoyant and active. In this situation typically the heat or fluids of the body aren't circulating properly and so they stagnate, resulting in various damp signs. This is termed "false cold."

Signs: feelings of fullness, tendency towards heaviness, lack of appetite, heavy joints, distention or soreness in the chest, head, flank or abdomen, oozing ulcers, copious discharges which are clear to white, runny, copious, turbid, cloudy or sticky, slowness, nausea, watery stools, lassitude, edema, bloatedness, runny light colored diarrhea or vaginal discharge, no desire to drink even if there is thirst, lack of sensation or taste.

Treatment Principle: Dry the dampness and tonify the Yang with warming and drying stimulants, diuretics, expectorants, diaphoretics, laxatives, carminatives, analgesics, astringents, nervines, antispasmodics, emetics, emmenagogues and vulneraries.

DEFICIENT YANG

When Yang is deficient there is a lack of energy and heat in the body, resulting in tiredness and coldness together.

Signs: cold limbs, slow deep pulse, frequent urination, impotence, low energy, lowered immunity, puffy tongue and face, undigested food in the stool, aversion to cold, little desire to move or speak, lack of appetite, night time urination, low libido, infertility.

Treatment Principle: Tonify the Yang to eliminate coldness and any possible dampness, and strengthen the energy. Use Yang tonics with warming carminatives, stimulants, emmenagogues, diuretics, nervines, antispasmodics, astringents, expectorants and energy tonics.

EXCESS YANG

This is a condition of Excess Heat in the body which was previously described under the Internal and External Heat categories.

OVERALL

Combinations of the above conditions can also occur, and most mixed symptoms come under this. They include half external-half internal, half excess-half deficient, half cold-half hot symptoms. These kinds of conditions are treated with harmonization therapy. This therapy is one of using integrated approaches such as varied combinations of detoxification and tonification, cooling and warming, internal and external applied simultaneously as seems appropriate.

Further, sometimes the Cold and Hot symptoms can be confused. If someone has Cold symptoms, for example, it may be due to an Excess of Coldness (Excess Yin) or a Deficiency of Heat (Deficient Yang). Or if someone has Heat symptoms, it may be due to an Excess of Heat (Excess Yang) or a Deficiency of Coldness (Deficient Yin). To see which it is, there must be three or more signs in one of the corresponding categories.

Determining the cause and nature of illness can be complicated. It can also involve more principles than those discussed here, such as stagnant blood and energy, energy moving in the wrong direction and so forth. Yet, what has been given can definitely help the identification of many illness conditions and indicate the proper treatment direction. Knowing this and the energy of herbs can help one look for the appropriate therapeutic herbal approach for correcting the condition found.

Having a model for approaching herbal healing energetically deepens Western herbology and transports it into a new arena. Rather than just using one or two aspects of an herb, such as its properties and chemical constituents, all of its components are valued and considered to comprise its total energetic effect. Likewise, rather than just looking at and treating disease in a person, all the contributing factors which cause that disease are evaluated.

Then by matching the appropriate herbal energies to the disease causing factors, the true underlying cause of the illness is treated. Although this approach is based on ancient principles, it is a leap toward future herbal therapy which incorporates Western herbalism into an energetic point of view and treats the whole person effectively.

Location	State	Energy	Result	Treatment Category
Internal	Deficient	Cold	Deficient Yang	*Yang tonics with warming* stimulants, emmenagogues, carminatives, nervines, antispasmodics, diuretics, astringents, expectorants, energy tonics
Internal	Deficient	Hot	Deficient Yin	*Yin tonics with cooling* demulcents, alteratives, nervines, antispasmodics, hemostats, laxatives, blood tonics with *rest*
Internal	Excess	Cold	Excess Yin	*Warming* stimulants, carminatives, diaphoretics, analgesics, diuretics, laxatives, expectorants, astringents, nervines, emetics, antispasmodics, emmenagogues

Location	State	Energy	Result	Treatment Category
Internal	Excess	Hot	Excess Yang	*Cooling* alteratives, analgesics, antibiotics, antpyretics, antispasmodics, nervines, cholagogues, demulcents, emollients, diaphoretics, diuretics, hemostats, expectorants, febrifuges, laxatives
External	Deficient	Cold	Deficient Yang	A little yang tonics with *warming* diaphoretics, expectorants, stimulants, nervines, astringents, vulneraries with *rest*
External	Deficient	Hot	Deficient Yin	A little yin tonics with *cooling* diaphoretics, expectorants, alteratives, antispasmodics, hemostats, demulcents, emollients, vulneraries, nervines with *rest*
External	Excess	Cold	Excess Yin	*Warming* diaphoretics, stimulants, expectorants, astringents, vulneraries, laxatives, antispasmodics, nervines, carminatives
External	Excess	Hot	Excess Yang	*Cooling* diaphoretics, expectorants, febrifuges, antipyretics, alteratives, antibiotics, demulcents, emollients, analgesics, antispasmodics, nervines, hemostatics

Herbal Energetics in
Clinical Practice

Michael Moore

Purpose

People get sick. By the time they are in their twenties they usually start to get sick in predictable ways. The constitutional approaches outlined in this essay are meant to offer a way to strengthen the person who gets sick by supporting inherited and acquired weaknesses, lessening the effects of habitual stress and correcting habitual fluid imbalances. They are not meant to directly treat disorders, but to strengthen the person with chronic disorders according to his or her nature. I am not being coy or delicate here, improving between the lines that these approaches are for disease. These approaches are intended to strengthen the *person* who gets sick, not to deal with the illness.

One of the basic premises of stress is that once a pattern of chronic disease or weakness has been set up, any stress can contribute to the imbalance. Homeostasis is the state of being in balance, locally and throughout the body, accomplished by controlling our internal and external environment through nerves, hormones, fluid movement, all reacting to many feedback mechanisms. In the broad sense, we only lose homeostasis when we die. Stated another way, we have a fixed amount of life energy to expend in a given day…call it $100. If running our body costs $45 in life energy (or chi or blood transport surface area) in 24 hours, we have $55 to spare. We may expend $30 on our work, $10 on our relationships, $5 wasted in agitation over the evening news, $5 on a brief argument with our mate, and fall asleep without overspending. If it is Friday, we may get blotto on bourbon at our local swillery, costing us $15 in life energy, overspend ourselves, wake up Saturday with a headache from hell and sloth reflexes, and maintain second-day homeostasis by moving carefully, methodically and with great fragility. We have maintained our metabolic balance by getting semi-sick the next day, expending few $, allowing the liver to have the balance of money to clean up after ourselves. If we had osteoarthritis, however, we might have ended up with a *bad* day Saturday...our chronic disease manifested by an acute episode. If we had strengthened the body, made it less expensive (say, $30 a day for upkeep), we might not have had an acute arthritis attack...or maybe not had the hangover...or maybe not even have needed the release of demon rum at all. Breaking up a relationship, moving, losing a job, a death in the family, a tax audit, all are expenses which, added on to normal life, can contribute to chronic disease. I don't have any herbs to offer for breaking up, but methods of constitutional strengthening outlined here will definitely decrease the cost of living, helpful in supportive treatment for chronic disease.

The problem of treatment in chronic disease is two-fold. First there is the difficulty of the honeymoon period; the arthritis responds to a direct approach for awhile, then comes back and the primary therapy becomes ineffective. You try another approach and it too wears out. More often than not, neither approach will work well again. If you are an M.D., you wince as you gradually have to increase the strength and iatrogenesis-potential of the meds. If you are an herbalist or an acupuncturist, you wince as, one by one, your best therapies wear off.

Secondly, there is the simple problem of chronic disease; it begins as a functional disorder (thermostat settings off, things subtly out of balance) and, after recurring acute episodes, can become organic (things broken, scarred, not factory original, busted). The idea of supporting your therapy with a constitutional methodology is that your main stuff will work longer since the person is healthier, the acute episodes get further apart (they don't overspend as often) and the functional disorder is less likely to become organic, as the body has more time to reorder itself between episodes.

Once again, the purpose of this approach is to strengthen the person in a rational and non-toxic fashion, while you do your main stuff. The main focus of both the Traditional Chinese Medicine and Ayurvedic Medicine approaches is the same: strengthen the person, *then* treat their problem. Of course they work. They diagnose imbalances, have therapies that make the homeostasis easier and they help people. *TCM and Ayurvedic practitioners like and gently and bemusedly approve* of our use of herbs and diet, but they regularly and emphatically tell us, "Fine, good work, but *you have no tonics*...how can you take yourself so seriously when you ain't got no philosophy of us...just gentler medicines than the M.D. has." The format of use here is an attempt (and a good one) to supply several parameters to evaluate the strengths and weaknesses of a patient, a body of tonic herbs to strengthen the weaknesses and (sometimes) to cool the excesses, and a chart outlining the effects of all major herbal medicines on the organ systems to avoid unwanted synergism.

ORGAN SYSTEM ENERGETICS

This is the primary approach in constitutional evaluation. In setting up patterns of excess and deficiency, the starting point is the primary physiologic function of the organ system. Herbs effect absorption, metabolism, fluid transport and excretion; the important aspect here is function (physiology), not structure (anatomy). In energetic support of chronic imbalances you want to strengthen the function of systems in order to avoid impairment of structure. Excess means that that organ system is overfunctioning, usually from hormonal or neurologic causes. More often than not, the excess in one organ system is paid for by a deficiency or suppression in another system. The simplest way for the body to stimulate one system is mechanical; more arterial blood is pumped in by vasodilation, sometimes with concurrent hormone or neuro-hormone stimulation of the same system. If the body stimulates one system through normal channels (no pathology), it will decrease blood supply and metabolism to other systems. To suppress an excess function often entails some form of drug effect. Drug effect tends to build up resistance and tolerance; further, direct sedation of an excess is more often than not likely to suppress the structure, whereas the ideal would be to decrease the need for excess function. If you have essential hypertension, it is usually because you *need* a harder working heart in order to be homeostatic. Without lessening stress or changing body energetics, suppressing cardiovascular excess in essential hypertension with a drug leaves the need for homeostatic accommodation intact but takes the most able system out of the game. Other systems (renal or liver, as an example) must make less efficient changes, eventually weakening them.

The ideal, of course, is to place a helping hand into the limbic system, hypothalamus, even the genetic code. The best balance for a person is of the person's making. Lacking that, we take the organs suppressed by stress and habit, stimulate them physiologically with herbs, and deflect life energy from those functions that are chronically hyperactive. This isn't the same as endogenous balance. It is, after all, just another external manipulation. But, of course, it is a manipulation by inference, not by direct suppression. Use defines form; use an organ or function or tissue and it becomes stronger, better organized and better fed. It grows more mitochondria, draws more blood, elaborates better neuro-peptides, elbows out a larger place in the physiologic pecking order of the body-colony...gets stronger. Stimulating the deficient upper intestinal tract with herbs will never be the same as having, by nature, a strong upper G.I. But, in an imperfect world, helping those depressed functions to strengthen will, in time, retrain them to become stronger. It ain't the real thing, but it will do for starters.

Another starting premise for organ system evaluation is: don't try to judge the system involved in the main complaint. If the patient has a peptic ulcer, Tagamet, antacids, cabbage juice, whatever, *that* is the primary therapy. If the person has progressed to the point of an overt chronic disease, ignore it in a constitutional context and try to balance out everything else. In this example, ignore Upper GI and try to tonify everything else *but* the stomach. Then the primary therapy, of whatever modality, will have a more fertile ground, a less expensive homeostasis with less cost of living and more probability of extended success.

UPPER INTESTINAL TRACT

Outline of function. Saliva is secreted in response to chewing, taste, visual and olfactory stimulation. It is partially mucoid, viscous and thick (to mix with food and lubricate swallowing), partially thin and watery (to alkalize mouth, inhibit bacteria and begin starch digestion). Stomach secretions are also stimulated, muscle coats relaxed to ease swallowing and stomach filling, proteins for B12 carrying and absorption secreted. The bottom of the stomach secretes protein-digesting acid into a small volume of food, separated by constriction from undigested food above, and is ejected into the duodenum of the small intestine. Hormones secreted in the stomach and duodenum stimulate the pancreas and gall bladder to evacuate together into the food leaving the stomach. These hormones neutralize the acidity, make soap to emulsify fats, and inject enzymes for protein, fat and further carbohydrate digestion. If fats are still unemulsified, the stomach is inhibited hormonally. Further enzymes and secretions are aided by glands in the upper small intestine. Digestion has been set up and continues methodically down the intestinal tract.

Upper GI deficiency symptoms are a dry mouth, usually with a history of gum and teeth problems. The person has a coated tongue and bad breath first thing in the morning and seldom eats breakfast. He/she often does not finish meals or may intentionally eat to calm down, often has indigestion or a sense of excess fullness after eating and has trouble with evening meals. The stomach, like the mouth, has deficient or slow secretions, with erratic tone and peristalsis and sometimes there is difficulty in swallowing. The slow evacuation of the stomach results in poor coordination of pancreatic and gall bladder secretion, which in turn results in poor digestion of fats and inhibition of subsequent stomach evacuations. This induces an extended retention of food in the stomach with resultant fermentation, smelly burps and frequent problems with food sensitivities and food combinations. Consequently, the person probably doesn't too many proteins and fats, and if food-educated, may (understandably) have a rigid and articulate approach as to what can/can't be eaten. Heavy, long-term use of alcohol can induce deficiency symptoms whereas cigarette smoking may have been instinctively picked up in the first place because it helped stimulate upper GI functions that were weak. To counter this deficiency, *Herbs to stimulate may be given,* either to excite by reflex as a bitter tonic taken just before meals, increasing both mouth and gastric juices to encourage better function, or to stimulate function by exciting membrane secretions or increasing blood supply to the mouth, stomach and pancreas.

Upper GI excess symptoms are a moist mouth and oversecreting stomach *in the presence of food,* often with a pointy, red-tipped tongue (even to the extent of a sore tip), and an exaggerated and rapid evacuation of the stomach and bowels in the morning. The person can (seemingly) eat anything, often preferring high protein and fat foods. If the person has any tendency to chronic nausea, it is in the mornings or just before a delayed meal. *Herbs to cool* are astringent (acting locally as a vaso-constrictor, decreasing inflammation), protectant (coating the mucosa) or anesthetic to the muscle coats and mucosa. Generally, a difficult imbalance to modify directly with herbs (except in gastric ulcers), it is easier to overstimulate accidentally, so avoid using other tonic herbs with the side effect of strong upper GI stimulus. It is a reactive condition. Low doses of *Rheum* (rhubarb) work as well as anything.

LOWER INTESTINAL TRACT

Outline of function. After passing through much of the small intestine under almost total local control (and therefore subject to little stress potential from the autonomics and CNS), with lipids absorbed primarily into the lymph system and carbohydrates and proteins digested and absorbed into the portal blood (from capillaries in the intestines, into the portal system and portal vein and then back out into capillaries in the liver…a way of isolating all intestinal venous blood and its wildly varying constituents from general circulation until the liver has picked through it), the digesting food (chyme) passes the lower ileum. Here very complex substances are absorbed, such as B12, folic acid, some essential fatty acids, vitamins A, D and E, and the bile acids originally secreted in the duodenum for fat emulsifying. The chyme, now exhausted of usable substances, is squirted into the cecum of the large intestine, where the intestinal flora break down the chyme further (now called feces) and release for absorption some folic acid and vitamin K. The large intestine (colon) then sets about reabsorbing the sodium, chloride and water that was secreted into the food in the upper GI, along with gases made in the cecum, adding mucus to lubricate the feces and bicarbonate and potassium to raise the pH to alkaline. In the descending colon, formed feces are passed into the rectum (usually from reflex when the stomach is filled) and the defecation reflex (parasympathetic) is followed by conscious defecation.

Lower GI deficiency symptoms are either constipation, with poor stimulation of colon function, overdehydration of feces, extended transit time and the long-term tendency to overlook the defecation reflex (usually of short duration and not repeated for several hours), or the more complex syndrome of fat malabsorption with episodes of steatorrhea. Like the first, the latter is the result of upper GI deficiency, but usually in the person that chronically consumes fats in excess of their digestive capacity. The lipids are poorly set up for emulsification in the stomach and duodenum, the fat bubbles are poorly absorbed into the lymph system, much more is taken into the liver (thickening the portal blood and slowing the liver), and the rest passing raw into the cecum. Intestinal flora reflects the stuff it's fed, and lipid-digesting bacteria, rare in the normal cecum, proliferate with undigested fats. The small intestine is nearly sterile, the decum is a stomach-like cultural vat, and the juncture of the two is heavily protected with lymph nodes and specialized defense organs…the appendix in the cecum and the Peyer's Patches of the lower ileum. With the change in flora, the whole area becomes moderately inflamed and becomes impaired. Fat is sometimes excreted in the feces and in some persons the deficiency may vacillate between constipation and loose stools (Irritable Bowel Syndrome). With impaired drainage of blood from the lower GI into the portal system and the liver, venous drainage from the descending colon and even transverse colon has to bypass into smaller collateral veins that drain into general circulation. These veins become congested and hemorrhoids, varicose veins in the inner thighs and general pelvic congestion is the result. Further, the rather noxious metabolites from the lower colon are not removed by the liver first; they go into general circulation. In both types, the liver plays an important role and in both types the efficiency of upper GI function must be improved before any approach helps the lower.

Herbs to stimulate increase bile, pancreatic and succus entericus secretions (for both types of deficiency), and for the constipative type may increase peristalsis by direct irritation, vasodilation or parasympathetic stimulation.

Lower GI excess symptoms are rapid transit of food through the GI tract (usually 20 hours or less) with dark soft stools and heightened defecation reflex (eat a meal, get the urge shortly after). The beginning of a bowel movement is formed, the major part is semi-formed, and the whole process is quick (no magazine reading here). *Herbs to cool* sedate plexus nerves in muscle walls or parasympathetic excess, cool the thyroid, or act as simple astringents.

LIVER

Outline of function. The liver is responsible for synthesizing most blood proteins, including globulins, albumin, heparin, fibrinogen and prothrombin, a variety of specialized carrier proteins, and maintaining the balance between the breaking down and building up of the labile protein resources of the body. It detoxifies a large share of the body's metabolites, and maintains the balance of fats and carbohydrates, storing glucose as glycogen, feeding the brain and other tissues' glucose under the stimulus of glucagon (from the pancreas), adrenalin (adrenal medulla) and cortisol (adrenal cortex). Further, it synthesizes cholesterol and other building and storage fats, increases building materials for growth (under the stimulus of pituitary somatotropin, gonad hormones and some adrenocortical steroids) and in general maintains the ebb and flow of catabolism (breaking down) and anabolism (building up). Broadly speaking, during the day it lets things out, while sleeping it builds things back up again for the following day. It breaks down aging red blood cells, holds some storage iron and ships off the rest of the hemoglobin in carrier form to the bone marrow to make more red blood cells. Further, it takes all the blood from the pancreas, spleen and the entire intestinal tract, sorts through it, organizes, stores and feeds the blood, cleaning out the junk with its great array of resident white blood cells (liver macrophages or Kupffer Cells), and organizing with its enzyme-rich hepatocytes. All this metabolism in the liver creates waste products many of which are excreted into the liver's own sort of urine, the bile. Bile contains special cholesterols called bile acids, and when mixed into the duodenum with pancreatic alkali makes the soap that emulsifies food fat for digestion. The bile from the liver is stored in the gall bladder where it is concentrated and dehydrated into a thick liquid, capable of very efficient fat digestion when needed. Liver bile can also drain past the gallbladder to empty directly into the duodenum. Unrecyclable hemoglobin is excreted in the bile as bilirubin and colors the feces brown, while bile itself acts as a stimulus to peristalsis in the colon.

Liver deficiency symptoms are dry skin and mucosa, atopic allergies in the skin, sinuses and bronchial mucosa, and generally poor fat and protein metabolism and appetite. There is a tendency for labile blood sugar levels and an overall catabolic homeostasis, with yinny sweet foods preferred to yangy fats and proteins. Most folks with blood sugar problems, allergies and constipation are liver deficient. It can be acquired later in life with viral hepatitis, heavy drinking and extended contact with solvents. *Herbs to stimulate* increase liver metabolism by exciting hepatocyte enzyme production, increasing bile synthesis and liver cleansing, improving fat absorption into the lymph and taking the lipid load off the portal blood and liver, or increase blood supply by dilating the hepatic artery.

Liver excess symptoms are moist, oily skin, rapid defense response with quick fever and sweating, fat and protein cravings with a general anabolic excess; in middle age tending to elevated cholesterols, hyperuricemia and essential hypertension. The usual causes are adrenocortical stress, with elevated testosterone and progesterone, but also may be caused by thyroid stress, in which case there is general tachycardia and disruption of sleep patterns. *Herbs to cool* tend to increase blood buffering of nitrogenous retention with electrolytes, increase bile secretion without stimulating liver metabolism or aid in sodium loss/potassium retention. In reality, diet is the most important approach, decreasing proteins and fats, and increasing those green and red things hated by liver excess folks. A trip to a salad bar by a liver excess is an excuse to eat blue cheese dressing; hard people to change.

KIDNEYS

Outline of function. The kidneys take the arterial blood from the renal arteries squeeze it through half a million little filter tubes (the nephrons) which separate the blood into thick protein sludge and watery serum. The serum passes lymph-like through the tubules, allowing all the important constituents to be absorbed back into the sludge until the exiting blood is restored and cleaned. A minute amount of fluid (containing waste solutes) is passed out into the pelvis and ureters as urine. The result is that sodium or potassium is retained (under the influence of the adrenal cortex), water is retained or not (the pituitary) and the balance between acid and alkaline is maintained. Further, the reactivity and constriction of blood vessels and the heart is potentiated by kidney proteins, acted on by the liver, allowing blood to flow to the brain when we stand, to back off when we sit, etc. Basically, the kidneys control blood volume, quality and dispersal, with urine facilitating this and not the primary function. The kidneys are organs that hold in far more than they let out.

Kidney deficiency symptoms are frequent, dilute and pale urination (often at night), flushing, thirst and sometimes low blood pressure. Orthostatic hypotension is common…you stand up and the blood stays somewhere around your solar plexus, gradually surging up to your brain. There is a tendency to react poorly to sudden changes in temperature and humidity, with short-term water retention and headaches. The urine is often neutral or alkaline. *Herbs to stimulate* either strengthen or stimulate kidney nephrons, improve renal blood supply that is often diminished in adrenal stress and improve hormonal stimulation. With kidney deficiency and increased volume or urine, there is less fluid surplus for the skin, intestines, and lungs; this is further defined later.

Kidney excess symptoms are sodium and water retention, essential hypertension (increased blood volume), concentrated acidic urine, warm moist skin (under any circumstance), and orthostatic hypertension (you stand up quickly and it feels like your ears are going to bleed). *Herbs to cool* either dilate renal arteries, relax the limbic system and the hypothalamus, decrease tubular reabsorption of sodium and therefore increase the volume of the urine since water follows sodium, or decreases water reabsorption by altering osmosis in the nephrons, with sodium following. As in liver excess, food is very important here, decreasing protein in the diet and increasing foods high in electrolytes and minerals. The same hormonal stresses are also involved.

REPRODUCTIVE

Outline of function—women. This is easiest to define through the estrus cycle. At ovulation (day 14–15) FSH (follicle-stimulating hormone) is secreted by the pituitary (controlled by the hypothalamus of the brain), and a now fully matured egg is popped from an ovary, the initiation of next month's egg begins (the one that will mature and pop in 28 more days), and the newly emptied follicle seals off to form the corpus luteum, the temporary endocrine gland that makes progesterone. The newly initiated egg follicle will be the source of estrogen for 4 weeks (until its egg pops and it starts making progesterone), and both the old follicle (progesterone) and the new follicle (estrogen) will secrete under the influence of another pituitary hormone, LH (luteinizing hormone). LH drops two or three days before menses, the corpus luteum falls apart (no more progesterone for that cycle), and the estrogen from the new follicle stops. Menses begins (day one); a few days later LH is surged up by the pituitary until estrogen levels are high enough to trigger LH depression and FSH secretion, triggering ovulation and another follicle to mature (day 14–15). Estrogen triggers growth of the uterine lining and some breast tissue after menses (the proliferative phase) and the dominance of progesterone after ovulation (the secretory phase) results in secretory organization and the increase in blood supply to the tissues stimulated by estrogen earlier. Progesterone, a testosterone relative, increases fat and protein metabolism, red blood cell synthesis and insulin sensitivity. When menstruation starts, the flow has been set up by the secretory phase so that there is heparin (anticoagulant), lysozyme (anti-microbial) and thin mucus to aid the dissolution of the thickened uterine lining. The fluid retention of the progesterone phase (particularly in the breasts) is reduced and urine production slightly increased. Estrogen is yinny, progesterone yangy, and women (in their reproductive years) go through four-week cycles of contraction and expansion.

Outline of function—men. Testosterone is the dominant reproductive hormone and the only important one in the bloodstream. It is secreted by the Leydig cells of the testes (stimulated by LH) and is moderated in the testes by the Sertoli cells, which secrete estradiol and androgens locally (stimulated by FSH) and can inhibit LH and therefore testosterone. This ebb and flow between the Leydig and Sertoli cells constitutes the male equivalent of the estrogen-progesterone ambivalence in women, and the balance of yin and yang in the testes maintains fertility, prostate health and prevents testosterone overdominance in the body.

Reproductive deficiency in women includes regularly long cycles (30 days or more), erratic cycles and menses that start slowly with cramping and spotting that extend too long. Deficiency can also include frequent vaginal or uterine inflammation or congestion, cervical erosion or history of class II or III pap smears and herpes flareups around the time of menstruation. Since liver deficiency is often concurrent, the anabolic peak of days 21–24 is handled poorly, with a sense of heaviness, malabsorption and pelvic congestion from portal blood engorgement. In men, deficiency is characterized by benign prostatic hypertrophy before age 45, difficulty in maintaining erection in appropriate circumstances (sometimes) and a low sperm count together with dry skin. Frequent use of alcohol, cannabis and cocaine can induce an acquired deficiency. *Herbs to stimulate* (in both sexes) increase utilization of steroids, improve pelvic circulation, or affect the hypothalamus/pituitary relationship.

Reproductive excess symptoms in women are a short estrus cycle, signs of estrogen excess after ovulation such as hypoglycemia, excess water retention and sore breasts as early as a week before menses. Excess symptoms in men include recent increases in skin and scalp oiliness in the absence of recent alcohol or solvent exposure. Regular alcohol consumption can mimic excess in both sexes, regular cannabis use can mimic excess in women.

RESPIRATORY SYSTEM

Outline of function. The lungs expand and contract under the action of the diaphragm, intercostal muscles and abdominal muscles, and are controlled by the central nervous system and both sections of the autonomics. The main volume of air stays static and warm, never leaving the lungs except under stress. The bronchi of the lungs expand (letting more air in) and contract (letting less air in), depending on the carbon dioxide buildup in the blood. The blood piped into it from the heart (venous blood) and back to the heart (arterial) is similarly controlled, all to maintain a balance between waste gas (CO_2) and needed gas (O_2), and acid and alkaline pH. The main body of lung air is static, and the differences between internal and external gases diffuse through this body, with inhaled air being as little as a pint in volume or several quarts (in physical activity). The air is inhaled through the nose and sinuses, cleaning and moistening the air. The upper respiratory system, larynx, trachea and bronchi are all lined with mucus, flowing up and out to clean the membranes, cilia to move the mucus and, deep in the meat foam, many macrophages to protect the most delicate parts of the lungs from bacteria and particles that manage to penetrate that deeply. Sympathetic adrenergic nerves dilate the bronchi and increase the bore (physical activity, stress). Parasympathetic nerves contract the bronchi and stimulate moistening mucus secretions (resting).

Respiratory deficiency symptoms are shortness of breath, dry respiratory membranes with poor expectoration and frequent yawning. The person guards breathing, with labile respiration (sometimes shallow and fast, other times with deep sighs) reflecting emotions…sort of respiratory non-verbal communication, and he/she has frequent lung problems. Respiratory deficient people often smoke tobacco as an instinctive response to its respiratory stimulation but usually quit after several years because it is by nature too irritating. Those that continue smoking gravitate not to its respiratory effects but its stimulation of GI tract and liver functions, as well as a simple addictiveness. *Herbs that stimulate* effect an increase in cardiopulmonary circulation efficiency, oppose the adrenalin stress that is often associated with deficiency by increasing parasympathetic function, or generally increase secretions of mucus, activity of cilia or lymph and serous movement in the lungs.

Respiratory excess symptoms are few except for a tendency to hyperventilate under stress, have active and excessive expectoration, and have cardio-pulmonary excess concurrent with thyroid stress and a general increase in metabolic rate. *Herbs to cool* (although usually not important) mimic sympathetic function or decrease thyroid excess. By and large in excess, cooling liver and mucus membrane function or cardiovascular excess will take care of the limited secondary effects of respiratory heat.

CARDIOVASCULAR SYSTEM

Outline of function. The heart pumps arterial blood out from the left ventricle into the aorta and thence out through the major arteries, into arterials and out into the capillary beds where nutrients surge out into the tissues as serum/lymph, feeding cells and picking up waste products. Some of the fluid, containing complex and solid waste, flows into the lymph capillaries and into the lymph system. The rest, containing soluble and gas waste, filters back into the venous blood, to return through venules and veins, meeting up with its missing fluid (lymph) in the subclavian veins, into the right atrium of the heart, the right ventricle, and out into the lungs to discharge CO_2 and pick up oxygen, back to the right atrium, right ventricle, and so forth. Under physical stress, adrenalin and sympathetic nerves increase the heart output and pump more blood to the skeletal muscles, drawing it from the viscera. At rest, the heart works more slowly and blood returns to the viscera. The kidneys and liver, together with the brain and autonomic systems, control constriction and relaxation of major arteries. Local circulation into the skin and mucosa is under more local control. Together, these mechanisms maintain an even rate of feeding and cleansing, taking substances in excess to where they are deficient, always trying to balance the constantly created imbalances of life. To speed up metabolism to an organ or tissue, more arterial blood goes there. To slow down metabolism, blood supply diminishes. Although the control systems for homeostasis are unimaginably complex, when push comes to shove, more blood/more life force, less blood/less life force, and the cardiovascular system causes and responds to these changes.

Cardiovascular deficiency symptoms are cold hands and feet, dry skin and mucosa, and a thready, shallow pulse that is usually quick and easily compressed. The skin flushes and blanches under environmental and emotional stimulus and there is a general tendency towards peripheral vasoconstriction. *Herbs to stimulate* either increase the force and efficiency of cardiac output, increase the resilience of arterial walls, stimulate parasympathetic energy or act as simple vasodilators.

Cardiovascular excess symptoms are warm skin, bounding pulse and strong and easy secretions and excretions, usually concurrent with varying degrees of essential hypertension with excess blood and interstitial fluid. Blood viscosity may be high, due either to increased chylomicrons (transport fats) from the liver and lymph or a general high level of blood proteins. Simply lowering the blood pressure without decreasing either blood volume or viscosity is to suppress the effect without altering the cause. This often means working on the kidney and liver excess that is the usual cause. *Herbs to cool* generally support parasympathetic or cholinergic energies, sedate the heart and major arteries or act as sodium leaching diuretics.

LYMPH/IMMUNE SYSTEM

Outline of function. From the heart to the smallest capillary, the CVS is lined with endothelial cells that maintain a strong charge which repels blood proteins and corpuscles towards the center of the blood, allowing (in the capillaries) the serum to separate and flow out through the crypts between the capillary cells and into the interstitial fluid (actually a starch hydrogel). The old axiom holds that blood feeds the lymph and lymph feeds the cells. Most of this fluid is reabsorbed back into the capillaries as they leave the tissue and drain into the venous blood, but some, carrying disorganized junk too large to fit back into the blood vessels, drains into open-ended lymph capillaries, which in turn join to form lymph vessels (complete with valves). This is the back-alley garbage collecting system of the circulatory system. As the lymph vessels move into the center of the body, the lymph passes through nodes where the junk is digested and sorted through to check for bacteria, toxins and known antigens. In the small intestines, lymph capillaries absorb dietary fat that has been organized by the intestinal wall, carrying it out of the bloodstream for slower metabolism. The lymph drains into a large vessel, the thoracic duct, which, after many hours of perusal and cleansing, finally drains the lymph back into the venous blood where it belongs. The immune responses are partially carried on in the lymph, the blood and the tissues. These can be separated into innate and acquired immunity. Innate immunity is nonspecific and genetically programmed, consisting of reactions that induce inflammation, induce pagocytosis (white blood cells eating bad stuff) and some chemical responses. This is carried out by the granulocytes—neutrophils, basophils, mast cells, macrophages and eosinophils. Acquired immunity is a learned memory bank of previously encountered bad news, held mostly in the lymph nodes, and manifested by a whole other group of white blood cells called lymphocytes. When microorganisms or large toxins are digested by macrophages, large chunks of digested protein are worn on their membranes and, if previously encountered, lymphocytes are cloned to directly respond to and kill the organism, or to make antibodies out of immunoglobulins as specific "antidotes" (antibodies) for the foreign molecules. Well organized lymph drainage into lymph tissue results in a quick acquired immunity response and speeds up the cleaning of debris from tissues that undergo innate immunity responses, such as in a contusion. Although grossly oversimplified, this is the main stuff pertinent to managing subclinical imbalances.

Lymph/immune deficiency symptoms are mainly those associated with chronic moderate immunodeficiency like slow recuperation, slow healing of injuries and bruises, frequent low-level infections in high-stress tissues such as the respiratory mucosa and skin, and cold and flu symptoms that come and go for a month or more. Underlying causes can be a diet poor in protein, constant and subtle infections that never go away and drain immunologic energy (such as "slow" viruses, candidiasis and sinus infections), and depressions and frustrations. Allergies that persist and induce hypersensitivities to other agents are also symptoms of deficiency. *Herbs to stimulate* increase efficiency of lymph transport, the bone marrow proliferation of neutrophil while blood cells, liver catabolism of immune waste products, phagocytosis by innate immunity white blood cells and overall synthesis of blood immunoglobulins and complement proteins by the liver. Most allergies have as a base an acquired immunity underpinning (antibody response to Juniper pollen, for example) and, if the chemicals produced by the response are not removed from the blood by the liver in an orderly fashion, then the chemicals induce a cascade of unnecessary innate immunity reactions, so stimulation of liver protein metabolism is often necessary.

Lymph/immune excess, although sometimes a pathology as in some autoimmune disorders, seems to have little constitutional importance. Or perhaps I just don't know.

SKIN/MUCOSA

Outline of function: skin. This is the protective covering that connects with the mucosa (the inside skin) like the outside of a doughnut. It cools and heats the blood by sweating, conduction and vasodilation/vasocon-striction, provides a major surface of excretion for waste products, both in sweat and sebaceous fats (sometimes equal to the kidneys), and acts in many ways as the first defense immunologically. It is heavily protected by the granulocytes of innate immunity and is capable of rapid shifts of arterial and venous blood and lymph, to both defend the surface and to protect the fluids by sending them deeper into the body. It contains many sensory organs and is responsible for monitoring our direct environment.

Outline of function: mucosa. This is the protective covering that connects with the skin at the entrances of the body and protects it from the external environment that enters into the body (respiratory and digestive) or when there is possible physical access (urinary tract, repro-ductive, etc.). Even though these tissues are often buried deep in the body, they, like the external skin, face the outside and drain outwards. Since the body organizes waste products in order to excrete them (often to the nearest outside surface), mucus is excretory as well as secretory. Mucus protects the mucosa, taking the place of the dead but flexible squamous epithelium that covers external skin, and when the mucosa is irritated, the mucus increases to protect. The cells below the slime are alive and absorption is possible (as in the intestinal tract) much more rapidly than through the skin. Mucous membranes are therefore highly permeable whereas skin covering is much less so, but the outside and the inside are a continuous cover; if the outside is dry, the inside usually is also. If there are skin allergies, there will be similar reactions in the mucosa. If the person is moist and sweaty, their mucosa will be hypersecretory. As well as their skin heals, so does their mucosa. There are, however, different neurologic and circulatory responses affecting the two skins and they may sometimes need different evaluations.

Skin/mucosa deficiency symptoms are often caused by liver defi-ciency. With tonifying the liver there is some vasodilation and secretory stimulus needed for the skins. Dry flaky skin with cracks and fissures, eczema and strange rough spots are typical, as are frequent mouth, rectal and vaginal sores or inflammation. *Herbs that stimulate* generally increase arteriole or blood supply, stimulate cholinergic sympathetic and parasympathetic enervation of secretory functions, or support the liver to make better quality proteins and fats for cell regeneration. Remember, you need to stimulate blood constituents for rebuilding, blood availability to the tissues and secretory and excretory secretions from the skins.

Skin/mucosa excess symptoms are greasy, oily skin, often with adolescent type acne (acne vulgaris). There is hypertrophy in often-used membranes, such as keratosis pilaris, and a tendency to ingrown hair or even hydrosis. All the skin is oily, not just the face, and all the skin is moist, not just the face, neck, hands and feet (an adrenalin-induced sweat). The person has warm, radiant heat and often a strong body scent. Mosquitoes love them. *Herbs to cool* are sedative to skin nerves or decrease liver excitability. Skin/mucosa excess is usually dependent on reproductive, liver and kidney excess and hard to affect directly.

MUSCLE/SKELETAL

Outline of function. The evaluations exclude the importance of bones in blood cell formation and mineral metabolism, but deal with their structural importance as anchors for tendons and muscles. With muscles (speaking here of skeletal or voluntary muscles only), their tone is set by spinal chord nerves and reflexes, the brain, sympathetic adrenergic nerves; their blood supply (and therefore available energy) is controlled by autonomic nerves and adrenalin. They store glucose for fuel as glycogen; after physical activity, their stored fuels exhausted, they are fed by glucose from the liver, facilitated by insulin from the pancreas. The more often they are used, the greater their tone when at rest, and the more resting blood they receive. In physical activity, their increased blood supply is drawn mainly from the viscera; at rest, digestive, metabolic and reproductive functions recover blood supply (and energy).

Muscle/skeletal deficiency symptoms are subtle except for joint aches and a sense of weakness in the shoulder or legs. A telling sign is very pronounced lethargy after eating. Deficiency symptoms are sometimes found in adrenalin stress. Those with very excessive liver and GI functions usually show deficiency in the muscle-skeletal energy. Those with muscle-skeletal excess usually have deficiencies in liver, kidney, GI and reproductive energy. Much joint and muscle pain, particularly dull-ache chronic stuff, seems to have little constitutional implication and needs to be treated separately. *Herbs to stimulate* are sympathetic and motor nerve tonics or help to increase blood flow to the muscles and joints.

Muscle/skeletal excess symptoms are tight muscles and tendons in the neck, back and legs. The person often needs massage, hot tubs and body work, as the skeletal muscles are both overstimulated when used and hypertonic and taut at rest. The most pronounced excess is in the muscles most affected by adrenalin, those of the neck, shoulders, intercostals, lower back and legs. Other muscle excesses are caused by emotional guarding, with the brain and spinal cord defensively overstimulating some muscles that protect parts of the body that are being offended. This may show up as abdominal hypertonicity (guarding reproductive functions), arms and shoulder hypertonicity (guarding the head or chest), upper back hypertonicity (from a protective or submissive slump or over-large breasts) and so forth. These are hard to treat with herbs and need rolfing or chiropractic. *Herbs to cool* oppose adrenergic stress, disperse blood to the viscera or act as simple muscle relaxers.

Remember, in organ system constitutional evaluations, the herbs need to be tonic. If the herbs cause distress they are wrong, unless there is a clear healing crisis in the primary (disease) problem…and don't overestimate this probability, since most worsening of symptoms is a worsening of the disease and not beneficial. Any formula that induces a new problem is simply wrong. Don't try to treat imbalances that are barely evident and don't try to use an herb for *everything* (the best herbs help several systems at once). Conversely, if the primary problem is aggravated by herbs meant to strengthen everything else, you *are* on the right track, just lower the dosage or substitute with less potent ones.

PATTERNS OF STRESS

We are capable of immense changes in our internal and external environments. We have brains that remember the past, react to the present and evaluate implications and future potential, then hold an internal ad hoc committee meeting (our limbic system) where we decide, given the physical state of our bodies as a further perimeter, how we feel. Our hypothalamus, the decide-and-act part of the limbic system, then sets our various stress thermostats to respond to the presumed order of the day, using both the pituitary hormones and its own hormones to control the body. As we are animals that specialize in this uniquely complex array of stress reactions and automanipulations, we do what we can do, easily setting up patterns of neurohormonal manipulations that become habit, tending to drive our body and psyche in the ways we learn early in life are our innate strengths. We learn to manipulate our metabolisms and energies in excess of physical need, skim off the cream to meet job and life requirements, and let the body soak in the remaining stresses. It is easier to release substances into the bloodstream than it is to put them back if they are not needed. It is easier to stimulate a stress reaction than it is to undo it when there is no outlet. Most of us live physically sheltered lives in well-controlled environments and our stress reactions, being largely physical, are usually redundant. The basic neurohormonal patterns of stress are rather predictable and I lump them into adrenalin (catabolic) stress, adrenocortical (anabolic) stress and thyroid stress. Although these patterns are observed more specifically in the organ system energetics and are more easily modified than innate stress patterns, they need to be understood and sometimes they can be modified. If a person is a thyroid stress type and, besides their primary disorder, has no specific organ system weakness, the stress response can often be helped by *lycopus* or *leonurus* alone, without having to address specifically the effects of thyroid excess on the organs, since they are all predictably responding to thyroid elevation. Generally speaking, in chronic disease it often helps to modify not only the organ imbalances but also the stress patterns; without overt disease I usually leave the stress patterns alone and deal with the organ system imbalances.

Adrenalin stress results from the consistent reliance on epinephrine or flight-or-fight responses to get through the day; it is the most common type. It would take pages of *very* boring discussion to describe the process, but the more we use nerve pathways and neuro-effector junctions, the easier it is, the more dominant they get, and the stronger the organ and tissue changes they induce become. As most adrenalin responses (sympathetic adrenergic) are opposed by other nerves (parasympathetic cholinergic mostly), adrenalin dominance also becomes parasympathetic suppression. This results in the following predictable patterns: GI, liver, kidney, skin/mucosa deficiencies and central nervous system and muscle/skeletal excess. *Herbs to cool* increase parasympathetic strength or relax the hypothalamus and decrease its stress manipulation. Since the brain has such a high rate of metabolism (25% of blood sugar and oxygen is consumed by it), any shifts in blood chemistry or nutritional deficiencies show up there first as CNS (central nervous system) irritability and hypersensitivity, long before less reactive organs have symptoms. Always check the diet and blood proteins and fats first, then use herbs.

Adrenocortical (anabolic) stress results from excess reliance on adrenal cortical and gonad steroids (testosterone, progesterone) and somatotropin, the pituitary hormone that stimulates protein metabolism. The consequence is over-production of structural and storage proteins and fats, essential hypertension and elevated blood lipids. The cause is limbic system stress, the pituitary induces it, and this is just the way some people instinctively stress themselves. These are the predictable patterns: liver, kidney, reproductive, cardiovascular and skin/mucosa excess. *Herbs to cool* help to modify hypothalamus stress, lessen liver anabolism or add alkali to the blood. Unlike adrenalin or thyroid stress, this is tough to deal with directly, as there are no direct deficiencies to stimulate. Help by organ system or fluid energetics.

Thyroid stress is not to be confused with thyrotoxicosis or Graves disease, real pathologies, but instead is a pattern of stress a few people use. It is the only one I have seen acquired through excess coffee, amphetamine or cocaine use, as well as the usual hypothalamus/pituitary axis. These people use their metabolic rate as their stress response. Superficially they seem like adrenalin types, but their skin is warm and moist and their intestinal tract is one a lion would envy. Mild tachycardia is nearly always present, even first thing in the morning, and they sometimes have a mild pseudo-lethargy during the day, with troubled, short sleep. These are the predictable patterns: GI, liver, cardiovascular, lymph/immune and skin/mucosa excess, kidney and muscle/skeletal deficiency. *Herbs to cool* relax the hypothalamus or mildly decrease thyroid response to thyroid stimulating hormone from the pituitary.

Thyroid stress: depressive. Unlike the other two stress types, where there is actually increased strength in the target tissues, thyroid stress is ongoing, with functions affected only so long as the pituitary responds to the hypothalamus. Many thyroid stress people manifest a sort of manic-depressive duality. If they respond to agitation with elevated metabolism, they may respond to depression with a decrease of thyroid stimulation. It is difficult to see, unless they have been in excess during extended periods in the past. Predictable patterns are: GI, liver, lymph/immune and skin/mucosa deficient. They have sluggish eyes and pasty skin. *Herbs to stimulate* act on the hypothalamus primarily, although some central nervous stimulation is often helpful.

FLUID ENERGETICS

This is still another parameter of imbalance. It is the least complex but it is an approach that by itself is often sufficient. The basic premise is this: land animals must carry their ocean with them. We evolved in the ocean, developed methods of controlling potassium, sodium and chloride across membranes to maintain metabolism and life (using solutes in the water), and, along with land plants, we must now carry the ocean in our membranes, controlling these electrolytes (particularly sodium), bathing our cells outside like they were single-celled organisms in the sea. The ocean feeds and cleanses them, and the colony/body must excrete the wastes while maintaining the ocean.

We excrete in the neighborhood of a quart of salty waste-water a day, through the kidneys, the outside skin, the mucosa and through the lungs. When one surface excretes more than it should, the others suffer. Rebalancing the fluid excretions helps maintain better homeostasis and more efficient waste removal.

Skin deficiency results from adrenalin stress or thyroid depression. The surplus fluids are going out through the kidneys (kidney deficiency), and being diminished in the skin, mucosa and usually the lungs. Treat for kidney deficiency and the stress type.

Mucosa deficiency is most noticeable as upper and lower GI deficiency, with surplus fluids going out the kidneys. The skin is usually dry as well, the lungs' fluid energetics are variable and the best approach is to stimulate the GI and the liver bile secretions.

Kidney excess is found in adrenocortical stress people, with the surplus fluids cleansing the skin, mucosa and lungs but being held back by the kidney excess. This needs to be dealt with by treating the kidney excess with sodium/water leaching diuretics, cooling the liver and using the herbs that relax the hypothalamus. The person usually needs to increase dietary minerals (especially calcium) and decrease dietary animal fats and proteins.

Lung deficiency is almost always the result of adrenalin stress and the increase in respiration and dehydration caused by a brittle cardiopulmonary adrenergic stimulus. This is best approached by treating for kidney deficiency and adrenalin stress, perhaps adding some *Asclepias tuberosa* as well.

All membranes over-secreting is the result of thyroid stress and usually is helped by treating that imbalance alone. If the person is adrenocortical stressed but with seeming kidney deficiency, this is often the sign of the anabolic excess burnout with early symptoms of adult-onset insulin-resistant diabetes, so have the blood sugars checked first.

All membranes under-secreting is usually found in thyroid stress depression and treating that is the best approach. If it is found in an adrenalin stress person with diminished kidney production (and some recent enema), have kidney function tests performed; it may be early warning symptoms of renal failure or iatrogenic responses to prescription drugs.

PRIMARY HERBS FOR USE IN CONSTITUTIONAL TREATMENT

ORGAN SYSTEM ENERGETICS

Upper G.I.—Deficiency. Bitter Stimulants: Agave, Aletris, Artemisia spp., Berberis, Cnicus, Coptis, Frasera, Gentiana, Mahonia, Menyanthes, Ptelea. Functional Stimulants: Angelica, Anthemus, Aristolochia (all), Capsicum, Panax quinquefolium, Xanthoxylum.

Upper G.I.—Excess. Astringents: Erigeron, Geranium, Juglans, Myrica, Rubus, Salvia. Protectants: Acacia, Althea, Glycyrrhiza, Prosopis, Symphytum. Anesthetic/Sedative: Dioscorea, Foeniculum, Garrya, Humulus, Mirabilis, Nepeta, Pluchea, Verbesina.

Lower G.I.—Deficiency. Constipative Type: Cassia, Glycyrrhiza, Menyanthes, Podophyllum, Rhamnus, Rumex. Congestive Type: Aristolochia (all), Chionanthus, Collinsonia, Euonymus, Fouqueria, Rumex.

Lower G.I.—Excess. Acacia, Erigeron, Garrya, Geranium, Lycopus (thyroid), Myrica, Prosopis, Rheum.

Liver—Deficiency. Metabolic/Biliary Stimulant: Aloe, Asclepias tuberosa, Berberis, Brickellia, Chelidonium, Chelone, Euonymus, Iris, Leptandra, Linaria, Mahonia, Menyanthes, Phytolacca, Silybum. Lipid/Portal Stimulant: Aristolochia (all), Iris, Larrea, Rumex. Arterial Stimulant: Aristolochia (all), Leptandra, Podophyllum, Xanthoxylum.

Liver—Excess. Buffering Cooler: Medicago, Trifolium, Urtica. Anabolic Cooler: Arctium, Harpagophytum, Lycopus, Silybum, Tribulus. Biliary Cooler: Artemisia vulgaris, Bidens, Coralorrhiza, Erigeron, Taraxacum.

Kidney—Deficiency. Angelica sinensis (Dong Quai), Capsella, Equisetum, Glycyrrhiza, Panax (all), Vaccinium.

Kidney—Excess. Metabolic Cooler: Asclepias (all), Harpagophytum, Iris, Tribulus, Vinca. Diuretic Cooler: Arctium, Capsella, Erigeron, Equisetum, Taraxacum.

Lower Urinary—Deficiency: Capsella, Eryngium, Verbascum Root.

Lower Urinary—Excess: Agropyron, Althea, Piper methysticum, Serenoa.

Reproductive—Deficiency. Anabolic Stimulant: Angelica sinensis, Caulophyllum, Glycyrrhiza, Paeonia, Panax (all). Circulatory Stimulant: Aristolochia (all), Asclepias asperula, Cimicifuga, Collinsonia, Corynanthe,

Fouqueria, Phytolacca, Ptychopetalum, Solanum dulcamara. Hypothalamus/Pituitary Stimulant: Anemone, Gossypium, Leonurus, Turnera, Vitex.

Reproductive—Excess. Functional Cooler: Dioscorea, Mitchella, Oenothera Seed, Trillium, Viburnum. Anabolic Cooler: Eleutherococcus, Tribulus, Vitex.

Respiratory—Deficiency. Circulatory Stimulant: Aconitum (cured Chinese), Copaiba, Eriodictyon. Guaiacum, Stillingia. Parasympathetic Stimulant: Anemone, Asclepias (all), Lobelia, Polygala, Sanguinaria. Secretory Stimulant: Aralia racemosa, Asclepias (all), Drosera, Ligusticum porteri, Polygala, Sanguinaria.

Respiratory—Excess. Functional Cooler: Equisetum, Glycyrrhiza, Grindelia, Prunus, Verbascum. Thyroid Cooler: Lycopus.

Cardiovascular—Deficiency. Cardiac/Arterial Stimulant: Aconitum (cured Chinese), Apocynum, Asclepias asperula, Cereus (Selenicereus), Cola, Convallaria. Parasymp/Vasodilator: Anemone, Aristolochia (all), Bryonia, Ginkgo, Guaiacum, Leonurus, Stillingia, Xanthoxylum, Zingiber.

Cardiovascular—Excess. Cholinergic Cooling: Crataegus, Chrysanthemum parthenium, Leonurus, Lycopus (thyroid), Passiflora, Veratrum, Viscum. Diuretic: Arctium, Taraxacum, Tribulus, Vinca.

Lymph/Immune—Deficiency. Althea, Anemopsis, Aristolochia (all), Baptisia, Bursera, Ceanothus, Commiphora, Echinacea (all), Fouqueria, Guauacum, Phytolacca, Polymnia, Stillingia, Thuja.

Lymph/Immune—Excess. Erigeron, Leucanthemum, Scutellaria, Tribulus.

Skin/Mucosa—Deficiency. Vascular Stimulant: Aristolochia, Asclepias (all), Calendula, Capsicum, Guaiacum, Hydrastis, Stillingia, Xanthoxylum. Liver Stimulant: Guaiacum, Mahonia, Panax (all).

Skin/Mucosa—Excess. Nerve Cooling: Ambrosia, Encelia, Ephedra, Euphrasia, Krameria, Urtica. Liver Cooling: Arctium, Erigeron, Euphrasia, Taraxacum, Tribulus.

Muscle/Skeletal—Deficiency. Motor Stimulant: Aconitum (cured Chinese), Aesculus hippocastanum, Caffea, Cola, Lophophora, Paullinia, Sumbul. Vascular Stimulant: Anemone, Aristolochia serpentaria, Arnica, Oplopanax, Panax (all).

Muscle/Skeletal—Excess. Adrenergic Cooling: Avena, Harpagophytum, Lobelia, Yucca. Muscle Relaxant: Aconitum, Cimicifuga, Cypripedium, Gelsemium, Lobelia, Passiflora, Populus, Scutellaria.

PATTERNS OF STRESS

Adrenalin Stress. Parasympathomimetic: Anemone, Cimicifuga,

Hypericum, Lobelia, Piscidia, Scutellaria, Verbena. Hypothalamic: Avena, Eleutherococcus, Oplopanax, Panax (uncured).

Adrenocortical Stress: Hypothalamic: Aralia (all), Eleutherococcus, Oplopanax, Panax quinquefolium. Anabolic Cooling: Arctium, Medicago, Taraxacum, Trifolium, Tribulus, Urtica.

Thyroid Stress: Leonurus, Lycopus.

Thyroid Depression. Anemone, Aristolochia serpentaria, Centella asiatica, Mahonia, Phytolacca Berries.

FLUID ENERGETICS

Skin Deficiency: See Kidney Deficiency, Adrenalin Stress, Thyroid Depression

Mucosa Deficiency: Upper GI and Lower GI Deficiency, Liver Deficiency

Kidney Excess: See Kidney Excess, Adrenocortical Stress

Lung Deficiency: See Kidney Deficiency, Adrenalin Stress, add Asclepias tuberosa, Lobelia, Polygala, Stillingia.

The Contribution of Herbalism to Western Holistic Practice

DAVID HOFFMAN

A new understanding of health, wholeness and disease is appearing within the dominant culture of the Western world. It is a multifaceted change in both attitude and approach, and is often referred to as Holistic Medicine. Questions are being raised about every aspect of medicine, from the nature of health and disease to appropriate therapeutic techniques. All of which is the exploration of the new paradigm, a change in the patterns of belief and perception that our culture has about itself. This development of new patterns of expectation and explanation is, of course, affecting the field of medicine.

What then is health from the context of this new paradigm? The World Health Organization has the clearest definition, its simplicity highlighting its profound relevance:

Health is more than simply the absence of illness. It is the active state of physical, emotional, mental and social well-being.

This is a wonderfully precise encapsulation of the perspectives of holistic medicine. This approach to medicine starts from the assumption that health is a positive and active state, that it is an inherent characteristic of whole and integrated human beings. From a holistic standpoint, a person is not a patient with a disease syndrome but a whole being. This wholeness necessitates the therapist appreciating the mental, emotional, spiritual, social and environmental aspects of their patients' lives, as well as the physical. A holistic practitioner, of whatever specific therapy, has a deep respect for the individual's inherent capacity for self-healing. This enables a relationship of active partnership in the healing process rather than of expert and passive recipient.

Relating to the whole person is, of course, not new. It is an inherent part of the healer's heritage. From the teachings of Hippocrates onward, caring support of the patient is a goal that every doctor, every herbalist, every nurse, is guided towards by their teachers. Naming and emphasizing holistic medicine today is an attempt to correct the tendency in modern medicine to equate health care with the treatment of a "disease entity." It does not pre-define any medical technique or theory, rather it is a context in which the whole person is considered, their physical health as well as mental/emotional state, relationships and life in the world. A medical doctor can be holistic, as can a medical herbalist or osteopath. This perspective emphasizes the uniqueness of the individual, for whilst acknowledging physical, emotional, mental and spiritual aspects, the importance of tailoring treatment to meet the individual's broad needs is fundamental. As holistic medicine sees health as a positive state of well being and not simply the absence of disease, it emphasizes the promotion of health and the prevention of disease, mobilizing the individual's innate capacity for self-healing.

Herbal medicine fits well into this emerging holistic paradigm. It is a healing technique in tune with nature and has been described as ecological healing because of its basis in the shared ecological and evolutionary heritage with the plant kingdom.

A common idea amongst holistically orientated therapists is that a human being is a self-healing individual and at best all a medical practitioner can do is facilitate this profound inner process. Addressing pathology is relatively straightforward, but health is much more than the absence of disease, it is an active state of well-being. Self-healing is a birthright of all—at the core of what it means to be human is a spark of the divine that moves us towards wholeness and fulfillment. It does not negate the importance of medicine and the healing arts, but provides a broad context within which to view them. The individual is enmeshed in a therapeutic ecology, embraced by a range of healing modalities. I am calling it an ecology because the various components are in relationship with each other and the wider world.

Such therapeutic relationships point to the possibilities of mutual support. This may take the form of compensating for any weaknesses within a particular therapy; for example, homeopathic remedies will not put a fractured arm into a splint. From a more positive perspective, cooperation can lead to synergistic support, with the whole of any treatment program being more than the sum of its parts. A geodesic relationship develops where extraordinary potential and strength can flow from cooperation between the therapies. Differences can now lead to a celebration of the richness of therapeutic diversity and no longer be a cause for acrimonious debate and conflict.

A key insight for the practitioner is knowing the limits of both their therapy and themselves. It should be evident that a well qualified practitioner is skilled in their chosen healing art, but a true holistic healer will be thinking beyond their training and focusing on the needs of the sick person. This, however, raises questions about educational standards which cannot be meaningfully explored here. Suffice it to say that an M.D. who attends a short training in acupuncture is no more an Acupuncturist than a Chiropractor who attends a workshop on herbs becomes a Medical Herbalist.

The various therapies are simply different modalities within the broad spectrum of medicine. With the rapidly changing situation amongst the healing professions, it would be a mistake to talk of Medical Herbalism as a form of alternative medicine. Is it an alternative to Acupuncture, Osteopathy or Psychiatry? Of course not; they complement each other creating a complex of relationships where the whole is much more than the sum of the parts. In light of the unique strengths and weaknesses each approach offers, mutual support and cooperation is the way forward towards a truly holistic health service. All medical modalities are complementary within the perspective of the patient's needs.

Language often blocks communication and shared endeavor in medicine. Apparent vocabulary and jargon disparities may mask fundamental agreements of ideas and approach. On the other hand, lack of clarity obscures important differences in both guiding principles and technique. There is an all too common dogmatic attachment to words and specific formulations of belief, opinion and theory. If the "correct" words or phrases are not used then the speaker must be wrong!

Entrenched confrontation between dedicated allopathic practitioners and dedicated holistic practitioners becomes irrelevant when seen in the context of therapeutic ecology. Open-mindedness and tolerance should be characteristics common to all involved in health care, whether as practitioners, researchers, or patients. Medical modalities that have their foundations outside of the biomedical model should not be ignored or discounted simply because they exemplify a different belief system. They should be respected as an enrichment of possibilities and not a challenge to the status quo.

What then is the contribution of Medical Herbalism to this healing framework? The potential is great, both as a primary therapy and as a support for others. The only real problems are the assumptions of practitioners about the role herbs can play, assumptions which are the result of inadequate training or clinical experience. All too often they are relegated to a symptomatic relief role, "safe" drug alternatives. In other words, the problem is that the herbs work! Working at this level obscures the tonic healing possibilities.

An enduring strength of herbalism is its strong foundation in traditional healing, while at the same time being part of modern science and medicine. Paradoxically, herbalism is both a simple and staggeringly complex therapy. Its simplicity is reflected in the case of picking Cleavers from the hedgerow. Its complexity is seen when trying to grasp processes that underlie the multitude of biochemical interactions between all of a plant's chemical constituents and the metabolic basis of human physiology. The degree and depth of interaction are breathtaking.

This leads to the question of how to use medicinal plants holistically? There is nothing inherent in a plant that defines the way it should be used, and with the wealth of herbs that share our planet, some coherent selection criteria is essential to guide herbalists in their healing work. Over half a million plants present themselves as possible healing remedies. The British Medical Herbalist routinely uses 250, while in China the Herbal practitioner has about 2000 easily available of which 250 or so are commonly used in clinical practice. Some set of guidelines is obviously being applied to whittle down 500,000 to a more manageable figure, but what are they? There are a number of ways to group relevant criteria, but three categories are helpful in Western herbalism.

- Assessment of the herb's impact upon the body and mind.
- Using herbs within the context of a system of some kind.
- Non-therapeutic criteria such as aesthetics, economics and ecol ogy.

Applying these three sets of criteria facilitates the formulation of treatments that can be wholly specific for an individual's unique needs as well as environmentally sensitive and economically reasonable.

ASSESSMENT OF THE HERB'S IMPACT

The herbal remedies of the world vary in strength from potentially lethal poisons to gentle remedies that might be considered foods. The holistically orientated herbalist works with the underlying idea that the body is self-healing and that the therapist simply supports this innate healing process. Thus the tonic herbs become of paramount importance, as this is exactly what they do. A characteristic of tonics is that they are all gentle remedies that have a mild yet profound effect upon the body. Not all herbal remedies are tonics, of course, with many having a powerful impact upon human physiology. These must be used with the greatest respect, reserving their use for those times of illness when strong medicine is required. Identifying the intensity of impact upon an individual is a useful selection criteria. The remedies may be categorized in the following way:

1. Normalizers—Remedies that nurture and nourish the body in some way that supports inherent processes of growth, health and renewal. These are the tonics and are often seen as "herbal foods." Nettle (*Urtica dioica*) and Oats (*Avena sativa*) are excellent examples.

2. Effectors—Remedies that have an observable impact upon the body, providing medicines for the whole range of human illness. Two groups can be identified:

- Whole plant actions, where the effects are the result of the whole plant impacting the human body. Specific constituents may have known effects, but the observable results are more than simply the sum of such chemicals. Consider the anti-inflammatory herb meadowsweet (*Filipendula ulmaria*).
- Specific active chemicals, where the effect is due to a chemical whose impact is so overpowering upon the human body that whole plant effects are not usually seen. Due to the presence of such chemicals they are potentially poisonous if taken at the wrong dose or in the wrong way. The cardio-active herb foxglove (*Digitalis* spp.) and the opium poppy (*Papaver somnifera*) are examples.

The normalizing tonics play a role in ensuring that the individual is at his/her personal peak of health and vitality. The quality of such a state of well-being will vary from person to person, but everyone will sense an improvement in their experience of life. They may also be used to ward off a specific health problem or a family weakness. By selecting remedies that act as tonics for the organ or body system that is the site for recurrent illness or genetic weakness, it is possible to do some impressive preventive work. Of the many examples consider hawthorn (*Crataegus* spp.) for the heart; mullein (*Verbascum thapsus*) and elecampane (*Inula helenium*) for the respiratory system; oats for the nervous system; nettles for the skin and musculoskeletal system. Such remedies will usually have some associated action that will further indicate their best use. Whenever possible, the herbalist will focus on the use of such remedies and will use stronger effectors only if absolutely necessary. The chemically-based effectors are hardly used at all. They are, however, the foundation of modern allopathic medicine.

USING HERBS WITHIN THE CONTEXT OF A THERAPEUTIC SYSTEM

Since the very beginnings of medicine there has been a striving to make sense of the human body, the ills that assail it and the healing remedies used to treat it. This has led to many models or systems of medicine, most of which are only found now in texts on the history of medicine. The use of herbs has been repeatedly organized and then reorganized into systems that reflect the prevailing world view of the time and culture. Today is no exception, especially with the herbal renaissance in full flood.

Herbalism has much to offer holistic medicine when used within the context of a coherent philosophical system. Such systems work with intellectual, conceptual models of the nature of a human being and the nature of the disease process. This description of health and human wholeness is simply a subset of that culture's model of the nature of the world itself. They may be an overly reductionist interpretation of the biomedical model of western medicine or the more holistic medical systems of China and India. The ancient medical systems of the world are profoundly holistic in both diagnosis and therapeutics, a direct result of their focused expression of spiritually whole and integrated cultural world views. This is often the attraction to western herbalists. The holistic strengths of such non-reductionist systems appear to fulfill the deep need experienced by Western practitioners for a holistic approach that is meaningful, practical and relevant.

Recognizing the fundamental role played by such all-encompassing cultural perspectives highlights the need for a Western context for holistic medicine. Acceptance of the Western biomedical model as a useful interpretation of the body does not then mean that the analytical and reductionist approach that characterizes modern allopathic medicine is the only option. Many possibilities arise if the biomedical model is used as a basis for treating the whole person and not simply the disease.

However, this also leads to the frustration that plagues Western health care professionals when they initially explore holistic medicine. There is yet to be written a definitive text on Western holistic medicine, a guide for the practitioner that clearly illuminates these new perspectives, but there is a maelstrom of activity amongst holistic practitioners, exploring and applying the new ideas. For some this is just too frustrating, leading to an abandonment of the endeavor or a turning to one of the oriental systems. For others this is a very exciting time, as the unclarity is an aspect of the flowering of new ideas. It is a time of flux, where many new insights arise and old ideas are reassessed, discarded or embraced anew. Though there may be no clear holistic context yet defined for Western medicine, many of the different approaches in the wide field of health care have achieved much in that direction.

Herbal medicine has a unique contribution to make in this time of change. As a healing modality it is inherently holistic in that its very nature is ecological. The use of plants links both patient and practitioner into their environment in profound ways, facilitating a healing process that could be seen as therapeutic ecology. Such an herbal contribution is but one part of the mosaic that will be Western holistic healing. The application of such ideas is developed below.

Non-Therapeutic Criteria

Applying appropriate therapeutic criteria may sometimes lead to a list of equally relevant remedies. To help further in the selection process there are a number of non-therapeutic factors that can be taken into account. These are aesthetic, economic and environmental.

Economic Criteria

Herbs should be free. Nature does not impose a financial levy as they grow wild and free. There may be environmental costs to take into account, but that is another matter. When possible, use common and inexpensive herbs. Expensive, rare or imported plants may not be any better in a particular case than common and not very glamorous species. The fast-developing herb industry has a financial stake in the promotion of expensive "new wonder herbs" from exotic parts of the world. Remember that Hoboken or Rohnert Park are exotic locales to most of the world!

Environmental Criteria

Seeing ecological relationships as having a bearing on the healing arts can lead to some important insights. The choice of the most relevant therapy should be based on the needs of the individual concerned; however, Donne's insight that "no man is an island" becomes crucial here. In a world where the environmental impact humans has become life threatening, the broader implications of health practices must be taken into account. There is not the space here to explore these vital concerns in the depth needed, but consider these points. What are the environmental repercussions of using a specific remedy or treatment? What is the ecological impact of wildcrafting a specific species? How does organic cultivation compare with agri-industrial methods? What are the costs of transportation and packaging from various sources? Such issues are diverse and complex, but of fundamental importance.

AESTHETIC CRITERIA

There is no reason for herbal medicines to always taste unpleasant! When the choice arises take into account taste, aroma and visual appeal. These factors are a matter of personal taste, but it is fine to select from the list of herbs that results from applying therapeutic criteria based upon personal aesthetic preference. An example is a cough remedy widely used in France, composed of the flowers of herbs that are expectorant, demulcent and anti-tussive. It is straightforward to make an herbal cough mixture that works well, but such effective combinations are often composed of unpleasant tasting plants. The same therapeutic results are achieved with the flower mixture, but in addition there is a wonderful aroma, a delicate taste and beautiful color.

Let us consider a model that enables a prescription to be formulated that addresses the needs of the whole person. Any herbal component must be used in the context of addressing non-herbal factors such as diet, lifestyle, emotional, mental and spiritual factors. All of which must take place in a socio/economic context. Such a model provides the practitioner with the possibility of identifying and addressing a whole range of factors, from symptoms and disease pathology to constitution and whole body toning. This model is not new but rather a formulation of well-established and proven approaches described in holistic terms. There is little that is truly new in such an ancient field as herbalism! This model assumes that the practitioner has a firm grasp of human physiology and "disease" process. It is based upon a five-stage process:

1. Herbal actions—The core of the model is the application of an understanding of herbal actions to human physiology. Obviously, selection of actions that are suitable for a specific person will depend on accurate diagnosis. The following stages are worked through:

   a. Select some diagnostic procedure and identify what physiological process to address and the way in which to address it.
   b. Select what actions are appropriate to achieve stage 1.
   c. Select herbs based on their range of primary and secondary actions, thus ensuring the "best fit."

2. System tonics—The phytotherapist can take advantage of the fact that some herbs show a tonic affinity for certain organs, body systems or even specific types of tissue. Such herbs can be used freely and safely

without thinking of them as "medicines." During illness the system tonics will enhance the health of the organ or system concerned when combined with remedies selected for their specific actions. They are especially useful where a tendency towards illness is recognized but no overt disease is present, opening the possibility of overcoming a weakness that could lead to disease later in life.

3. Specific remedies for the illness—The wealth of herbal knowledge that has been garnered over many generations is rich in plants that are traditionally considered specific in the treatment of certain diseases or symptoms. Even though holistic healing aims at going beyond symptomatic therapy, this knowledge deserves great respect. Knowledge of such specific remedies can add much to a prescription based on actions and system support.

4. Herbal biochemistry—Increasing attention is being given to the pharmacology of plant constituents. This has led to the development of many lifesaving drugs, but is very limited as an approach to using whole plants. In the hands of an experienced herbalist, such knowledge can add to the healing possibilities, but not as much as is often thought.

5. Intuition—There is a flowering of intuitive rapport between herbalists and their plants. Intuition has a special role to play in healing and the unique relationship between plant and person augments it well.

As examples of this approach let us consider treatments for hypertension and osteo-arthritis. There is not enough space to discuss these in the depth they require so attention will be placed on the application of this model. The broader context of treatment must always address nutritional, structural and psychological factors. Lifestyle, environmental and social issues must also be considered if possible.

HYPERTENSION

This common problem usually responds well to herbal medicine. However, how do the insights of holism get applied to the herbal aspects, so that the individual is treated rather than a set formula for hypertension be prescribed? A differentiation must be made between elevated blood pressure with no obvious medical cause (essential hypertension), and that due to an underlying pathology such as kidney, endocrinological or cerebral disease. Here we are concerned with essential hypertension.

Hypotensives, remedies that reduce elevated blood pressure, are the core of any treatment. However, this is a description of observed result rather than an insight into the mechanism of action. Examination of an herb's other actions illuminates the way in which the blood pressure is lowered. Here is a brief listing of those used most commonly in European phytotherapy:

Black Cohosh	*Cimicifuga racemosa*
Black haw	*Viburnum prunifolium*
Cramp Bark	*Wiburnum opulus*
Fenugreek	*Trigonelum foenogrekum*
Garlic	*Allium sativa*
Hawthorn	*Crataegus* spp.
Linden	*Tilia* spp.
Mistletoe (European)	*Viscum alba*
Motherwort	*Leonurus cardiaca*
Nettles	*Urtica dioica*
Onion	*Allium cepa*
Parsley	*Petroselinum crispum*
Passion flower	*Passiflora incarnata*
Scullcap	*Scutellaria* spp.
Valerian	*Valeriana officinalis*
Vervain	*Verbena officinalis*
Yarrow	*Achillea millefolia*

Part of the great potential of herbs in the hands of a holistically orientated practitioner is the multifactorial nature of their impact upon the body. Rarely does a plant have but one action. Through a grasp of the whole action picture of a plant the possibilities of formulating prescriptions that address the individual's unique needs becomes apparent. The secondary actions of these hypotensives are:

Alterative: Black Cohosh, Garlic

Anti-Catharral: Fenugreek, Garlic, Onion

Anti-Inflammatory: Black Cohosh, Blue Cohosh, Buckwheat, Valerian

Anti-Microbial: Garlic, Onion, Yarrow

Anti-Spasmodic: Black Cohosh, Black Haw, Cramp Bark, Garlic, Linden, Motherwort, Passion flower, Scullcap, Valerian, Vervain

Astringent: Black Haw, Cramp Bark, Linden, Nettles, Yarrow

Bitter: Yarrow

Cardian Tonic: Hawthorn, Motherwort

Carminative: Parsley, Valerian

Demulcent: Fenugreek

Diaphoretic: Garlic, Linden, Onion, Vervain, Yarrow

Diuretic: Linden, Nettles, Parsley, yarrow

Emmenagogue: Black Cohosh, Motherwort, Parsley
Expectorant: Fenugreek, Garlic, Onion, Parsley
Galactagogue: Fenugreek
Hepatic: Onion, Vervain
Laxative: Vervain
Tonic: Black Cohosh, Fenugreek, Garlic, Hawthorn, Nettles, Onion,
      Scullcap
Vulnerary: Fenugreek, Onion

The first stage of applying the model outlined above is to identify what actions are indicated for the processes behind this disease.

Hypotensives are, of course, indicated. Selection from the brief listing given above should be based upon their secondary actions.

Cardiac tonics play a fundamental role in strengthening and toning the whole CV system when under such literal pressure. Used in the correct way they facilitate beneficial changes in both the pattern and volume of cardiac output.

Peripheral Vaso-dilators will lessen high resistance within the peripheral blood vessels, thus increasing the total volume of the system and so lowering the pressure within it.

Diuretics help remove any excessive build-up of water in the body and overcome any decreased renal blood flow that might accompany the hypertension.

Vascular tonics will help nourish the tissue of the arteries and veins.

Nervines address the tension and anxiety that will be associated with any stress component in the patient's etiology. There will also be an increase in tension due to hypertension itself, which will be eased with the appropriate nervine. As most nervines are also anti-spasmodic the following applies for them as well.

Anti-spasmodics will ease peripheral resistance to blood flow by gently relaxing both the muscles that the vessels pass through and the muscular coat of the vessels themselves.

SPECIFIC REMEDIES:

A number of herbs have a reputation of being specific for hypertension, usually working because of their impact on at least one of the processes involved in the condition's development. From a British perspective the most important remedy is Hawthorn, followed by Linden.

One possible prescription for essential hypertension might be:

Crataegus spp.	2 parts
Tilia spp.	1 part
Achillea millefolium	1 part
Viburmum opulus	1 part
Valeriana officinalis	1 part to 5 ml of tincture 3 times a day
Allium sativum	should be used as a dietary supplement.

All of these remedies are hypotensives but a review of their secondary actions show that this prescription supplies:

- hypotensive *Crataegus* spp., *Tilia* spp., *Achillea millefolium, Viburnum opulus, Valeriana officinalis*
- cardiac tonic *Crataegus* spp., *Tilia* spp.
- diuretic *Achillea millefolium, Crataegus* spp., *Tilia* spp.
- anti-spasmodic *Tilia* spp., *Viburnum opulus, Valeriana officinalis*
- vascular tonics *Crataegus* spp., *Tilia* spp., *Achillea millefolium*
- nervine relaxant *Tilia* spp., *Virburnum opulus, Valeriana officinalis*

Other plants would come to mind depending upon the individual's specific symptom picture. For example, if headaches are part of the picture of the patient's hypertension then include wood betony (*Stachys betonica*) as part of the prescription. If there is tachycardia associated add Motherwort (*Leonurus cardiaca*). Stress as a factor would indicate increasing the nervine content and possibly including an adaptogen. Thus:

A possible prescription for Hypertension with stress as a major factor:

Crataegus spp.	2 parts
Tilia spp.	1 part
Achillea millefolium	1 part
Eleutherococcus senticosus	1 part
Scutellaria laterifolia	1 part
Viburnum opulus	1 part
Valeriana officinalis	1 part to 5 ml of tincture 3 times a day
Allium sativum	should be used as a dietary supplement.

A possible prescription for Hypertension with associate headache:

Crataegus spp.	2 parts
Tilia spp.	1 part
Achillea millefolium	1 part

Viburnum opulus	1 part
Stachys betonica	2 parts to 5 ml of tincture 3 times a day
Allium sativum	should be used as a dietary supplement.

From here it is possible to fine-tune an individual's medications to address their unique situation. The possibilities are as endless as people are diverse. From depression, debility, digestive problems, to bronchitis or PMS, the phytotherapist's formulation can readily embrace their treatment.

A possible prescription for Hypertension with debility:

Crataegus spp.	2 parts
Tilia spp.	1 part
Achillea millefolium	1 part
Viburnum opulus	1 part
Artemisia vulgaris	1 part to 5 ml of tincture 3 times a day
Allium sativum	should be used as a dietary supplement.

A possible prescription for Hypertension with bronchitis (exact proportions will depend upon the relative severity of the associated symptom picture):

Crataegus spp.	2 parts
Tilia spp.	1 part
Achillea millefolium	1 part
Marrubium vulgare	1 part
Viburnum opulus	1 part
Verbascum thapsis	1 part to 5 ml of tincture 3 times a day
Allium sativum	should be used as a dietary supplement.

A possible prescription for Hypertension with PreMenstrual Syndrome:

Crataegus spp.	2 parts
Tilia spp.	1 part
Achillea millefolium	1 part
Scutellaria laterifolia	1 part
Scutellaria laterifolia	1 part
Viburmum opulus	1 part
Valeriana officinalis	1 part
Vitex agnus-castis	1 part to 5 ml of tincture 3 times a day
Allium sativum	should be used as a dietary supplement.

BROADER CONTEXT OF TREATMENT:

There are a plethora of factors that have been identified as being important in the cause and treatment of essential hypertension. However it must be remembered that causation is always multifactorial and statements about alcohol or calcium are often too simplistic. For example, one study failed to show any association between heavy coffee consumption and long-term hypertension. Such coffee drinkers tend to be heavy smokers as well and this in turn may be associated with a lower body weight and thus a lower blood pressure—but with increased risk of heart attack! Lifestyle can often be the key in reversing this condition. Exercise, massage and other approaches to the body are important as are relaxation techniques and meditation. The nature of the individual's work, relationships, world view, self image, diet, etc. all may contribute to hypertension, creating a challenging job for the practitioner!

OSTEO-ARTHRITIS

Osteo-arthritis, the commonest form of arthritis, affects one out of every six Americans, including 80% of persons over the age of seventy. It is a condition that responds well to herbs if used within a treatment regime that addresses diet, lifestyle, etc.

The herbal traditions of the world abound in "Anti-Rheumatics." These are remedies that have been observed improving the patient's experience of rheumatic problems. That is not to say that they have a specific effect upon the disease or even necessarily upon the musculo/skeletal tissue itself. It is a description of outcome rather than process, and as such is very limited in its applicability, unless the processes at play for each herb are understood.

The activity of these herbs can be explained as an expression of a more broadly relevant action. Those that facilitate a real healing of the problem can usually be identified as alteratives, diuretics or some other systemically beneficial action. The anti-inflammatory ones usually simply reduce the symptom picture, and as desirable as this is, it does not indicate a beneficial change in the disease process. An exception to this last point would be where an active inflammation is worsening the pathological changes to bone tissue. Of course such connections between actions and results cannot always be worked out. If you want predictable, reductionist cause and effect, become an accountant! A review of the anti-rheumatics commonly used in Europe reveals these actions:

Anti-Inflammatories: Angelica (*Angelica archangelica*), celery seed (*Apium graveolens*), birch (*Betula* spp.), wild yam (*Dioscorea villosa*), meadowsweet (*Filipendula ulmaria*), wintergreen (*Gaultheria procumbens*), guaiacum (*Guaiacum officinale*), devil's claw (*Harpagophytum procumbens*), bogbean (*Menyanthes trifoliata*), white poplar (*Populus tremuloides*), willow bark (*Salix* spp.).

Alteratives: Burdock (*Arctium lappa*), mountain grape (*Berberis aquifolium*), guaiacum (*Guaiacum officinale*), devil's claw (*Harpagophytum procumbens*), blue flag (*Iris versicolor*), bogbean (*Menyanthes trifoliata*), poke (*Phytolacca decandra; Rumex crispus*), sarsaparilla (*Smilax* spp.), nettles (*Urtica dioica*).

Diuretics: Celery seed (*Apium graveolens*), yarrow (*Achillea millefolium*), bearberry (*Arctostaphylos uva-ursi*), boneset (*Eupatorium perfoliatum*), parsley (*Petroselinum sativum*), dandelion (*Taraxacum officinalis*).

Circulatory Stimulants: Horseradish (*Armoracia lapathifolia*), mustard (*Brassica* spp.), cayenne (*Capsicum minimum*), bayberry (*Myrica cerifera*), rosemary (*Rosemarinum officinalis*), prickly ash (*Zanthoxylum americanum*), ginger (*Zingiber officinale*).

Anti-Spasmodics: Black cohosh (*Cimicifuga racemosa*), cramp bark (*Viburnum opulus*).

Applying the model to osteo-arthritis, these actions might be indicated for the processes underlying this condition:

Anti-Rheumatics are indicated, but their selection must be based upon a sound therapeutic rationale.

Anti-Inflammatories are fundamental as their use will not only ease the symptom picture but help to stop the degenerative changes to bony tissue. In O.A., the salicylate-based herbs are helpful.

Alteratives are the key to any attempt at transforming the systemic problem (if present). If the O.A. has its roots in physical wear and tear they will not be quite as effective.

Anti-Spasmodics lessen the impact of friction through relaxing the muscular envelope around joints.

Circulatory Stimulants help the healing process by increasing peripheral blood flow, thus facilitating all the work this amazing tissue fulfills.

Rubefacients can be useful for local stimulation of circulation and inflammation reduction.

Analgesics may ease discomfort, but must not replace appropriate treatment.

Diuretics help the kidney do its cleansing work.

Nervines will usually be relevant because of the many ways in which a stressed patient can benefit from such support. The relaxants also act as anti-spasmodics and the tonics will help the person deal with the constant stress of the pain and discomfort.

Other actions: bitters, hepatics, expectorants, emmenagogues, etc....For example, the whole digestive process must be working well and not damaged by side effect reactions to non-steroidal anti-inflammatories.

SYSTEM SUPPORT:

In addition to musculo/skeletal attention, the digestive system needs special care. Beyond that it will depend upon the individual's specific case. Always remember the general principles of good elimination, without resorting to strenuous "purging and puking."

SPECIFIC REMEDIES:

Both *Menyhanthes trifoliata* and *Harpagophytum procumbens* could be considered as specifics. However, the multi-factorial causation must be remembered, highlighting the unlikelihood of one specific. *Urtica dioica* is a traditional remedy throughout Europe, used internally and externally. This external use, with fresh raw leaf, is not a treatment for the fainthearted!

One possible prescription:

Menyanthes trifoliata	2 parts
Filipendula ulmaria	1-1/2 parts
Cimicifuga racemosa	1 part
Zanthoxylum americanum	1 part
Apium graveolens	1 part
Angelica archangelica	1 part
Achillea millefolium	1 part in tincture to 5 ml three times a day

External treatments as indicated.

If there is any associated stomach irritation due to the harshness of the *Menyanthes,* then add *Althaea.* In this combination we are combining antirheumatics that provide a range of relevant actions:

- alterative remedies—*Menyanthes trifoliata, Cimicifuga racemosa*
- salicylate anti-inflammatories—*Filipendula ulmaria*
- general anti-inflammatories—*Angelica archangelica, Menyanthes trifoliata, Cimicifuga racemosa*
- nervine anti-spasmodics—*Cimicifuga racemosa and Apium graveolens*

- peripheral vaso-dilator—*Zanthoxylum americanum*
- diuretics—*Apium graveolens, Achillea millefolium*
- carminative and intestinal anti-inflammatories—*Angelica, archangelica, Apium graveolens*
- bitter tonics—*Menyanthes trifoliata, Achillea millefolium*

CONCLUSION

Herbal medicine can make a profound contribution to Western medicine, especially when used in a holistic context. It provides a unique interface between patient and the living world. As a relevant and effective therapy it has much to offer medical treatment, but also finds relevance as part of humanity's reacknowledgement of the rest of the living world.

Above all else, Herbalism is the medicine of belonging, the direct experience of the whole healing the part. Our world blesses us with herbs, with leaves of life. In the face of blind abuse of nature, we discover remedies that can help us survive the impact of humanity's mistakes. To heal ourselves we must know ourselves, and all of ecology, spirituality, intuition and common sense tells us that we are all one. If our world is sick and poisoned then so are we. If the forests are being destroyed, then we die a little with each felling. Every whale that is respected blesses us. Each river cleaned and renewed, flows through our veins and renews us.

Humanity is being faced with the realities of a shared planet. This may take the form of a drought caused by the greenhouse effect, pollution-induced birth defects or the purgatory of human overpopulation. On the other hand it may be the dawning recognition that the intimate embrace of our world is a healing force moving humanity towards a transformation of our relationship with the earth, ourselves and each other. The medieval herbalist and Christian mystic Hildegard Von Bingan, talks of "viriditas," the greening power. The healing offered so abundantly and freely by the plant kingdom is indeed a greening of the human condition, pointing to the reality of a new springtime. Humanity is awakening and finally becoming present within the biosphere, vibrantly alive, eyes wide open with hearts that feel the love of the Whales and the Redwoods, minds revivified, filled with the vision of a healed world and ready for the challenges ahead.

Herbalism abounds with opportunities to experience the reality of the healing presence of nature, whether in treating disease or in hugging a tree. Approaching herbalism from its array of diverse and divergent components illuminates a field of human endeavor that is a wonderful weaving of the miraculous and the mundane. It is a therapy that encompasses anthraquinone laxatives, the spiritual ecstasy of the Amazonian shaman and the beauty of the flower. The limits to what might be called the the path of the herbalist are only those imposed by parochial vision and constipated imagination!

It has been said that without vision the people die. Without a personal vision, life becomes a slow process of degeneration and decay, and without some social vision civilization rapidly disintegrates. Such life-affirming vision of humanity's place within the family of Planet Earth is rapidly illuminating our culture. Herbalism, with its reverence for life and bridging between plants and people, is at the heart of this transformation.

Traditional European Medicine and Transcultural Polymedicine:
A Western Clinical Model of Herbal Medicine from Traditional Chinese Medicine, Ayurveda and Traditional European Medicine

CHRISTOPHER HOBBS

Throughout the history of human civilization, cross-cultural influence has been a remarkably enriching process, particularly in medicine.[1,2,3,4] Such is the case with medicine today, which is experiencing a major evolutionary movement—the influence and power of industrial medicine has peaked and we are now realizing this old order, "old paradigm" medicine, has been a major contributor to environmental destruction. One need not look too far to see that industrial wastes from the manufacture of synthetic drugs and the use of hi-tech medical diagnostic devices, such as X-ray and radiation treatment machines are not environmentally sound. This is not to say that all technological medicine is worthless and should be discarded. Advancements in gene repair and replacements of body parts that have been injured or diseased are remarkable achievements. However, embracing a more simple, environmentally-responsible, less technologically-oriented person-contact medicine can by no means be counted as a regression in the overall health of the people or the planet.

The new "Environmental Medicine" or "Eco-Medicine" (or holistic medicine as it is being called) will contain elements of both technological medicine and allopathy and will incorporate various world cultural healing systems. The medical office of the future will incorporate two distinct kinds of practitioners—one or more trained in treating pathology (an allopathic doctor, for instance) and one or more trained in health—i.e. helping patients or clients increase levels of wellness and maintain a high level of health such as naturopathic physicians, chiropractors, acupuncturists, herbalists and spiritual healers.

Foremost among medical systems that are influencing the industrial, allopathic, drug-oriented model at present are Traditional Chinese Medicine and Traditional European Medicine (TEM). I have coined this last name, based on the ancient Western traditional system of therapeutics using herbs and nature-cure (water, foods and other natural therapies).

These medical systems are medical arts and sciences very much resonant with eco-medicine, in the sense that they embrace the human interaction with the cycles and seasons of nature. TEM has changed considerably over the centuries; in the last 100 years, it has embraced the industrial, allopathic model profoundly. However, in the last 10 years under the influence of the holistic health movement and "herbal renaissance," it is changing once again.

Other influential healing systems include Ayurveda, the ancient Indian medical system, as well as Native American herbalism, Tibetan medicine and Unani medicine. It is not the purpose of this present work to review the history of TCM, or any of the other cultural medical systems mentioned, but the reader is referred to the reference section for further reading.[5,6,7,8,9]

Today, as the planet shrinks we are seeing the emergence of a "planetary medical model," which may be the medicine of the future, combining the best of all three major ancient medical systems. Although TCM has been touted as the most intact and usable healing system, it is obvious that Ayurveda also has much to offer. TEM has been severely fragmented and disorganized for many centuries, and in some Western industrial countries, has atrophied as a viable clinical system. It is my belief, however, that this system has been meeting the needs of the people for over 3,000 years and will continue to do so. It only needs a super-structure in which to bring it into artistic coherence and modern practical application. All the pieces are present—the four elements, the humors, the temperaments, herbalism, nature-cure (including hydrotherapy and diet therapy) and the fine-pointed understanding of the physical laws of nature (including physics and chemistry) which can be drawn into a practical clinical system. This essay is an attempt to continue the conversation in this process. Since the nature of my work has been primarily to explore the wealth of practice and experience that comprises Traditional European Medicine, and the influences of the other systems upon it, the reader is also referred to the reference list (which is comprehensive) for further study on the history of herbalism. This list has been compiled from the Institute for Natural Products (INPR) Library. As an avid collector of old herbals, materia medicas, pharmacopeias, dispensatories, writings in ethnomedicine and other works on the history of health and medicine, I have brought together a library of over 2500 books, some original works going back to the 1500's, also including modern translations and reviews of the most important works on ancient herbalism as well as an extensive collection of journal articles on the ethnobotany of the Native American peoples and the history of herbalism. Additionally, my ongoing work is to translate previously unavailable books and articles from the original German and French, of which there is a wealth (such as Gerhard Madaus' *Handbook of Biological Medicine* in 3 volumes and *Hagar's Handbook* in 7 volumes.)

THE COMMON ROOTS OF TRADITIONAL HEALING SYSTEMS

As the planetary sociosphere becomes smaller, it is interesting as well as useful and practical to compare the beginnings of medical thought and practice with what is evolving today in modern holistic medicine. It is easy to delineate the common roots in widespread world cultural medical systems; for instance of Egyptian, Greek, East Indian and Traditional Chinese Medical systems. In the ancient medicine of the Egyptians and Greeks, a system of medical and herbal energetics, diagnosis and practice was widely used and discussed. For instance, common diagnostic techniques in TCM then, as now, included determining the quality, regularity and strength of the pulse, the quality, color, texture and coating of the tongue, physiognomy and lifestyle habits and patterns. Energetic properties such as taste, texture and biochannel energy activation were noted for various herbal medicines.

INDIVIDUAL CONSTITUTION (INDIVIDUAL BIOTYPE)

It was recognized early in the written history of medicine that the constitution or unique nature of the individual was of importance for determining the causes and outcome of illness. The significance of the individual constitution in diagnosis and the course of illness has been recognized in all ancient systems of medicine. In an important Hippocratic work, *Epidemics I* (Chapter 23), we read *"Then we must consider the patient, what food is given...the conditions of climate and locality...the patient's customs, mode of life, pursuits and age, and that 'the nature of man in general and of each individual and the characteristics of each disease' must be taken into account."*

In TCM and Ayurveda, constitutional types are well developed and an integral and indispensable part of the systems. See Dharmananda, Kaptchuk, Dash and Sharma for further reading.

PULSE DIAGNOSIS

The value of the pulse in diagnosis was known by the Egyptians (Castiglioni, 50) and the Hippocratic writers, about 450 B.C., but it was Praxagoras of Cos (ca. 300 B.C.) that first wrote extensively of it (Lloyd, 31).

Galen (ca. 131–201 A.D.), one of the most renowned and prolific of the ancient medical practitioners, wrote down his extensively developed "pulse lore," where he described pulse attributes such as "broad," "long," "deep," "shallow" and "small," much the same as developed in TCM (Clendening, 42–3).

FIVE-ELEMENT THEORY AND THE FOUR QUALITIES

Another common feature of TCM and TEM is five-element theory and temperature attributes in constitutional diagnosis and in herbal energetics. Five-element theory is often stated to be of Chinese origin (Veith, 18), though similar systems can be seen from the Vedic scriptures, the formative document of the Indian system of medicine, Ayurveda, as well as TEM. The five elements as given in the *Nei Ching* (Veith) are water, fire, wood, metal and earth.

In TEM, the doctrine of four elements arose in the century before Hippocrates (5th–4th century B.C.). Medical writers of this period often spoke of more elements than fire, air, water and earth, and also of more qualities than four, but were strongly influenced by the "mystic number 4" of Phythagoras (530 B.C.) and his followers. Galen describes 4 elements (Siegel, 145), which he mentions as being written of by Aristotle (ca. 360 B.C.) and even earlier, Hippocrates (455 B.C.). Interestingly, an additional element, wood, is also mentioned as consisting of air and earth. This element is also present in TCM, but it is difficult to determine if this is an artifact of a very early common system.

Galen (2nd century A.D.) brought the four element theory of TEM to its fullest expression. In Galen's writings, which remained a dominant influence for nearly 1700 years, one finds that the four elements consisted of different combinations of the four essential qualities from which they are made. The four *primary qualities* are hot and cold, dry and moist.

Thus

Water is cold and moist,
Air is hot and moist,
Fire is hot and dry,
Earth is cold and dry.

These closely correspond with the "5 climates" of cold, heat, dryness,

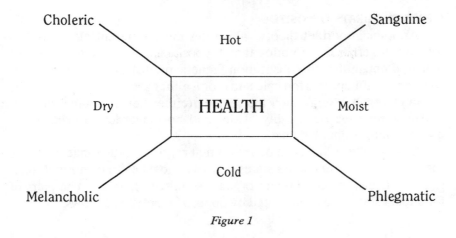

Figure 1

moisture and wind in TCM (Veith, 117). In TCM as in TEM, the elements corresponded to the seasons. Thus, Autumn was considered a cold and dry season, spring, warm and moist, summer, hot and dry and winter, cold and moist.

Figure 1 represents these concepts in graphical form, adding the four humors (blood, mucus, yellow bile and black bile) and four classical TEM constitutional types which are choleric, sanguine, phlegmatic and melancholic.

Although I see value in exploring and developing the four traditional constitutional types, the entire theoretical basis of the four humors needs to be reworked or dropped—it is too simplistic and does not fit for today's practice. For instance, there are obviously many more "humors" that have been identified today, including the various hormones, digestive enzymes and immune substances. It is possible that three main humors, blood, bile and mucus and a number of secondary humors such as hormones, various immune substances, and prostaglandins, might be useful.

It is my belief that any completely workable and fully operational clinical system of TEM needs to be integrated with (but not dominated by) modern scientific understanding of health, physiology and disease. Although some would like to see a return to more simple and traditional healing ways, it is unlikely that this will come to replace scientific medicine. Hopefully, these traditional ways of healing will influence and help infuse current medical thinking with the heart of healing. Meanwhile, it is probable that traditional medical systems will continue to grow in influence.

OPPOSITE TREATS OPPOSITE

Another important theory, which ties these different elements and qualities together is the notion that "opposite treats opposite." In other words, if one, either by constitution (genetic predisposition), or by environmental influences is too cold and moist, either generally or in a specific organ or organ system, then the remedy (either herbal, animal or mineral) should have the quality of dry and hot, in order to bring these qualities into proper balance.

Graphically, a circle can be drawn that represents the range of values for these pairs of functional states that will allow health or normal functioning of cells, tissues, organs, organ systems or organism. The pairs of functional states are represented by opposite arrows, as follows:

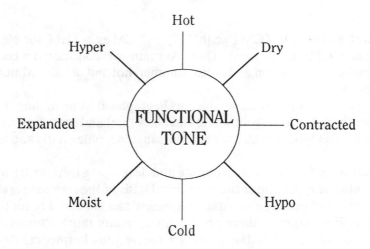

If one looks into these opposite qualities of "states of being," it is easy to add any pair that describes the usual conditions of cells, tissues, organs, organ systems or the complete organism, including:

Expanded/Contracted
Hyper/Hypo
Dispersed/Congested
Flexible/Rigid
Stimulate/Depress
Soothe/Irritate

This system of pairs of opposites is still commonly used in English medical herbalism and is today influential in holistic thought. When these opposite functional states are dynamically poised within a range of values that create optimum health, I use the word "functional tone." A rather erudite way of defining tone is a "dynamic state of functional readiness to fulfill biogenetic potential." Or, in other words, a cell, tissue, organ, organ system or organism is at maximum ability to do its job—that which it was designed to do or that which it grew into being to accomplish. This may be difficult to determine because of the "randomness" of life and health.

In TEM, then, the most important beginning concepts are that of "opposites treat opposites" and the energetic qualities of the medicines, whether they are herbs or nature-cure (hydrotherapy, breathing, diet, etc.).

It is interesting that some writers on medicine and disease, if their perspective is strictly allopathic, tend to talk of the energetics of medicines and constitutional theory, common threads of the medical thought of most human cultures, as archaic (if they are charitable).

MODERN TRANSCULTURAL POLYMEDICINE—A SYSTEM OF CLINICAL HERBALISM

After reviewing the common bonds and origins between three major medical systems, TEM, TCM and Ayurveda, I will now present my own very preliminary vision of a practical system incorporating some of the elements of the ancient systems, interpreted and expanded to encompass a more modern understanding of physiology, biochemistry and current thinking in health and disease. This model will be presented in two parts:

I. That having to do with the individual in health and illness

II. The actions of the herbs or drugs or interaction between the individual and the remedy

INDIVIDUAL HEALTH AND ILLNESS

A. Any discussion about the individual concerning health, illness, imbalance, failure to adapt to environmental change (*environmental stress*) or failure to "let go" of destructive family patterns, such as alcoholism (*ancestral stress*) must include 5 distinct aspects of our being:

1. Spirit: The highest, finest vibrational and everlasting essence.

2. Astral: Our "guardian angel," spirit guide or conscience.

3. Emotional: The medium that connects the higher bodies with the physical body—feelings or knowledge that comes from higher realms affect us consciously as "intuition."

4. Mental: Symbolic, articulate ideas that organize the physical world

so that we can live in it.

5. Physical: Our tangible casing, vehicle for being in the physical world—a temple for exquisitely unique spirits.

These 5 "bodies" are all fully integrated in the healthy individual as part of the *human coalition* or *human organization,* but one or more can be imbalanced by ancestral stress, "collective unconsciousness" (racial stress) or physical environmental factors (environmental stress).

Rudolf Steiner and Anthroposophy take a slightly different view of the human organization,[10,11,12] though this system has had its influence on my thinking, along with that of Dr. Randolph Stone, the founder of Polarity Therapy. In Anthroposophy, the four elements of the human include the Ego or Human spirit, which is listed as a heat-organism, the soul body or astral body, an air organism, the etheric body, a water-organism and the physical body, which is associated with the earth element. Generally, the two systems relate to each other in this way:

TEM	Anthroposophy	Element
Spirit	Etheric	Ether
Astral	Etheric	Air
Emotional	Astral	Water
Mental	Ego	Fire
Physical	Physical	Earth

All 5 bodies need nourishment to flourish, examples of which follow:

1. Spirit: Communion with nature or God (a myth created by people to symbolize the infinite, timeless bliss-reality) through meditation, etc.

2. Astral: Dreaming, trance, astral travel.

3. Emotional: Appreciation, touching, expressions of caring, art (painting, music).

4. Mental: Enlightened conversation, concepts, profound understanding of "reality" through the mind, art.

5. Physical: Nourishing, high vitality food, physical exercise, sex, abundant breath, etc.

All 5 bodies need to eliminate wastes from assimilation, utilization of "nutrients" and metabolism:

1. Spirit: Communion with God

2. Astral: Dreaming

3. Emotional: Positive discharge of negative and excessive emotions through crying, laughing, projection, etc.

4. Mental: "Talking things out" with a receptive friend, public speak-

ing, etc.

5. Physical: Elimination of physical wastes through the skin, bowels and urine.

In the medicine of the future, diagnosis and application of remedies will focus to a much greater extent than at present on other aspects of our being than the physical. The physical is the most obvious—it is where our awareness is attached in disease, illness, pleasure and pain at the present state of planetary vibrational evolution. Most treatments today start with the physical body, but increasingly, during present and future cultural shifts, we will become aware that the higher vibrational bodies have a more powerful effect on our well-being and health. It is easier and requires less energy to create an immediate and lasting change in a person's health/illness patterns by working with the higher vibrational bodies, but we are not used to working with them and often fail to notice when they are imbalanced. When working with vibrational bodies, it is also easier to do harm if the remedies are misdirected, wrong for the individual or used with personal attachment. Just as we look back on the blood-letting and mercurial preparations of 100 years ago as being primitive and barbaric, so will the people of 100 years from now look on our medicine with disbelief.

B. Individuals may exhibit 3 main functional states of imbalance on a cellular, organ, system or personal level—and these affect all 5 bodies.

1. Deficiency
   A lack of nourishment, nutrient assimilation, information, functional energy or vitality.
2. Stagnancy
   There are sufficient energy reserves (vitality) in the individual, but they are temporarily inaccessible—they encounter too much resistance within a system to be effective.
3. Excess
   Energy, movement, nutritive force is too great for the specific individual, a system, or bioenergetic channel to function maximally or even normally.

Diagnosis

During the process of diagnosis, one must determine the person's ancestral constitution and state of present health, as influenced by *environmental* and *ancestral stress*. Once these factors are discovered, the proper regime, remedies and influences can be initiated, discussed and offered in the form of medicines, changes of living habits, etc., whereby a more perfect state of functional environmental resonance and individual biogenetic fulfillment and expression (health) can be achieved.

THE EFFECTS OF HERBS OR DRUGS, OR THE CO-EFFECTS BETWEEN PLANTS AND INDIVIDUALS

Herbal remedies, especially patent (manufactured) remedies, are popular because they require the least amount of energy output by the individual to implement, yet create a positive change. In many cases, all that is required of the individual is to swallow pills or take drops of a liquid extract several times daily. Compare this with the amount of energy that is required to change one's ancestral or cultural habit patterns (such as diet and attitude about other people), change the level of physical activity or exercise, begin inward contemplation, imbibe new knowledge or work with a psychologist or other practitioner of the persona, intellect or emotions. Much more commitment and energy is required for these latter working therapies—energy that may not be available to the individual during a specific time period.

THE QUALITIES OR ENERGETICS OF HERBS

All herbs have inherent qualities, both biochemical and energetic, determining how they will interact with an individual. These general qualities have also been called "herbal energetics." For a well-researched and concise explanation of these qualities of herbs in TCM, see the introduction in Bensky and Gamble. In the present system of TEM, they can be divided into several classes:

The Spirit of the herb:	which of the 5 bodies the herb mainly treats
The Will of the herb:	the strength or tonifying/forcing nature of the herb
Its Effect:	cleansing, balancing or building
Its Affinity:	the organ systems in which it is most active
Taste:	the energetic flavor potential
The Quality of the remedy:	temperature and moistness

REMEDIES TO TREAT THE 5 BODIES (I CALL THIS THE *SPIRIT* OF THE HERB):

1. Spiritual: Communion (being aware of our ultimate sameness with a plant or plant spirit, or all plants and nature).
2. Astral: Interaction with spirit guides, plant and nature spirits

3. Emotional: Bach flower remedies, gem elixirs, aromatherapy, placebo
4. Mental: Bach flower remedies, gem elixirs, aromatherapy, homeopathic medicines, placebo
5. Physical: Herbal remedies

One would then say that St. John's wort has an *emotional* and *physical* spirit, because it is often used to treat physical ailments such as ulcers, but also it is used to treat mild depression. In ancient times, St. John's wort was also considered to have an *Astral* spirit, as a magic and protecting plant, and it was often hung in dwellings or carried on one's person to protect against "pernicious influences."

THE 3 KINDS OF MEDICINES (I CALL THIS THE *WILL*) OF THE HERB.

1. Tonics: Nourish specific cells, tissues, organs and the whole individual. Often used for long periods of time. These remedies help focus and *call forth* the biogenetic potential or *vitality* of the individual for use such as enabling the immune system, nerve function or hormonal balance and vigor.

Tonics are very gentle and slow stimulants *and* they provide nutrients that the body can use, such as vitamins, minerals and many other constituents like plant pigments, such as anthocyanins or flavinoids. Large quantities can be given without harm of overstressing cells, tissues, organs or body systems.

Most importantly, the therapeutic and toxic doses are very far apart—giving a large margin of safety. For this reason, these herbs are called "superior" herbs in TCM. The tonics are remedies that are well-tolerated, do not force the body to change and have a slow, nourishing and normalizing effect on body systems, imparting strength and tone. In TEM, these medicines were called "alteratives," "roborants" or even "tonics." The most famous example in this category is ginseng.

2. Specifics: They have a specific job to do for a limited time (up to three 10-day cycles is common); they "fine-tune" biochemical processes, move energy or regulate energy in the *bioenergetic channels* to help remove stagnancy and redistribute energy in excess conditions. These herbs are moderately active stimulants that must be given in lesser amounts and for shorter periods before over-stimulation and unwanted side-effects occur. One to several therapeutic cycles of 10 days on and 2 or 3 days off is usually adequate. The therapeutic and toxic doses are closer together than in the tonics, but there is still a good margin of safety in most cases.

Specifics are remedies that gently move or "adjust" a process in the body, whether it be hormonal, nervous or in immune function—they are catalysts or assisting remedies. These generally work by stimulating a process—one of the best examples here is echinacea, which stimulates immune cell function and thus confers heightened resistance to pathogenic influences (infections). The specific remedies are generally used only as needed, usually for up to 2 or 3 weeks at most. Other common examples of *specific* herbs are goldenseal, osha, and pau d'arco.

3. Heroics (forcing remedies): They blast through energy blocks and dramatically move or inhibit energy in the bioenergetic channels. For use by practitioners that know their action and dangers when there are seriously imbalanced energies in the individual, especially when the constitution is generally sound. These are strong and highly irritating, causing dramatic changes to occur. They must be used very carefully because there is not much difference between a toxic and therapeutic dose.

These herbs are "heroic" remedies that when properly used, are taken for a very short time to overcome refusal of the body and its processes to change (stuckness). Examples are digitalis (foxglove), belladonna (nightshade) and rauvolfia. Many allopathic, synthetic industrial "drugs" fall into this category. Synthetically-derived compounds such as xanax, tetracycline and aspirin are examples of drugs that are very purified, concentrated and penetrating and have the potential for very profound side-effects. In fact, many hours are spent in medical school just learning how to recognize and manage the side-effects of allopathic drugs.

4. Protective and Cleansing: These are herbs that remove wastes and pollutants from tissues and organs, only minimally affecting the actual processes of the body. Examples are ionic substances such as pectin and soluble and insoluble fibers. Perhaps plant pigments, such as "bioflavinoids," that simply accumulate in the tissues near the skin and can help reduce damage from such agents as ultra-violet light from the sun can be included in this category.

Thus one would say that ginseng generally has a *tonic* will or simply is *tonic,* whereas goldenseal has a specific will (or is *specific*) and *Digitalis* has a forcing will (or is *forcing*).

Amounts

How much of an herb or herb formula is given is almost as important as its intrinsic nature. In practice, one will often find that a small amount of a *specific* herb or herb combination is tonic, more of it will be specific, and even more will be toxic. By definition, even large amounts of a tonic herb or herb formula should not become specific or toxic, but eventually could become so after protracted use.

THE 3 MAJOR EFFECTS:

1. Cleansing—purifying, removing obstructions, rendering bioenergy channels more efficient for carrying energy and nutrients (more dense energy). Nutrients and energy are all types of information.

2. Balancing—restoring and maintaining tone, functional balance, homeostasis, harmony—*pairs of functional opposites* are all balanced.

3. Building—providing essential information of varying vibrational frequencies, such as encouragement (emotional, mental), tonic foods and herbs (physical), etc.

AFFINITY

Herbs also have a greater effect on some tissues and organs of the body over others. I call this characteristic the herb's *affinity*.

For instance, by tradition and scientific investigation, hawthorn has an affinity for the heart, dandelion has an affinity for the liver and Yerba Santa has an affinity for the upper respiratory tract. Herbs can have primary and secondary affinities.

ORGAN SYSTEMS

In TCM, there are a number of organs that sustain bodily activity. These are the yin organs, heart, lungs, spleen, liver and kidneys. The Yang organs include the gall bladder, stomach, small intestine, large intestine, bladder and triple burner.

TEM recognizes the heart, lungs, stomach, intestines, liver, gall bladder, sexual organs, the ductless glands (thymus, pituitary, pineal, thyroid, parathyroids, adrenals, testes, ovaries), sexual organs, spleen and lymph nodes.

I propose that in TEM, a more traditional and useful view than separating each and every organ is to combine them into systems. Modern physiology texts and holistic texts alike often take this view. Thus, the major 12 systems of the body:

Cardiovascular (CV) includes the heart, veins, arteries and capillaries, bone marrow and blood.
Digestive (DG) includes the liver and gall bladder, stomach, small and large intestine, pancreas.
Glandular (GL) includes the ductless glands.

Immune (IM) includes effector cells (T-cells, B-cells, etc.), the bone marrow, thymus, spleen, lymph nodes, lymph vessels and mucous membranes—the "secretory immune system."

Integumentary (IN) skin, hair, nails.

Microflora (MF) includes microorganisms that flourish inside our large and lower small intestine, skin, oral cavity and mucous membranes—this may be the largest active "system" in the body.

Muscular (MS) includes the muscles, tendons and ligaments.

Nervous (NV) includes the brain, spinal cord, nerves, ganglia and synapses.

Respiratory (RY) includes the nasal passages, sinuses, bronchi and lungs.

Sexual (SX) includes the ovaries, uterus and breasts or testes and prostate.

Skeletal (SK) includes the bones and teeth.

Urinary (UR) includes the kidneys, ureter, bladder and urethra.

An herb can have a specific affinity for one or more organ systems, just as herbs have affinities for organs in TCM or Ayurveda. In TEM, if an herb has traditionally been associated with an organ, the herb will probably affect other organs in the same system. For instance, uva-ursi affects all parts of the urinary tract, not just the bladder or kidneys.

TASTE

"The ethereal spirit receives its nourishment from the air and the body receives its nourishment from the flavors." (Veith)

Modern science has helped us to bring herbalism into the modern age with such tools as HPLC (high-pressure liquid chromatography) and TLC (thin-layer chromatography). This technology provides a way to look inside a plant and see what "energetic principles" might be present, as symbolized by biochemical structures—the constituents or secondary metabolites. This is a fascinating and useful view, helping us to determine the identity of an unknown plant powder, for instance, or how growing conditions might effect the strength of a plant. Toxic chemicals can be observed in new species without the risk of much trial and error, as our ancestors had to do.

However, despite the complexity and usefulness of these modern devices, the herbalist has a far more sensitive and complex "technology" with them at all times—the sense of taste and smell. With these, the identity, energetics (taste or temperature, etc.), possible toxicity and therapeutic action can sometimes be determined, depending on how "educated" and sensitive these sensory perceptions are.

Although the physical evaluation with our taste buds provides clues to an herb's taste or flavor, it is really the effect that is most important. In other words, it is likely that a salty-tasting herb has a salty effect in the body, and this holds true for the other flavors. However, just because an herb doesn't immediately taste salty or sweet or sour doesn't absolutely rule out that the herb doesn't have this property in the body. For instance, the herb *Ephedra sinensis,* ma huang, is considered to have a pungent and warm nature (Yeung, 27—Bensky and Gamble), but it actually tastes slightly sweet and astringent. It is the alkaloid, ephedrine, that gives it a warm nature, by increasing respiration, heart rate and blood pressure, helping to create heat by the movement of the blood.

Additionally, tastes have a *primary* and *secondary* characteristic. For instance, acrid has an immediate effect of stimulating digestive gastric and intestinal acid and enzyme production, but eventually may affect many parts of the body, including the circulation to the periphery (hands and feet), the activity of the liver, nerve function, heart activity and elimination from the kidneys and bowels. Not all bitter herbs contain the same chemical constituent types and obviously they don't have the same effect in the body. That's why the tastes of an herb offer only a guideline and approximation to an herb's overall therapeutic activity in the long-term.

In TCM and Ayurveda, there are traditionally 5 primary flavors:

Sweet, sour, salty, pungent (often equated with acrid or spicy) and bitter. Additionally, one finds the "taste" of bland (the absence of all flavor) added in some texts, as well as astringent. Furthermore, pungent is sometimes separated into "pungent-cold" or "spicy-cool" and "pungent-warm." Examples of the first are peppermint, vitex fruits and chrysanthemum—these herbs are used to clear wind-heat conditions such as the common cold or headaches. The second category is characterized by angelica, cinnamon twig, fresh ginger and garlic, which are used to resolve phlegm and warm the lungs for rheumatic pain and chronic bronchitis.

In the system of TCM, the taste of an herb often determines its therapeutic effects. Bensky and Gamble give the following correspondences:

Acrid	disperses and moves	lungs	yang
Sweet	tonifies, harmonizes, sometimes moistening	spleen	yang
Bitter	drains and dries	heart	yin
Sour	drains, prevents abnormal leakage of fluids or energy	liver	yin

| Salty | drains, purges, softens | kidneys | yin |
| Bland | seeps and drains, leeches dampness, promotes urination | — | yang |

One can also find this correspondence for astringent:

| Astringent | drains and dries | none given | none given |

Taking into consideration that every taste must fit into the overall system and cannot be expected to stand alone, I propose the following flavor characteristics in TEM.

THE 6 MAJOR FLAVORS AND THEIR PROPERTIES IN TEM:

Flavor	Primary Functions	Primary Systems
Acrid (spicy-warm)	penetrates, disperses, removes stagnancy	CV, UR, RY
Sweet	nourishes, harmonizes, tonifies, energy sparing	DG, IM, GL, MS, MF
Bitter	dries, stimulates assimilation, expands, removes weakness (all in small amounts)	IM, DG, NV, CV
Sour	cleanses, cools, regulates pH	UR, DG, NV
Salty	moisturizes, strengthens nerves (in moderate amounts)	CV, UR, IN, NV
Aromatic (spicy-cool)	cools interior, warms exterior, treats the surface	DG, NV, RY, UR

THE 2 MINOR FLAVOR QUALITIES:

Flavor	Primary Functions	Primary Systems
Astringent	draws and removes moisture, cooling	DG, UR, MF, IN
Demulcent	cools, moistens	DG, UR, RY, MF, IN

A thorough search of the historic literature of TEM discloses the above 8 flavors in all, in one form or another. Some of these are often called by different names. I propose that demulcent is more complex than a simple quality like hot and cold, moist and dry; it therefore becomes a secondary "flavor quality." I also propose that astringent is not a primary flavor and is not usually considered to be one—it is more of a flavor experience than a true flavor like bitter. Therefore, I place it in opposition to demulcent, as the second *flavor quality*. Demulcent softens, moisturizes, relaxes and cools. Astringent hardens, dries, tenses and warms.

The 8 flavors in TEM are determined from old European traditions, especially as described in the Western herbals from Dioscorides (ca. 70 A.D.) until the 19th century. Besides their long tradition in TEM, they are supported by modern scientific work. These correspondences are also given in Table 2.

Most of the primary flavors match exactly across the 3 systems, except "aromatic." The word aromatic comes from the major characteristic of these herbs—many of them have an aromatic odor and this odor affects the perception of taste. This taste generally corresponds to "spicy-cool" in TCM. These herbs are well-represented in the Mint family (*Labiatae*) with such herbs as the mints, thyme, oregano and basil; and the Parsley family (*Umbeliferae*) with such herbs as cilantro and dill-greens. The seeds of Umbeliferae members usually fall into the category of pungent, because they are more penetrating and dispersing.

TEM	TCM	Ayurveda	20th Century Science-Examples
Primary Flavors			
Bitter	Bitter	Bitter	sesquiterpenes—anti-inflammatory
Sweet	Sweet	Sweet	sugars—glucose source, nourishes nervous system, digestion (by saving vital energy spent in creating enzymes to break down and process foods)
Pungent	Pungent-warm	Pungent	resins—irritants, increases blood flow, stimulates nerve endings (counter-irritant), affects organs and tissues by reflex action, penetrates, anti-microbial
Aromatic	Pungent-cool	—	monoterpenoids—warms surface mucous membranes and "treats the surface," draws blood, immune activity and energy up, cooling interior

TEM	TCM	Ayurveda	20th Century Science-Examples
Salty	Salty	Salty	mineral ions—enhances nerve transmission, regulates water flow in and out of cells, regulates pH plant acids (i.e. citric, maleic)—

Secondary Flavor Qualities

Astringent	Astringent	Astringent	phenolic compounds (tannins)— antiviral effect, precipitates proteins, removes water
Demulcent	—	—	mucopolysaccharides, gums— inhibits prostaglandin synthesis (anti-inflammatory), coats mucous membranes, offering mechanical protection, replaces body's mucus, may activate surface immune system

EXAMPLES OF WESTERN HERBS

Bitter
: Virginia snakeroot, gentian, artichoke leaves, horehound

Sweet
: Yams, barley, spring dandelion root, Jerusalem artichoke, dates

Pungent
: Ginger, pine bark or pitch, prickly ash, angelica seed and root

Aromatic
: Peppermint, spearmint, cilantro, fennel leaves, thyme

Salty
: Celery, angelica leaves, sea vegetables (bladderwrack), parsley

Sour
: Lemon, new growth of conifers, dock leaves, sheep sorrel

Astringent
: Oak (new growth), oak galls, witch hazel, wild geranium root

Demulcent
: Marshmallow root, common mallow greens, sassafras leaves

Obviously, in most plant medicines, one can detect a combination of flavors, rather than a pure taste. Often taste will predominate, but it is usually easy to detect a second or third flavor, if one "looks" for it.

BITTER:

Bitter is a flavor that is not much favored by Americans. Many cultures enjoy it, however, and feel unbalanced if they do not get it every day. Nowhere else is the outcome of our jaded modern taste more evident than in our avoidance of bitter and the lust for sweet and salt.

Energy

Bitter is cooling, stimulating to bile and other digestive secretions; small amounts are tonic and nourishing to the yin; large amounts are debilitating and contracting.

Examples

Many green wild herbs are bitter (such as Mugwort or horehound), especially after flowering. Many roots are bitter in the late summer and early fall (such as Dandelion). After the first freeze, the sweet principle develops and the bitter is reduced.

Indications

Many people who need bitter the most, react to it strongly. Bitter in small tonic amounts should be taken 1/2 to 1 hour before meals to strengthen digestion, open and cool the liver, stimulate bile for better fat digestion and improve the nutrition of the body in deficiency diseases (use with sweet).

SWEET

Most Americans have excessively sweet blood which encourages heat and various infections. This is due to the large amount of refined sugar and refined fruit juices that are consumed. For optimum health, natural sweets, such as sub-acid whole fruit (applies, pears), well-chewed grains and sprouted beans should be used.

Energy

Sweet may be taken in the form of squash, baked yams, carrots, burdock and other roots and tubers during the winter to nourish and warm the body. Tonic sweet herbs, such as ginseng (which is also bitter) or rehmannia are used to support the nourishment and glands of the body. Tends to be warming.

Humans and all animals crave sweet foods. Foods that are sweet but not excessively refined are helpful and economical for the body's generation of energy, warmth, motion and thinking capacity.

Examples

Sweet herbs include jujube, dates, raisins, various rice products such as amasake, sprouted legumes, winter and spring roots such as burdock, dandelion and chicory, salsify and Jerusalem artichokes which contain fructose.

Indications

For degenerative diseases, weakened yin, to support the nutrition of the body. Has a beneficial effect on the hormones, nerves, muscles. Sweet is associated with the digestive organs, the pancreas and the muscles.

ACRID (SPICY)

Some people are highly attracted to acrid. Think of chile peppers, mustard, horseradish and watercress. Acrid stimulates heat in the interior and removes stagnancy in tissues, organs, systems and bioenergetic channels. Tonic to the digestion (in moderate amounts) brings blood and nourishment to internal organs. Readjusts the energy of the body (when out of balance, as in colds, flu). Also activates other remedies and helps with absorption. Stimulates metabolism, the "lower" passions and the circulation. Dispels stagnancy, congestion, expands.

Energy

Warming, stimulating—taken where there is stagnancy, lack of blood flow to areas of the body, due to coldness or under certain conditions, excess stress stimulating the sympathetic nervous system.

Examples

Hot peppers, angelica, aralia, osha, ginger, prickly ash, mustard, Umbelliferae members such as fennel and cardamom, conifers (pitch) and other aromatic or resinous plants.

Indications

Colds, flu, poor digestion, poor circulation, fear of the cold, deficiency, sluggish organs, etc.

SALTY

Most people in modern industrial societies have too much salt in their diet. Besides being poured out of the salt shaker, it is hidden in many processed foods. We need small amounts of natural salt, but excessive amounts can throw the body's electrolyte balance off, adversely affecting the fluid balance of the body, nerve transmission, put an extra strain on the heart, lungs and kidneys and create an environment where the cells of the body cannot function properly.

ENERGY

Can be moisturizing or drying to tissues, depending on the amount. It will strongly affect the moisture balance of the body. It has a specific action on the nervous system and glands, over-stimulating them when taken in large amounts. Tends to be warming, stimulating and promotes yang. In excessive amounts, creates dampness and coldness.

Examples

All sea vegetables, such as kelp, bladderwrack, wakame, etc. Many desert and seashore green plants. Native Americans burned these to make a salty addition to food. Organic celery and other wild Umbeliferae (such as *Angelica* spp.) are good sources of natural balanced salt.

Indications

Dryness in the body, poor or weakened nerve function, deficient yang.

SOUR

Most people like sour tastes in moderation, especially if combined with sweet. On a hot summer day, there is nothing like a good glass of lemonade, and most people recognize that it is cooling.

Energy

Sour is deeply cooling, refreshing (in tonic amounts), cleansing, clearing and detoxifying. It combines well with sweet. The liver is the organ associated with sour, being cleansed and nourished by tonic amounts. The electrolyte balance of the body can also be affected (alkaline/acid balance), which must be maintained within a narrow range. If this balance is lost, bacterial infections, excessive heat, poor nerve function, etc., can result.

Examples

Oxalis, or sour grass in the redwoods, lemon grass, lemons, Douglas Fir tips, pine tips, unripe fruits (sour and bitter or astringent), sheep sorrel, docks, etc.

Indications

Excess heat in the body, to enhance elimination, to clear persistent infections such as impetigo, candida infection, rank odors in the body.

AROMATIC

The word aromatic does not usually indicate a taste per se, but I am considering it as such in this system of herbal energetics. It corresponds to spicy-cool in TCM. It indicates a taste that also involves the sense of smell and comes from plant constituents that are rich in volatile oils.

Energy

Aromatic plants "warm the surface" and "cool the interior" (peppermint is an example). They bring blood to the mucous membranes, are mildly antibiotic and anti-fungal, dispel gas in the digestive tract, relax the sphincter of oddi and generally warm and tone the digestive tract, upper respiratory tract and urinary tract. In Chinese medicine, plants from this class are known to help lower fevers and smooth the flow of chi.

Examples

The families that are most abundant in these compounds are the Mint family, parsley family and Eucalyptus family. Plants such as peppermint, spearmint, dill, fennel greens and eucalyptus are all aromatic.

ASTRINGENT

Astringent is one of two *flavor qualities,* and is familiar to most people as a prominent flavor in black and green tea, especially when steeped too long. If one brews a cup of peppermint tea and leaves it in the water overnight, it becomes quite astringent. Astringent draws tissues in (contracts) and dries.

Energy

Astringent warms, tightens. Chemical compounds called tannins are usually associated with this taste. These are water-soluble and have been found in scientific tests to be anti-viral and bacterial, thus cooling.

Examples

All parts of the oak, willow bark, young twigs and "oak apples" which are galls (up to 50% tannic acid). Many young growing tips of shrubs are astringent. Also *Heuchera* (alum root).

Indications

Great for tightening the gums. Chew young oak twigs for anti-bacterial, toning effect on the gums—our chewing sticks. To slow diarrhea, to contract tissues such as mucous membranes that are too loose (hemorrhoids).

DEMULCENT

Demulcent, one of the two flavor qualities, is familiar to herbalists as the "slimy" quality of such herbs as comfrey, flax and the mallows.

Energy

The experience of demulcent is neutral, bland, usually tasteless, moisturizing and cooling. The molecules that create this type of action are giant sugar molecules, polysaccharides. More specifically, they are pectin, mucilage, muco-polysaccharides and gums. These substances soothe mucous membranes, replacing protective mucous as well as lowering inflammation, sometimes by inhibiting prostaglandins. Demulcent herbs are protective and cleansing.

Examples

The mallow family, Malvacceae is rich in mucilage. Plants such as marshmallow, garden mallow and hollyhock are examples. Other herbal sources of these demulcent agents are flax, chia, fenugreek and psyllium seeds, seaweeds, comfrey and plaintain.

Indications

For any infections, irritation or heat involving the mucous membranes. Urinary tract infections (cystitis, nephritis), upper respiratory tract infections (bronchitis, colds, flu, asthma) or digestive heat such as gastritis or colitis.

THE FOUR PRIMARY QUALITIES (TEMPERATURE AND MOISTURE)

Temperature is an important indicator of how an herb will affect a condition, organ, system or person. This energetic principle set is as important in TEM as it is in TCM and Ayurveda. For instance, in TCM, it is stated in chapter 74 of the *Yellow Emperor's Inner Classic* that "Hot diseases must be cooled, cold diseases must be warmed." Accordingly, herbs were given one of the temperature evaluations, cold, hot, warm, cool or neutral. TEM, Galen, and many writers on the materia medica and medicine throughout the following seventeen centuries ascribed various degrees of each temperature value, according to their intensity of effect. Thus, the four primary "humoral qualities" of moist, dry, warm and cold had varying degrees, depending on an individual herb's characteristics. The degrees were as follows:

1st degree = the herb works "unnoticed"

2nd degree = the herb works "openly"

3rd degree = the herb works "intensely" or "violently"

4th degree = the herb works "completely" or "destructively"

For instance, according to Culpeper, cinnamon is "hot and dry in the second degree," angelica is "hot and dry in the third degree," leeks are "hot and dry in the fourth degree," mallow leaves are "cold and moist in the first degree," chicory is "cold and dry in the second degree," and purslane, "cold and moist in the third degree."

In my view, the above system of "degrees" is unworkable and inappropriate for today. For most cases, the temperature characteristics of TCM with the additions of moist and dry are excellent indicators of one important aspect of the effects of the temperatures. Modifiers such as "slightly," or "intensely" are sufficient to provide all the gradation that is necessary in practical clinical work.

ENERGETICS OF SOME OFTEN-USED HERBS

Herb	Will	Primary Effect	Primary Affinity Organ System	Primary Tastes
Echinacea	specific	balancing	immune system	pungent cleansing
Goldenseal	specific	cleansing	mucous membranes, micro-circulation, digestion	bitter, astringent
Ginkgo	tonic	nourishing, protective	micro-circulation, immune system	sour, bitter astringent
Milk Thistle	tonic, protective	nourishing, protective	liver, spleen, kidneys	sweet, bitter, neutral
Astragalus	tonic, adaptogenic	nourishing	immune system	sweet, warm
Reishi	tonic	nourishing, protective	immune system, heart, blood sugar	sweet, warm
Cayenne	specific	balancing	mucous membranes, digestion, urinary tract	pungent
Licorice	tonic	balancing		sweet, neutral
Ginger	specific	balancing	cardiovascular	very pungent, hot
Rosemary	specific	balancing	digestion, nervous system	pungent warm
St. John's Wort	specific	protective	nervous system	bitter, sweet, cold
Eleuthero	tonic	protective, balancing	glandular system, immune system	sweet, neutral
Peppermint	specific	balancing	digestion	aromatic (pungent, cool)

REFERENCES

1. Castiglioni, A. 1947. *A History of Medicine,* 2nd ed. New York: Alfred A. Knopf.
2. Wilder, A. 1904. *History of Medicine.* Augusta, ME: Maine Farmer Publishing Co.
3. Clendening, L. 1942 (1960). *Source Book of Medical History.* New York: Dover Publications, Inc.
4. Gordon, B.L. 1959. *Medieval and Renaissance Medicine.* New York: Philosophical Library.
5. Ainslie, W. 1826. *Materia Medica.* London: Longman, Rees, Orme, Brown and Green. Reprinted by Periodical Expert Book Agency, Delhi (1979).
6. Veith, I. (tr.). 1972 (1949). *The Yellow Emperor's Classic of Internal Medicine.* Berkeley: University of California Press.
7. Bretschneider, E. 1895. *Botanicon Sinicum.* Hong Kong: Kelly & Walsh, Ltd.
8. Kleinman, A., *et al.* 1975. *Medicine in Chinese Cultures.* Washington: U.S. Department of Health, Education and Welfare (N.I.H.).
9. Bensky, D. and A. Gamble. 1986. *Chinese Herbal Medicine.* Seattle: Eastland Press.
10. Bott, V. 1984. *Anthroposophical Medicine.*Rochester, VT: Healing Arts Press.
11. Steiner, R. 1981. *Health and Illness.* Spring Valley, NY: The Anthroposophic Press.
12. King, F.X. 1986. *Rudolph Steiner and Holistic Medicine.* York Beach, ME: Nicolas-Hays, Inc.
13. Ebbell, B. (tr.). 1937. *The Papyrus Ebers.* London: Oxford University Press.
14. Dierbach, J.H. 1824 (1969). *Die Arzneimittel des Hippokrates.* Hildesheim: Georg Olms.
15. Hort, A. 1948. *Theophrastus: Enquiry into Plants.* Cambridge: Harvard University Press.
16. Jones, W.H.S. 1956. *Pliny: Natural History.* Cambridge: Harvard University Press.
17. Gunther, R.T. 1934. *The Greek Herbal of Dioscorides.* Oxford: Oxford University Press.
18. Levey, M. 1966. *The Medical Formulary or Agrabadhin of Al-Kindi.* Madison, WI: The University of Wisconsin Press.
19. Levey, M. & N. Al-Khaledy. 1967. *The Medical Formulary of Al-Samarqandi.* Philadelphia: University of Pennsylvania Press.
20. Cockayne, O. 1864. *Leechdoms, Wortcunning, and Starcraft.* London: Longman, Green, Longman, Roberts, and Green.
21. Madaus, G. 1938. *Handbook of Biological Medicine.* Reprinted by George Olms Verlag, NY (1976).
22. Pughe, J. (tr.) & J. Williams (ed.). 1861. *The Physicians of Myddvai.* London: Longman & Co.
23. Fordyn, P. (ed.). 1983. *The "experimentes of Cophon, The Leche of Salerne."* Brussels: Research Center of Mediaeval and Renaissance Studies.
24. *ibid.*

25. Larkey, S.V. & T. Pyles, trs. & eds. 1941. *An Herbal [1525]*. New York: Scholars' Facsimiles & Reprints.

26. Brunfels, O. 1532. *Kreüterbuch contrafayt*. Strasszburg: Schotten. Reprinted by Verlag Konrad Kölbl, München (1964).

27. Dodoens, R. 1586. *A New Herball, or Historie of Plants*. London: Ninian Newton.

28. Gerard, J. & Johnson, T. (ed.). 1633. *The Herbal or General History of Plants*. Reprinted by Dover Publications, New York (1975).

29. Parkinson, J. 1640. *Theatrum Botanicum: The Theater of Plants*. London: Tho. Cotes.

30. Urdang, G. 1944. *Pharmacopoeia Londinensis of 1618 reproduced in facsimile*. Madison: State Historical Society of Wisconsin.

31. James, R. 1747. *Pharmacopoeia Universalis*. London: J. Hodges, at the Looking-Glass.

32. Duncan, A. 1790. *The Edinburgh New Dispensatory*. Edinburgh: William Creech.

33. Cullen, W. 1802. *A Treatise of the Materia Medica*. New York: T. & J. Swords, etc.

34. Pereira, J. 1843. *The Elements of Materia Medica and Therapeutics*. Philadelphia: Lea & Blanchard.

35. Bartram, J. 1751. *Description, virtures and uses of sundry plants of these northern parts of America, and particularly of the newley discovered Indian cure for the venereal disease*. Philadelphia: Printed by B. Franklin and D. Hall.

36. Barton, B.S. 1810. *Collections for an Essay Towards a Materia Medica*. Philadelphia: Printed for Edward Earle and Co.

37. Bigelow, J. 1817–20. *American Medical Botany*. Boston: Cummings and Hilliard.

38. Eberle, J. 1834. *A Treatise of the Materia Medica and Therapeutics*. Philadelphia: Grigg & Elliot.

39. Griffith, R. 1847. *Medical Botany*. Philadelphia: Lea & Blanchard.

40. Gathercoal, E.N. & H.W. Youngken. 1942. *Check List of Native and Introduced Drug Plants in the United States*. Chicago: National Research Council.

41. *ibid.*

42. Felter, H.W. & J.U. Lloyd. 1898. *King's American Dispensatory*. Cincinnati: The Ohio Valley Co.

43. Smith, F.P. & G.A. Stuart. 1973. *Chinese Medicinal Herbs*. San Francisco: Georgetown Press.

44. Perry, L.M. 1980. *Medicinal Plants of East and Southeast Asia*. Cambridge: The MIT Press.

45. Ainslie, W. 1826. *Materia Indica*. Reprinted by Neeraj Publishing House, Delhi.

General References:

Castiglioni, A. & E.B. Krumbhaar (tr.). 1947. *A History of Medicine,* 2nd ed. New York: Alfred A. Knopf.

Clendening, L. 1960 (1942). *Source Book of Medical History*. New York: Dover Publications, Inc.

Dash, B. L. Kashyap. 1987 (1980). *Materia Medica of Ayurveda*. New Delhi:

Concept Publishing Company.

Dharmananda, S. 1986. *Your Nature, Your Health.* Portland: Institute for Traditional Medicine and Preventative Health Care.

Kaptchuk, T.J. 1983. *The Web That Has No Weaver.* New York: Congdon & Weed.

List, P.H. and L. Hörhammer. 1973. *Hagars Handbuch der Pharmazeutischen Praxis,* 7 vols. New York: Springer-Verlag.

Lloyd, G.E.R. 1978. *Hippocratic Writings.* NY: Viking Penguin.

Madaus, G. 1938. *Handbook of Biological Medicine,* 3 vols. (in German). Reprinted by Georg Olms Verlag, NY.

Siegel, R.E. 1968. *Galen's System of Physiology and Medicine.* New York: S. Karger.

Veith, I. 1966 (1949). *The Yellow Emperor's Classic of Internal Medicine.* Berkeley: University of California Press.

Efficacy vs. Effectiveness: Applying Scientific Trials to Clinical Practice

PAUL BERGNER

An herbal remedy "proven by science" may not actually be very effective in practice. Likewise, herbal medicines found ineffective or toxic in scientific trials may actually be quite valuable in another setting. The reason: the conditions, patients and materials used in scientific trials may not match the real-world conditions of the clinic.

This point was very well established during the formulation of West German drug laws during the 1970s. Proposals to require that the efficacy of all remedies be proven unequivocally before they could be sold to the public or used by doctors met strong opposition. Although it would seem that such an argument would pit scientists against "unscientific" practitioners of fringe disciplines, this was not the case. Arguments were presented against requiring strict proofs on scientific grounds. The concepts of "effects without efficacy" and "efficacy without effects" were introduced into the debate. "Efficacy" in U.S. FDA law means results observed during the controlled conditions of a scientific experiment. "Effects," according to the Germans, meant successful treatment in actual therapeutic situations. Opponents of strict standards proved with strong evidence that the two were not always related—substances proven effective in clinical trials may not work in actual practice, and substances disproved in trials may be otherwise effective. German legislators chose to accept reports of practitioners rather than require formal clinical trials for most remedies.

Although this may seem "unscientific," it is the same policy followed in the U.S. for surgical procedures, for which educational traditions and professional consensus are considered sufficient controls. Proofs of neither safety nor efficacy are required. A 1978 study by the U.S. office of

Technology Assessment, for instance, found definitive clinical trials showing safety or efficacy lacking for such common medical procedures as pap smears, chicken pox vaccination, mammography, skull X-rays, electronic fetal monitoring, coronary bypass surgery, tonsillectomy, appendectomy, hysterectomy and chemotherapy for lung cancer.

This "efficacy vs. effects" disparity applies to studies of herbal remedies as well as conventional drugs or medical procedures. Some reasons for the differences follow.

THE EXPERIMENTAL GROUP MAY NOT BE COMPARABLE TO A REAL PATIENT POPULATION.

Seventy percent of a patient group who had taken feverfew for long periods reported that it helped their migraine headaches. A group of seventeen patients from this group reported a 76% reduction in the frequency of migraines. The group was "self-selected," however. It included mostly people who had already found feverfew effective; those who found it ineffective had already dropped out of the group. A follow-up study which selected a more typical population found only a 23% reduction in migraines, about one headache a month less in people who had four or five attacks a month. It appears from the various trials that feverfew is clearly effective for only about a third of migraine patients, not the seventy percent reported by the first group.

TESTS ON AN ISOLATED CONSTITUENT MAY NOT APPLY TO THE WHOLE PLANT.

Herbalists rarely use isolated constituents in practice, while this is the most common form in animal and clinical trials. Experiments with isolated constituents are usually done in an academic setting, as the first step in the isolation or development of a pharmaceutical drug. Yet isolated individual saponins from ginseng often have properties that the whole plant does not. Individual ginseng saponins sometimes have entirely opposite pharmacological effects. And the group of flavonoids in ginkgo has properties that the individual flavonoids do not. Likewise, toxicology studies of isolated constituents may not apply to the whole plant. The constituent saffrole in sassafras, for instance, is carcinogenic in mice. It is insoluble in water, however, and is not present in sassafras tea. It was banned from public use in the U.S. not because of danger from the tea, but because soft-drink manufacturers used an alcohol extract for flavoring. Even the humble carrot is listed in one toxicology book as potentially abortive on the basis of isolated constituents from its seeds.

ANIMAL STUDIES MAY NOT APPLY TO HUMANS.

Scientists typically give potentially toxic plants to animals as a large percentage of the diet rather than in the small doses normally given to humans. Such large amounts may have entirely different effects than small doses. The National Cancer Institute recently stopped performing one such test after determining it could not predict carcinogenicity in humans. Thus neither the pyrrolizidine alkaloids in comfrey, nor the pesticide Alar may actually be carcinogenic in humans in normal amounts.

Hypericin from St. John's wort, taken orally by mice, was found to kill retroviruses in mice. Yet oral doses in humans appear incapable of producing the same blood levels that hypericin achieved in the mice, and appear not to influence the course of AIDS.

THE EXPERIMENTAL METHOD OF ADMINISTRATION MAY BE DIFFERENT FROM THAT USED IN PRACTICE.

Many Japanese studies of polysaccharides from ganoderma or shitake mushrooms administer these substances intravenously. Test results cannot automatically be applied to oral preparations, since polysaccharides are mostly destroyed in the digestive tract. Likewise, German studies of the effects of polysaccharides from echinacea in rats showed immunostimulating effects. In the U.S., many companies and writers (including this author) reported the research as if the polysaccharides were "the active ingredient." The high molecular weight polysaccharides in the German studies are in fact not present in the strong alcohol tinctures which established the clinical effectiveness of echinacea over the last hundred years.

THE PLANT FORM IN THE TRIAL MAY BE DIFFERENT FROM THAT USED IN MEDICAL PRACTICE.

Several clinical studies of feverfew tested either the fresh plant or a carefully assayed extract. A study of commercially available products in England, however, showed a wide divergence of clinical activity, and, for some products, none at all. Experimental results cannot be assumed to apply to commercial products. Likewise, a trial of feverfew in arthritis used dried, powdered and unassayed material and found it ineffective. Fresh material may in fact be effective. Similarly, many laboratory and clinical experiments use freeze-drying to standardize substances. These materials are kept in airtight or nitrogen-atmosphere containers, refrigerated and away from light. Test results cannot be assumed to apply to commercial products, even to commercial freeze-dried products, which are more susceptible than other materials to oxidation and loss of volatile components.

This is also true for toxicology studies. One found coltsfoot to be carcinogenic in mice. The plant buds, never used in actual practice, were fed to the mice in the trial. New leaf buds have extremely high concentrations of alkaloids, many times that of the leaf used in herbal practice. After investigation, the German government now allows coltsfoot to be sold commercially in spite of the negative studies in mice.

THE DOSE AND DURATION OF THE TRIAL MAY BE DIFFERENT FROM THAT IN CLINICAL PRACTICE.

Many herbal systems, including Chinese and Ayurvedic, recommend that some herbs be taken for long periods, anywhere from six weeks to two years, to effect a change in the deeper constitution. Scientific trials of longer than ten weeks, on the other hand, are rare. Several studies of ginseng found it ineffective as a tonic, but the studies were conducted over short periods. Ginseng is typically given for a month or more to judge its full effect. A study of the effectiveness of a homeopathic remedy for influenza showed only a modest, although significant, clinical "cure rate" after 48 hours. In practice, the 72–96 hour recovery rate may be more important. In the feverfew studies, a "traditional" dose of two leaves a day (about 80 mg) was found moderately effective. In actual medical practice in the U.S., doses up to seven times this amount have been given, with predictably strong effects.

STATISTICALLY SIGNIFICANT RESULTS MAY HAVE LITTLE CLINICAL RELEVANCE.

Statistical significance means that the results probably did not happen by chance, that there was a causative effect by the substance being tested. But "significance" does not mean that all your patients will find the herb significant in their terms. In the trial of nettles for hay fever, the nettles were proven to be more active than the placebo. Clinically the remedy was of benefit to only about half the patients and gave dramatic improvement to only one patient in six. For the homeopathic influenza remedy, 66% more people (39 of 228) taking the homeopathic remedy recovered from the flu within forty-eight hours compared with those taking the placebo (24 of 234). This sounds quite good and proves the presence of activity in the homeopathic substance. In practice, however, it means that if you gave the remedy to 228 consecutive patients, only fifteen more of them would be over their flu within 2 days than if you had given a placebo. That's only one in fifteen. The study criteria demanded complete recovery and did not measure decreased intensity of symptoms, but we can hardly call the homeopathic remedy a "cure" for influenza. A practitioner would have a hard time making a living helping only one patient in fifteen.

THE "PLACEBO" MAY NOT BE A PLACEBO.

Tests purporting to disprove the Feingold Diet, which possibly reduces hyperactivity by eliminating food additives, used a chocolate chip cookie as a "placebo." The wheat, chocolate, dairy, and possibly eggs in the cookie are all common allergens which may themselves cause mood changes. In a trial of nettles for hay fever, a milk sugar placebo was used. Milk is a common allergen, and the "placebo" may actually have an aggravating effect on the allergy.

Trial designs do not take "energetic" types into consideration.

It is common practice to sort the subjects of clinical trials by age, seriousness of condition, sex and so on. Then, the substance being tested is often found effective for one subgroup, but not the others. Patients are not sorted and tested according to parameters more relevant to herbal practice, such as hot or cold types, or conditions of excess or deficiency. A remedy found ineffective in a large group, may have actually been highly effective for an appropriate "energetic" subgroup.

A "negative placebo effect" may be at work in unblinded trials.

An unblinded British trial of ginkgo extract for tinnitus found very different results than those in better controlled trials in France. The British doctors who were skeptical about the potential of ginkgo, warned patients "not to get their hopes up" about the remedy, and this may have affected results. The power of suggestion is at least as powerful as some drug effects. In some trials of one placebo against another, for instance, the group that doctors thought was getting the active medicine show 5–10% more efficacy.

In some cases, experimenters have reversed the effect of a drug through suggestion. Women with morning sickness were given ipecac, which normally causes vomiting. When both the doctor and the woman thought it was a powerful anti-nausea substance, it actually effectively stopped the morning sickness, as measured both subjectively and objectively. A doctor's negative suggestion "not to get your hopes up" could be sufficient to negate or reduce the effectiveness of a remedy below statistically significant levels.

This influence may be at work even in controlled trials where prejudiced scientists know that an herbal substance is being tested. The designers of the homeopathy trial for influenza took measures to overcome this influence. The clinicians did not know they were testing a homeopathic remedy. *Lancet*, a British medical journal, commented favorably on the design, calling it "quadruple blind."

CONCLUSION

Clinical medicine is a combination of science and art. Science may prove an herb more effective than a placebo, but this rarely means universal effectiveness. The clinical artist must discover which patient it is effective for and apply the remedy in a context of overall healing.

Herbal practitioners may need a more sophisticated understanding of science to most effectively apply "scientifically proven" remedies. Not only are poorly designed trials used to "discredit" herbs, but herb marketers sometimes shamelessly misinterpret or overstate the results of favorable trials in order to better sell their product. To be empowered in an age of propaganda requires development of knowledge and critical faculties. The following questions will help determine how much a scientific trial can be applied to clinical realities.

1. What percentage of the trial group improved dramatically? This might be the portion of your patients who will be very pleased with your treatments.
2. Was the trial group typical of regular patients, or was there a negative or positive selection process?
3. What kind of patient improved? Old, young, early stage disease, etc.?
4. What kind and percentage of side effects were observed?

These are very general questions, and learning more details about clinical trials will lead to more refinement. An excellent book on the subject is *Studying a Study and Testing a Test: How to read the literature*, by Richard K. Riegelman.

Paul Bergner is editor of *Medical Herbalism: A Clinical Newsletter for the Herbal Practitioner.*

REFERENCES

1. Ferley, J.P. et al. "A Controlled Evaluation of a Homeopathic Preparation in the Treatment of Influenza-like Syndromes." *British Journal of Clinical Pharmacology*, 1989, 27, 329–335.

2. Kienle, G. *Arzneimittelsicherheit und Gesellschaft.* <D> p. 156. Stuttgart.

cited in: Unschult, PU "The issue of structured coexistence of scientific and alternative medical systems: a comparison of East and West German legislation." *Soc. Sci. Med.* 14(B):pp. 15–24.

3.   Mittman, P. "Randomized double-blind study of freeze-dried *Urtica dioica* in the treatment of allergic rhinitis." *Planta Medica*, 1990, 56:44–47.

4.   Murphy, J. J., Heptinstall, S., Mitchell, J. R. A. "Randomised double-blind placebo-controlled trial of feverfew in migraine prevention." *Lancet*, July 23, 1988. pp. 189–192.

5.   OTA: Office of Technology Assessment. "Assessing the efficacy and safety of medical technologies." National Technical Information Service. PB-286-929. 1978..

6.   Patrick, M., Heptinstall, S., Doherty, M. "Feverfew in rheumatoid arthritis: a double-blind, placebo-controlled study." *Annals of Rheumatic Disease* 1989; 48:547–549.

Herbal Toxicity and Contraindications

DR. MICHAEL TIERRA, O.M.D., L.AC.

With the increasing popularity and widespread use of herbs and herbal products, it is important for herbalists to develop a practical understanding of their toxicity and contraindications. Failing to do so will make the evolution and development of herbalism increasingly vulnerable to unsympathetic scientific research and consequent public scrutiny and legal restrictions.

There are two prevailing extremes regarding the safety of herbs: one is a scientific reductionist approach of evaluating herbal toxicity solely on the basis of isolated biochemical components. What usually occurs is that science determines that a particular chemical is toxic (and most of them are) and since the chemical is found to naturally occur as one of several components of an herb, the result is that the safety of the herb is in question.

The second extreme view centers around the belief that an herb is safe simply because it is a natural substance, or that it has been used for a long time and must therefore be safe, or finally, that one is not likely to experience adverse reactions by using the whole plant. While there are instances of truth for all these views, there are far too many exceptions for us to blindly accept their validity for all cases.

First let us differentiate between herbal toxicity and contraindication. An herb is toxic when it generally has a poisonous or harmful reaction to more or less all who use it. It is contraindicated when it is determined through diagnosis and analysis that it is likely to have a harmful reaction in a specific individual. We should realize, however, that if an herb that is contraindicated for a specific individual or condition is taken over a prolonged period of time, it can upset biological homeostasis to the extent that a toxic reaction is created.

One method of herbal classification for toxicity that herbalists need to agree upon is a method first outlined over 2000 years ago in China where "Shen Nung's Herbal" established the concept of properties, similar to Western classifications. In Shen Nung's Herbal 365 herbs were classified as superior (potent), average (mildly potent) and inferior (poisonous). The 120 superior herbs were considered as non-toxic and life supporting and have since been regarded as imperial quality. The 120 average herbs regarded as slightly toxic were used to provoke ministerial or active therapeutic functions, such as purgative, diuretic, diaphoretic, stimulant, blood moving and antispasmodic. The 125 inferior or toxic herbs had specific anti-pathogenic properties, such as anti-bacterial, anti-viral and anti-parasitical to name a few.

Let's see how this might work with Western herbs:

Superior	Average	Inferior
red clover	goldenseal	belladonna
yellow dock	cascara sagrada	aconite
nettles	comfrey	arnica
ginseng	coltsfoot	sanguinaria
angelica	sassafras	hyoscyamine
licorice	aristolochia	gelsemium
cinnamon	blue flag	squill
dandelion	chaparral	poke
burdock	myrrh	skunk cabbage
calendula	saffron	American mandrake

The list could go on but I propose that one task of the American Herbalist Guild, perhaps in combination with the British Medical Herbalists and The National Herbalists Association of Australia, is to develop a consensus agreement on how to officially classify the herbs we use. Perhaps this could be done by our submitting a list of herbs which we use regularly or would like to use if even seldomly, noting an S for superior, A for average or I for inferior beside each herb. These would be tabulated and later published in our respective journals. This list can be revised periodically according to our change of understanding. Its purpose is to offer some guidelines to fellow herbalists and the public on the relative safety of using herbs.

We must next distinguish between holistic herbalism and a more purely symptomatic approach that follows the allopathic medical model. Such a distinction is not intended to be qualitative because most herbalists and herbal systems use both. Holistic herbalism attempts to treat a complex of symptoms including the primary complaint along with adjusting dietary and lifestyle problems that could be creating the imbalance.

Western herbalism is holistic when it prescribes herbs based upon their primary and secondary properties as well as diet, lifestyle and emotional stress factors. For example, wild yam (*Dioscorea villosa*) is an herb that is primarily used for complaints of the liver and gallbladder. It is described as being a cholagogue which is an herb that aids the secretion of bile; an antispasmodic which relieves tension and spasms; anti-inflammatory which clears inflammation and anti-rheumatic which goes along with all its previous properties in aiding detoxification through the liver, relieving painful spasms and tension and reducing inflammation. As an antispasmodic, wild yam is quite different in its action from lobelia (*L. inflata*) or rue (*Ruta graveolens*). We determine this by reading all of its properties together as an indication of its herbal personality.

To take another example, willow bark (*Salix alba*) has analgesic pain-relieving properties probably because of the presence of salicylic acid, the active ingredient of aspirin. It is also antipyretic, which in traditional Chinese herbalism means that it has a cool or cold energy. Prescribing willow bark occasionally to relieve rheumatic pains and lower fevers, regardless of other symptomatic or constitutional factors, is its allopathic use. Using it specifically for fevers and pains caused by inflammation or excess heat and for generally hypermetabolic or yang-hot condition would be in accordance with holistic principles of Traditional Chinese Medicine.

Problems from using frequent and substantial doses of willow bark allopathically to relieve pain, irrespective of other symptoms and constitutional considerations, are eventually bound to occur. The same could be said for the use of licorice and comfrey roots or any other herb or vegetable that is used in a concentrated manner over a long period of time (a few weeks to months). If a problem persists and is only partially relieved with an herbal medicine, we must recognize the need to treat more according to holistic principles. An individual who has a vata-air constitution according to Ayurvedic medicine, or a yin-cold condition according to Chinese herbal medicine, is likely to experience an aggravation of symptoms from the use of an herb like willow, which has a cold, dry nature.

Still another example is the use of mahuang (*Ephedra sinensis*), which in Chinese medicine is classified as having a warm, dispersing energy. This is probably due to the presence of adrenaline-like compounds. Because of these properties, however, it can also be used as an occasional warming stimulant, like coffee for tiredness. Since it is not a tonic and does not build or increase energy but only stimulates and depletes innate bodily reserves, it would be contraindicated for heart conditions and hypertension. Holistically, mahuang is an acute acting herb useful for asthma, certain colds, flu and allergies as well as cold-damp rheumatic conditions.

Herbalists typically use herbs in formula to synergistically heighten a primary effect or to cancel or limit undesirable side effects. For instance, using a combination of echinacea, goldenseal, chaparral and garlic as an anti-inflammatory, anti-biotic and anti-viral formula is more effective than using echinacea alone. The reason for this is that while all these herbs have known alterative properties, echinacea may concentrate its effects upon certain physiological systems such as the lymph and blood, goldenseal works more on the liver and mucus systems, chaparral helps remove toxic residues from the cells and tissues of the body and garlic has mild warming properties, aiding digestion and assimilation and clearing inflammation from the lungs.

In Chinese herbalism, licorice is the most commonly used herb. It is called the "peacemaker," probably because it contains compounds that are similar to cortical steroids secreted by the adrenal glands. These are calming, anti-inflammatory hormones that relieve pain and irritation and also aid digestion and assimilation. Like cortisone, the side effect of taking too much licorice is fluid retention. For those with kidney related hypertension, taking licorice can aggravate their condition. For others, whose hypertension is caused by nervous tension and irritability, licorice will help to relieve the condition. However, because of its soothing effects and pleasantly sweet flavor, a small amount of licorice (perhaps 1 to 2 gms.) is added to 80% of the classical Chinese formulas because it is recognized that licorice tends to harmonize a formula, make it more agreeable and counteract the tendency towards a toxic reaction to either a single herb or a combination.

In making a formula more agreeable by adding a little licorice, honey or a pleasant tasting spice such as anise seed or mint, disagreeable side effects are often avoided, with the appropriate internal organs to be prepared to better utilize the therapeutic properties of herbal compounds. This is why the concept of using herbs as carriers, or what in Ayurveda is called *anupans,* is a useful concept of formulation. Honey is an anupan, or carrier, to the mucus and lymphatic systems, oil to the nervous systems and ghee, or clarified butter, to the liver, small intestine and circulatory systems. Barberry root is a carrier to the liver, huckleberry leaf to the spleen-pancreas and false unicorn to the female reproductive organs. Whatever action we wish to take on any of these specific areas of the body will be more effectively accomplished if we add a small amount of these specific organ reflex herbs in the formulation.

The total effect of herbs in the body is very complex. Mostly, this is described in terms of physiological modes of action, fundamentally synergistic and antagonistic. The combined action of herbs could augment or diminish the efficacy of the others and in some instances, could be potentially harmful.

Let's consider what these seven modes of action are:

1. *Isolation* where the specific herb is the only active component of the formula. Examples are when one might use licorice to treat a sore throat or feverfew to treat migraine headaches.

2. *Augmentation* where herbs of similar properties and actions are combined to augment or enhance the effects of each other. An example would be combining yarrow and lemon balm, both diaphoretics to stimulate sweating.

3. *Synergism* is where herbs of either similar or different properties are added to enhance the principal herb or action of a formula. An example is combining the mineral, calcium together with valerian to enhance its sedative effect.

4. *Antagonism* is where two herbs tend to neutralize each other. An example is the combination of a strongly cleansing cold herb, such as poke root, with a warm chi tonic herb such as ginseng.

5. *Counteraction* is where one herb is added to inhibit a particularly undesirable property of another. An example is adding a small amount of a warming antispasmodic, such as ginger root, with a purgative, such as cascara sagrada, to prevent painful gripping. Another example is combining a small amount of the cooling Chinese scullcap root to offset the warm nature of tang kuei for certain gynecological problems.

6. *Obstruction* is where an herb is added to neutralize the toxicity of another. Most commonly demulcent sweet herbs such as jujube date or licorice root, which is called the "peacemaker" herb, are added to complex herbal formulas to offset any possible negative reaction either from a single herb in the formula or a particular combination.

7. *Incompatibility* is where the particular combination of certain herbs results in toxicity.

The category of tonics generally cautions against taking tonic herbs during acute inflammatory states. The reason for this is that the strengthening properties of the tonics can give more strength to the pathogenic forces at the expense of the patient. In actual practice, however, this is often compromised with the principle of supporting the righteous energy.

An example of this is a discovery I have found with some individuals, that combining a small percentage of warming chi tonics such as ginseng, codonopsis or astragalus with at least 80% echinacea is effective in treating inflammatory conditions in individuals with chronic internal deficiencies.

In Traditional Chinese herbalism one studies the 18 incompatible and 19 antagonistic herbs. It is not necessary to outline what all of these are except to mention that one may not use ginseng with veratrum or licorice with seaweed. Combining these specific substances tends to render them as useless or toxic. Contrast this with Western herbalism, which apart from the standard legalistic "not to be taken by pregnant women,"[1] we have from Dr. Shook's *Advance Treatise in Herbology* (publ. by Trinity Press) to the teachings of the late Dr. Christopher and *Herbal Medication* (publ. by Fowler) of Priest and Priest, the only forbidden combination of high tannin containing herbs such as oak bark with iron or iron containing plants such as yellow dock.

The late 19th century eclectic herbalist, Dr. John M. Scudder in his books *Specific Diagnosis* and *Specific Medication* (republished by Eclectic Medical Publications, Portland, OR), warns against accepting a general pathological description of disease as a basis for herbal treatment. He outlines a complex system of differential diagnosis, evaluating tongue, pulse, complexion and various aspects of the patient's specific primary and secondary symptoms and constitution followed by a prescription of herbs and treatments according to these indications. By so doing, Scudder's work unwittingly becomes an amazing validation for Traditional Chinese Herbal Medicine and Ayurvedic herbalism in that he and the Eclectics were well on the way to independently discovering and formulating principles of differential diagnosis and treatment that were remarkably similar to that of the thousands-of-years-old systems of Traditional Chinese and Ayurvedic Medicine.

By studying the classifications of herbs in the Chinese Materia Medica and that of Western herbs presented in *Planetary Herbology,* herbal properties such as alteratives assume a much broader application and understanding when they are classified as *Heat clearing.* Western herbs that are classified as emmenagogues tend to be used mainly to regulate and treat female menstrual problems, yet under the Chinese category of

---

1. In fact many of the herbs that are standardly not recommended during pregnancy such as tang kuei (*Angelica sinensis*) are specifically indicated for some pregnant women who have symptoms of blood deficiency and anemia.

herbs that *regulate and move blood,* they assume a significantly broader application for the treatment of blood clots, acute pain and various circulatory disorders. There are also categories and properties that are not normally included in Western herbalism such as herbs that *calm the spirit.* These generally utilize heavier minerals such as the calcium carbonate found in oyster shells and the calcium of the ossified bones of prehistoric mammals (called "dragon bones") to serve as deep acting sedatives and calming agents.

The most important category unique to the Chinese Materia Medica are the tonics which include those properties which we in the West have come to recognize as "adatogenic" or immune potentiating. Unlike the West, which historically has only classified bitters that stimulate appetite and digestion as tonics, the Chinese classify *Chi Tonics* such as *Panax ginseng* and *Astragalus membranicus* as sweet and warm and therefore increasing vitality and energy, *Yang Tonics* such as *Epimedium grandiflorum* generate warmth, circulation and libido, *Blood Tonics* such as tang kuei (*Angelica sinensis*) which tonify blood and treat anemia, and *Yin Tonics* which strengthen body essence such as asparagus root (*Asparagus* off.) and *Rehmannia glutinosa.*

In traditional Chinese and Ayurvedic herbalism the diagnosis, treatment principles and herbal classification are a more integrated process. Because of this, each herb has specific indications of toxicity and the herb and its respective category have general contraindications based upon symptomatic and constitutional evaluations. For instance, based upon common sense, unless there is a special reason for doing so, one would not give purgative herbs to a patient with diarrhea, nor would diaphoretic herbs be given to a patient with a problem of weakness and involuntary sweating. This follows the basic tenet of Chinese herbalism which is to avoid giving hot natured herbs for hot or inflammatory hypermetabolic conditions and cold natured herbs for cold or hypometabolic conditions.

In actual practice there are many exceptions to this principle on the basis that herbs are also classified as primarily affecting specific organs and meridians. Thus, fresh ginger, for instance, affects the stomach and lung organs and meridians in the right instance, but could be combined with a cool natured herb such as dandelion root, which clears heat and congestion from the liver and urinary organs. However, herbs with a cold energy, such as willow bark, should not be given singly for yin-cold conditions and herbs with a hot energy such as cayenne pepper, should not be given alone for yang-hot conditions. The principles of herbal contraindications in Chinese herbal medicine offer particular insight for the practice of Western herbal formulary and the formulation of safer, more efficacious commercial herb products.

Some of the contraindications of Chinese herbalism are as follows:

1. Herbs that disperse the internal energy of the body to the surface, such as diaphoretics and stimulants, should not be given to individuals who are internally weak and deficient or already have complaints of external deficient or wasting heat (called Yin deficiency in Chinese medicine).

2. Herbs that purge heat (purgatives) should not be given to those who are internally cold. This contraindication provides a warning against the excessive use of laxatives. It also offers an important indication why cold natured laxatives such as cascara, senna or rhubarb may not work for certain individuals. Individuals complaining of constipation with internal coldness and deficiency may require another treatment strategy as their continued use of such cold natured laxatives will cause laxative dependency or possibly a more serious physiological imbalance.

3. Diuretics should not be given to individuals complaining of dryness.

4. Carminatives and Yang warming tonics should not be given to individuals who have acute or superficial heat (Yin deficiency as in AIDS or TB).

5. Alteratives, or heat clearing herbs with a bitter taste, can injure the stomach and cool the spleen. This means that they will eventually weaken the digestive system, ultimately giving rise to a wide variety of autoimmune and immune deficiency diseases with symptoms of food and environmental allergies, candidiasis, chronic fatigue syndrome and various other immune deficiency diseases.

6. Herbs with a wet or moist nature (demulcents), classified as Yin Tonics (asparagus root, rehmannia or the Western comfrey root, marshmallow root and Irish moss), can cause gastrointestinal stagnation and impair the digestion, symptoms of which may include bloating, nausea, gas and a feeling of heaviness.

THE QUESTION OF COMFREY

This suggests a possible basis for certain problems that could occur from the inappropriate and too frequent use of an herb like comfrey. Comfrey is a demulcent which increases the proliferation of cells in the body; as such, it would be classified as a Yin tonic in Chinese herbalism. This same propensity towards tissue proliferation could, in excess, be understood as congesting or stagnating, as reflected in the condition of liver veno-occlusive disease caused by pyrrolizidine alkaloids which are believed to be present in certain specimens of Russian comfrey (*Symphytum officinalis*). In this condition, the small and medium veins of the liver become obstructed, resulting in liver dysfunction, cirrhosis and death. Developing fetuses and small children may be particularly vulnerable since their tissues are in a fast proliferating growth cycle and comfrey may or may not be indicated.

One of the issues herbalists face is the threat that science, unwittingly serving the purposes of certain vested interests who fund it, such as the AMA and drug industry, can be invoked and used to discredit and ultimately ban the use of important medicinal herbs. This has already occurred with a number of empirically worthwhile and reasonably safe herbs such as sassafras,[2] banned by the FDA because of the presence of safrole.

Without debating the few cases implicating the controversial connection of comfrey with veno-occlusive disease, there are certain considerations that herbalists face. Veno-occlusive disease is, according to Traditional Chinese Herbalism, a disease of liver stagnation and congestion. Comfrey, as a demulcent herb with Yin tonic properties, is specifically contraindicated for conditions of liver stagnation and congestion. Using it symptomatically like a drug, three times a day on a regular basis in the form of "comfrey-pepsin" pills for chronic acute gastrointestinal problems, may invite the possibility of side effects and contraindications in certain individuals, especially those with liver stagnancy. According to herbalist Roy Upton, however, "Just as the risks of taking certain drugs are assessed and tolerated in favor of their potential greater health benefits, herbalists need to decide what degree of potential side effects may be tolerable in view of the potential benefits of using the herb."

I was recently given an outstanding article published in the *Canadian Journal of herbalism* (January, 1990) entitled "Comfrey: A Matter of Balance," by Richard De Sylva, CH. This article offers an herbalist's approach to the comfrey controversy.

Dr. De Sylva made many worthwhile points in his assessment of the research on comfrey, pyrrolizidine alkaloids and veno-occlusive disease in humans:

> "...the original research was seriously flawed. The laboratory rats that developed tumors on the liver were only six weeks old. At this age, quite a number of substances would be inappropriate for them to ingest. As well, the total amount of comfrey ingested formed 50% of their basic diet. This could be compared to human consumption of several platefuls of comfrey daily. This daily regimen did eventually cause tumors to grow on their livers

and proved only one of the standing laws of science: that every substance or chemical is a poison if we consume enough of it."

He further reiterates the Arndt-Schultz principle of pharmacology: a large amount will kill, a moderate amount will paralyze, and a small amount will stimulate—and goes on to say,

"...stimulation is needed by any cell, organ, gland, etc., to urge it onward in the performance of its function. It is necessary in the right amount and at the right times for overall system balance. It is this perspective that seems to be lost or ignored in assessing any herb for its potential damage to the organism."

The few cases implicating comfrey as the cause of liver veno-occlusive disease began with the assumptions that (1) certain people in third world countries have exhibited severe toxic reactions by accidentally ingesting the seeds of heliotrope, senecio and crotallaria, plants all known to contain dangerous amounts of pyrolizidene (P.A.'s) alkaloids, which contaminated their grain supply; (2) comfrey, along with borage and coltsfoot are members of the same family of plants in which pyrrolizidine alkaloids have been found (even though borage has been found to not contain any PAs); (3) small amounts of these alkaloids have been found in certain strains of Russian comfrey harvested at certain times of the year (the fresh young leaves of spring and early summer growth); (4) a number of six-week-old mice are fed a diet consisting of from 30 to 50% comfrey (probably a substance they naturally are not inclined to ingest) and develop liver tumors believed to be the direct result of their being fed comfrey; (5) comfrey is suspected to be hepato-toxic to humans who ingest it as tea or herb supplement; (6) an attempt is made (out of thousands of users, worldwide) to find cases of individuals who may have used comfrey and later develop some form of liver toxicity.

We can see from this that at least in relation to the exercise of the public's right to use herbs, the prevailing attitude of most scientific investigators and legal agencies is "guilty until proven innocent." Since it would take millions of dollars to run further tests on the safety of an herb like comfrey, a relative safety that most herbalists believe, based upon historical and personal usage, it is not likely to occur because of the lack of patentable economic incentives.

Other points which Richard made concerning comfrey deserve to be considered. First that the pyrrolizidine alkaloids found in comfrey are accompanied by an abundance of allantoin, a cell proliferant, calcium salts and a mucopolysacharride or mucilage, all of which are very nutritious to the cells. Thus, just as the lecithin in eggs serves to emulsify its cholesterol content when consumed, the allantoin in comfrey may serve to counteract the cell-inhibiting action of the pyrrolizidine alkaloids. Further, the pyrrolizidine alkaloid found in comfrey is in its "N-oxide" form, which unlike the form used in laboratory studies is "organic" and more likely to be degraded when digested in the human body.

Finally, De Sylva mentions how comfrey was analyzed for pyrrolizidine content by an independent United States company. Of three samples tested, one was returned as negative, the second with only trace amounts and the third with one part per million. From this, one could conclude that "using one teaspoon of comfrey leaves (3-5 grams), there is an infinitesimal amount of this alleged toxic substance"—so small that "even taking three cups of tea per day as a beverage or a therapeutic remedy is still not cause for alarm."

Even accepting the possibility of the alleged P.A.'s in comfrey root posing a hazard to one's healthy liver (which I do not believe is true of either all or the majority of livers), I would refer the reader to a comparison of relative toxicity taken by Dr. Jim Duke who is director of the U.S. Department of Agriculture. Based upon a system of determining relative carcinogenicities by comparing them to other well known and common foodstuffs, Dr. Duke arrived at a classification which he calls the burp index (Better Understanding of Relative Potencies) based on the statistical index developed by Drs. Bruce Ames and Lois Gold published in 1987 and again another publication in the same highly respected journal in 1989.

Dr.Duke's classification following the principles of the Ames index is as follows:

*BURP indices of some beverages**		
Relative carcinogenicity (BURP index)	**Beverage**	**Estimate based only on**
1	Tap water	Chloroform
10	Apple Juice	1, 1-dimethylhydrazine
25	Beer (before 1979)	Dimethylnitrosamine
125	Comfrey leaf tea	Symphyline
175	Diet cola	Saccharin
575	Root Beer (old fashioned)	Sairole
850	Basil tea (3 g. dry herb)	Estragole
7700	Cola	Formaldehyde
8000	Beer (modern)	Ethanol
18000	Wine	Ethanol

*Adapted from Ames et al and Ames and Gold

Another issue is the development of a kind of comfrey neurosis among herbalists and the public despite the personal experience of thousands who have successfully used comfrey in a variety of forms and preparations such as comfrey mucilage for dryness of the lung and sore throat, Comfrey Green Drink and the various teas, pills and preparations that herbalists and individuals have made using comfrey as a primary ingredient. It may be useful to consider a statement of Dr. Rudolf Weiss in his book *Herbal Medicine*, where he states, "Modern methods of chemical analysis are now so sophisticated, working in nano units (10 to the 9th power), that harmful substances will be found almost anywhere, with the result that we feel constantly threatened." Weiss himself seems rather cautious in accepting the recent scientific findings damning the use of comfrey.

If veno-occlusive disease was a significant threat to humans ingesting substantial amounts of comfrey, it would most surely have been apparent among the hundreds of herbalists both now and in the past who have regularly used it and given it to their patients. The fact is however, that comfrey neurosis has exposed a weakness in the theoretical understanding of Western herbalists and that weakness or deficiency is specifically involved with issues of appropriate use and specific contraindications.

SUMMARY

Historically, the primary use of herbs is based upon empirical knowledge as to whether or not a specific herb is efficacious. It has been demonstrated repeatedly that science is not always sympathetic nor refined enough to evaluate the validity of empirical evidence. Many herbs, like foods, have toxic potential and specific contraindications, and unless herbalists adopt a principle by which these are understood, there will always be questions about the practice of herbal medicine and use of herbs. Traditional systems like Chinese and Ayurvedic herbal medicine offer a time tested alternative medical model that differentiates between issues of herbal toxicity and contraindications not clearly defined in Western herbalism. It is time for Western herbalism to specifically offer a system of evaluating and testing the relative safety of herbs.

APPENDIX

THE AMERICAN HERBALIST GUILD

Join the American Herbalist Guild and support the future of Herbal Medicine in America. Since the Guild is a non-profit association, all membership fees are fully tax deductible. Membership entitles you to receive our quarterly journal, information and discount to our annual symposium and other workshops or seminars, attendance to our general meetings and the opportunity to confer and lobby with the voting membership concerning AHG policies.

There are five levels of membership:
1. Professional Herbalist
2. Student Membership
3. Associate Member
4. Benefactor
5. Corporate Sponsor

For information and application for membership in the AHG write:

American Herbalist Guild
Attn. Secretary
P.O. Box 1683
Soquel, California 95073

HERB SCHOOLS

California School of Herbal Studies
Box 39
Forestville, CA 95436
Faculty includes: James and Mindy Green, David Hoffmann, Amanda McQuade and others.

The following teachers also offer long-term studies and apprenticeship courses:

David Christopher
716 South 1550 East
Spanish Fork, UT 844660

Santa Cruz School of Herbal Medicine
Michael Tierra and Christopher Hobbs
Box 712
Santa Cruz, CA 95061

Offers a correspondence course and teaching program following the teachings of Dr. Christopher.

Christopher Hobbs
Box 742A
Capitola, CA 95010

Michael Moore
107 E. Broadway
Silver City, NM 88061

Santa Cruz Herbal Studies Program
Christopher Hobbs
Box 742A
Capitola, CA 95010

Dr. Michael Tierra
Box 712A
Santa Cruz, CA 95061

Herb Pharm
374 E. Fork Rd.
William, OR 97544
Ed Smith offers apprenticeship training.

Wise Women Herbal Medicine
Susun Weed
P.O. Box 64 AHA
Woodstock, NY 12448
Apprenticeships, workshops, correspondence courses.

David Winston
P.O. Box 458A

Bloomsbury, NJ 08804-0458
East Coast teacher, exemplifies Cherokee herbal medicine integrated
with Western and Chinese systems.

CORRESPONDENCE COURSES

Ayurvedic Correspondence Course by David Frawley
A comprehensive course in Ayurveda covering all the main aspects of
Ayurvedic Medicine. Explains Ayurveda as part of the science of Yoga by
David Frawley. The course has been approved by well-known doctors in
India.
P.O. Box 8357
Santa Fe, NM 87504-8357
(505) 983-9385

Dominion Herbal College
Correspondence course with 58 lessons and summer seminar facilities.
The oldest Canadian herbal training college, est. 1926.
7427 Kingsway
Burnaby, B.C. V3N 3C1
Canada
(604) 521-5822

The East West Herbal Correspondence Course
by Dr. Michael and Lesley Tierra
A comprehensive 36 lesson herb course that integrates the practice of
Western, Chinese and Ayurvedic Herbalism along with traditional nutrition, diagnostics and treatment protocol. For information write: East
West Herbal Correspondence Course, Box 712G, Santa Cruz, California
95061.

Herbal Studies Course by Jeanne Rose
A 36-lesson course with 1200 pages of valuable information. It is divided
into three sections: Seasonal Herbal, Medicinal Herbal, Reference Herbal,
with projects, tests and personal feedback. Write for information: 219
Carl St., San Francisco, CA 94117.

Therapeutic Herbalism by David Hoffmann, MNIMH
This course lays the foundation for the skilled use of herbal medicines,
going beyond simple symptomatic relief to show how they may be effec-

tive components of holistic therapy. It may be used: (1) as a cornerstone of developing a practice as a medical herbalist; (2) as a component within the practice of a practitioner of therapy; or (3) as an herbal foundation for personal health care. For course details, please write: 9304 Springhill School Rd., Sebastopol, CA 95436.

The Science and Art of Herbology Course by Rosemary Gladstar
This home study course is an excellent introduction to the way of herbs. Each lesson (a total of over 500 pages) covers medicinal herbology, plant identification, herbal preparation, gardening, natural cosmetics and herbal therapeutics for body systems. Written by Rosemary Gladstar, founder of the California School of Herbal Studies and Traditional Medicinal Herb Teas, Rosemary brings over 20 years experience to this course and personally answers homework, questions and correspondence. Certificate is awarded. Write Rosemary Gladstar, Box 420, East Barre, VT 05649.

Wild Rose College of Natural Healing
302, 1220 Kensington Rd. N.W.
Calgary, Alberta T2N 3P5
Canada
(408) 270-0936
This school is directed by Dr. Terry Willard, Ph.D. Nine months to two years part-time study (1600 hours planned). Classroom and correspondence courses.

HERBAL LIBRARY
The Lloyd's Library and Museum, 917 Plum St., Cincinnati, OH 45202. Ph. (513) 721-3707.

PUBLICATIONS AND BOOKS BY THE WRITERS
A Male Herbal by James Green, publ. by The Crossing Press.
Herbal Medicine Maker's Handbook also by James Green, available
through Simpler's Botanical Co., P.O. Box 39, Forestville, CA 95436.

Herbs and Things, The Herbal Body Book, The Herbal Food Book, Ask Jeanne Rose, Kitchen Cosmetics, The Modern Herbal, The Cosmetic Aromatherapy Book all by Jeanne Rose.

The Holistic Herbal by David Hoffmann, publ. by Findhorn Press.
The Holistic Herbal Way to Successful Stress Control by David Hoffmann, publ. by Thorsens.
The Herbal Handbook, A User's Guide to Medical Herbalism by David Hoffmann, publ. by Healing Arts Press.
The Herb User's Guide by David Hoffmann, publ. by Thorsons.
Welsh Herbal Medicine by David Hoffman, publ. by Abercastle.

Herbs, Actions and Systems: A Short Guide to Herbal Remedies, Relating Their Actions and Affinity for Body Systems by Amanda McQuade and David Hoffmann, publ. by California School of Herbal Studies, Box 39, Forestville, CA 95436.

Vitex: The Women's Herb; Echinacea: The Immune Herb; Milk Thistle: The Liver Herb; Ginkgo: The Elixir of Youth—four books written by Christopher Hobbs, publ. by Botanica Press, Box 742A, Capitola, CA 95010.

Medicinal Plants of the Mountains West and *Medicinal Plants of the Desert and Canyon West,* both by Michael Moore, publ. by Museum of New Mexico Press.

The School of Natural Healing by Dr. John R. Christopher, publ. by BiWorld.

Ayurvedic Healing: A Comprehensive Guide by David Frawley, publ. by Passage Press, Salt Lake City, Utah.
The Yoga of Herbs by David Frawley and Dr. Lad, publ. by Lotus Press.

The Way of Herbs by Michael Tierra, publ. by Pocket books.
The Natural Remedy Bible by Tierra and Lust, publ. by Pocket Books.
Planetary Herbology by Michael Tierra, publ. by Lotus Press.
Chinese Planetary Herbal Diagnosis by Michael and Lesley Tierra, self-published. All are available directly from East West Herbal Correspondence School, Box 712, Santa Cruz, CA 95061.

Herbs of Life by Lesley Tierra, publ. by The Crossing Press.

The following books are written by Bob Flaws:
*Nine Ounces: A Nine Part Program for the Prevention of AIDS in HIV
    Positive Persons*
The Treatment of Cancer by Integrated Chinese-Western Medicine
A Handbook of Traditional Chinese Dermatology
Turtletail and Other Tender Mercies: Traditional Chinese Pediatrics
*Endometriosis and Infertility and Traditional Chinese Medicine: A
    Laywoman's Guide*
*Scatology and The Gate of Life: The Role of the Large Intestine
In Immunity, an Integrated Chinese-Western Approach*
*Something Old, Something New: Essays on the TCM Description of West-
    ern Herbs, Pharmaceuticals, Vitamins and Minerals*

With Honora Wolfe:
Prince Wen Hui's Cook
All published by Blue Poppy Press.

HERBAL NEWSLETTERS

Medical Herbalism: A Clinical Newsletter for the Herbal Practitioner,
edited by Paul Bergner, P.O. Box 33080.

HerbalGram
P.O. Box 201660
Austin, TX 78720-1660
(512) 331-8868
Edited by Mark Blumenthal. All issues of this publication are beautiful,
authoritative and definite collectible material. They accept Visa and some
back issues are still available. Call 1-800-373-7105.

Herbal Perspectives by Roy Upton, P.O. Box 533, Soquel, CA 95073.

American Herb Association, edited by Kathi Keville, P.O. Box 1673,
Nevada City, CA 95959.

OUT-OF-THE-COUNTRY JOURNALS AND NEWSLETTERS:

Australian Journal of Medical Herbalism
P.O. Box 65
Kingsgrove, NSW 2208
Australia
The Canadian Journal of Herbalism: The Quarterly of the Ontario Herbalist's Association
11 Winthrop Place

HERBAL DATABASE PROGRAMS

Global Herb
A comprehensive library of herbal information listing over 700 herbs, formulas and other therapies.
PlanetHerb
Unifying planetary approaches to herbal healing based on Planetary Herbology. Describes 490+ herbs and formulas from Western countries, China and India. Comes complete with an editor to add your own herbs and data.
ProHerb
Based on 15 of the most authoritative references. Ideal for the store or office.
HomeHerb
A simple and inexpensive program ideal for home use.
Contact: Steve Blake, 5831 S. Highway 9, Felton, CA 95018, 408-335-9011

IBIS Interactive Body Mind Information System
A comprehensive data base linking Herbal, Acupuncture, Nutritional, Homeopathic and other modalities to the treatment of over 200 diseases. AMR'Ta, P.O. Box 14641, Portland, OR 97214, U.S. Toll free 1-800-484-4022 (code 0569)

THE CROSSING PRESS
publishes many books of
interest to people who need
more information about herbs.
For a free catalog,
please call (toll-free)
800 / 777 1048
Please specify a *health* catalog.